D1067501

Language in Psychotherapy

Strategies of Discovery

EMOTIONS, PERSONALITY, AND PSYCHOTHERAPY

Series Editors
Carroll E. Izard, *University of Delaware, Newark, Delaware*
and
Jerome L. Singer, *Yale University, New Haven, Connecticut*

THE EMOTIONAL BRAIN: Physiology, Neuroanatomy,
Psychology, and Emotion
    P. V. Simonov

EMOTIONS IN PERSONALITY AND PSYCHOPATHOLOGY
    Carroll E. Izard, ed.

FREUD AND MODERN PSYCHOLOGY, Volume 1: The Emotional
Basis of Mental Illness
    Helen Block Lewis

FREUD AND MODERN PSYCHOLOGY, Volume 2: The Emotional
Basis of Human Behavior
    Helen Block Lewis

GUIDED AFFECTIVE IMAGERY WITH CHILDREN AND ADOLESCENTS
    Hanscarl Leuner, Günther Horn, and Edda Klessmann

HUMAN EMOTIONS
    Carroll E. Izard

LANGUAGE IN PSYCHOTHERAPY: Strategies of Discovery
    Robert L. Russell

THE PERSONAL EXPERIENCE OF TIME
    Bernard S. Gorman and Alden E. Wessman, eds.

THE POWER OF HUMAN IMAGINATION: New Methods
in Psychotherapy
    Jerome L. Singer and Kenneth S. Pope, eds.

SHYNESS: Perspectives on Research and Treatment
    Warren H. Jones, Jonathan M. Cheek, and Stephen R. Briggs, eds.

THE STREAM OF CONSCIOUSNESS: Scientific Investigations into the
Flow of Human Experience
    Kenneth S. Pope and Jerome L. Singer, eds.

A Continuation Order Plan is available for this series. A continuation order will bring delivery
of each new volume immediately upon publication. Volumes are billed only upon actual ship-
ment. For further information please contact the publisher.

Language in Psychotherapy

Strategies of Discovery

Edited by

Robert L. Russell
New School for Social Research
New York, New York

Plenum Press • New York and London

Library of Congress Cataloging in Publication Data

Language in psychotherapy.

(Emotions, personality, and psychotherapy)
Includes bibliographies and index.
1. Psycholinguistics—Therapeutic use. 2. Psychotherapist and patient. 3. psychotherapy patients—Language. I. Russell, Robert L. II. Series. [DNLM: 1. Communication.
2. Physician—Patient Relations. 3.Psychotherapy—methods. WM 420 L287]
RC489.P73L36   1987   616.89'14   87-2511
ISBN 0-306-42422-3

© 1987 Plenum Press, New York
A Division of Plenum Publishing Corporation
233 Spring Street, New York, N.Y. 10013

Printed in the United States of America

Contributors

LOUIS A. GOTTSCHALK

Department of Psychiatry and Human Behavior, University of California at Irvine, Irvine, California

DONALD J. KIESLER

Department of Psychology, Virginia Commonwealth University, Richmond, Virginia

JULIUS LAFFAL

Department of Psychiatry, Yale University School of Medicine, New Haven, Connecticut

GEORGE F. MAHL

Departments of Psychiatry and Psychology, Yale University, New Haven, Connecticut

JOSEPH D. MATARAZZO

Department of Medical Psychology, Oregon Health Sciences University, Portland, Oregon

NAOMI M. MEARA

Department of Psychology, University of Notre Dame, Notre Dame, Indiana

MICHAEL J. PATTON

Department of Educational and Counseling Psychology, University of Tennessee, Knoxville, Tennessee

ROY D. PEA

Educational Communication and Technology Program, New York University, New York, New York

ROBERT L. RUSSELL

Department of Psychology, New School for Social Research, New York, New York

WILLIAM U. SNYDER

Department of Psychology, Ohio University, Athens, Ohio

WILLIAM B. STILES

Department of Psychology, Miami University, Oxford, Ohio

ARTHUR N. WIENS

Department of Medical Psychology, University of Oregon Health Sciences Center, Portland, Oregon

Preface

This book of original contributions presents investigations of psycho-therapautic interaction. While the methodological strategies and the-oretical orientations of these investigations are notably diverse, the utterance-by-utterance analysis of client-therapist dialogue provides a strong commonality of interest and a particularly productive perspective from which the process of psychotherapy can be illuminated. It is hoped that the contributions selected, and the problems with which they are occupied, will make evident the rich possibilities such a perspective has to offer.

It should be noted, however, that the present volume is not a com-pendium: any effort to be exhaustive would be thwarted by considera-tions of length alone. Thus, certain omissions were inevitable. It is hoped that the interested reader will use the extensive references to become acquainted with the works not here included.

Whatever effort I extended as editor and contributor to this volume could not have been undertaken without the lifelong spirit of support of my parents, Selma S. and Jay F. Russell. I dedicate my contribution to them.

ROBERT L. RUSSELL

Contents

Introduction

Robert L. Russell

When Anna O., an early patient of Breuer's and of considerable concern to Freud, naively labeled her treatment a form of talking cure (Breuer, 1981; Brill, 1972), she correctly anticipated what in popular opinion would be grasped—sometimes for ridicule, sometimes for praise—as an essential feature of psychotherapeutic care. Popular opinion, however, is not alone in attributing a pivotal position to the talk in psychotherapy: in comparison to the behavioral (i.e., proxemic or kinesic) or physiological constituents of psychotherapeutic interaction, the talk which transpires between therapist and client has consistently been in the critical limelight—in psychotherapy research, theory and practice. Today, the idea that a clinician's talk is instrumental in facilitating client change is as little contested as the idea that clients' talk can be a helpful indicator of their psychological well-being. The identification of what is said in psychotherapy with what is done in psychotherapy is, thus, a practice of professionals and nonprofessionals alike. Is this consensus in any way justified? How might its evidential base best be discovered? Can such queries, pursued empirically, reasonably hope to render clinical practices more efficacious, and in what ways? These are some of the questions the reader will want to put to the following chapters, each of which presents a distinct approach to the analysis of talk in psychotherapeutic settings.

By way of introduction, it may prove useful to point out that theoretical and practical estimates of the importance of talk in psychotherapy antedate systematic research on this topic by nearly a century.

ROBERT L. RUSSELL • Department of Psychology, New School for Social Research, 65 Fifth Avenue, New York, NY 10003.

Breuer and Freud (1981) were perhaps the first therapists to explicitly locate the curative treatment factors in characteristics of patient talk:

> we found, to our great surprise at first, that each individual hysterical symptom immediately and permanently disappeared when we had succeeded in bringing clearly to light the memory of the event by which it was provoked and in arousing its accompanying affect, and when the patient had described that event in the greatest possible detail and had put the affect into words. . . . The psychical process which originally took place must be repeated as vividly as possible; it must be brought back to its *status nascendi* and then given verbal utterance. (p. 7)

However accurate or circumspect Breuer and Freud's early curative triad (i.e., recollect, emote, verbalize) may be, it remained highly speculative and empirically unverifiable until the late 1930s and early 1940s, along with all other formulations of curative factors in terms of patient or therapist talk. The utilization of phonographic recordings to capture an objective representation of the talk in psychotherapy only became practicable then, and only then made possible systematic empirical investigations.

Armed with this new technology, psychotherapy researchers abandoned the use of session notes, case studies, and anecdotes as the preferred evidential bases for claims about the role of talk in psychotherapy. This new technology, it was hoped, would provide

> for the first time a sound basis for the investigation of therapeutic processes, and the teaching and improvement of psychotherapeutic techniques. . . . Psychotherapy can become a process based on known and tested principles, with tested techniques for implementing those principles. (Rogers, 1942, p. 434)

Unfortunately, those "known and tested principles" have been extremely elusive, and the payoff from research on client and therapist talk has not been as great as had been expected (Auld & Murray, 1955; Marsden, 1965, 1971).

The frustration of these early expectations can be accounted for by taking note of several factors. First, and perhaps foremost, even if the search for curative factors is restricted to the domain of client and therapist talk, the relevant phenomena to be investigated are forbiddingly numerous and complex. Language, and its deployment in interpersonal interactions, together constitute one of the highest cultural and intellectual achievements of our species, and any analysis of the forms and functions of language usage can expect to be a lengthy and arduous task, spanning across many individual research careers. Second, because of its complexity and universality (i.e., the pervasive importance of language behavior in almost all spheres of human interaction), the study of language and its use has been carried out in numerous disciplines (e.g., communication, linguistics, sociology, speech, psycho-linguistics, psychotherapy, developmental psychology, ethnography, and so on). Up until relatively recently, a sourcebook pointing the way to these various literatures, in particular to aspects of therapeutic communication, was lacking, making the going extremely difficult, especially for novices (Kiesler, 1973). But even if access is achieved, coordinating the different literatures, keeping abreast of current developments, building without reduplicating, all require time and effort that might otherwise be spent on research of a less demanding character. As Strupp (1973) notes:

> Content analysis in psychotherapy is an exceedingly difficult undertaking. It demands an unusual amount of patience, persistence, and dedication because the pay-offs are typically not spectacular or rewarding. (p. xv).

The first two pitfalls combine and contribute to a third, namely, the lack of truly programmatic research. This lack is prompted by the fact that granting agencies are not "terribly excited" by studies of psychotherapeutic talk, by the fact that progress is slow, and thus hazardous to beginning researchers, and by the fact that most graduate students choose, or are advised, not to pursue such research as topics for dissertations (see Kiesler, 1973, p. xvii; Strupp, 1973, p. xv). Marsden (1965) has summarized the resulting impact on the development of a cumulative research tradition:

> Despite the burgeoning of content-analysis studies of therapeutic interviews in the past two decades (Auld and Murray, 1955) one is struck by the relative infrequency with which any of these systems has resulted in more than an initial thrust at a given research problem. System after system has been developed and presented in one or two demonstration studies, only to lie buried in the literature, unused even by its author. Moreover, few variables or notions about therapeutic interviews have received anything approaching programmatic or extensive content-analysis investigation. This has resulted in redundancy; systems were developed with apparent unawareness that approaches to the same problem had already been reported. (p. 315)

In the twenty years since Marsden's assessment, studies concerning client and therapist talk have continued to appear in the literature at a prolific rate. Nevertheless, the accumulation of valid principles and the comparability of research findings have remained problematic (Russell, 1986; Russell & Stiles, 1979; Stiles, 1979). With so many obstacles, and with the expectancy of success in this area so often frustrated, it might well be asked why so much research energy is expended on it.

The fact of the matter is that there exists a general theoretical consensus that

> the crucial information [concerning the process of psychotherapeutic change] is somehow embedded in the verbal and nonverbal communications, and it

is the job of the researcher to impose order on the process in such a way that
meaningful answers emerge. (Strupp, 1973, p. xiii)

Since the time of Breuer and Freud, in fact, psychotherapy has been
formulated in one form or another as a "talking cure," that is, as a
process which may most profitably be viewed in terms of communicative expression (Forrester, 1980; Frank, 1961; MacCabe, 1981; Smith,
1978). This theoretical belief was explicitly formulated by Kiesler (1966)
as the "basic skeleton of a [research] paradigm for psychotherapy" (p.
132).

The patient communicates something; the therapist communicates something in response; the patient communicates and/or experiences something
different; and the therapist, patient, and others like the change (although
they may like it to different degrees, or for divergent reasons). What the
therapist communicates (the independent variables) is very likely multidimensional (and the patterning of this multidimensionality needs to be specified), and may be different at different phases of the interaction for different
kinds of patients. Similarly, what the patient communicates and/or experiences differently (the dependent variables) is likely multidimensional (and
the patterning of this multidimensionality needs to be clarified) and may be
different at distinct phases of the interaction. The enormous task of psychotherapy theory and research is that of filling in the variables of this paradigm.
(p. 130)

It is the promise associated with the "filling in" of this paradigm
(with some additions and emendations—see concluding chapter) which
continues to motivate research on client and therapist talk.

The selections of work included in this volume represent systematic, and in many ways, successful attempts to devise research strategies
profitably applicable to the analysis of the verbatim talk, and/or aspects
such as dysfluencies, silences, and interruptions associated with it,
which occur between clients and therapists. The strategic elements involved in these analyses concern the choice of the unit size selected for
study, the type of attribute in the speech sample isolated for coding, and
the type of coding procedures utilized in assigning units to appropriate
classificatory categories—in addition, of course, to the usual methodological decisions concerning subject selection and assignment, correlational or experimental design, and so on.

The reader will note that the studies included use a variety of unit
sizes (e.g., clause, sentence, thought unit, utterance), focus on different
attributes of the speech sample (e.g., semantic content, linguistic case
assignments, extralinguistic phenomena such as pauses, silences, dysfluencies, interactional categories), and utilize different coding procedures (e.g., requiring coders to score units to categories with or without making an inference about the speaker's characteristics, aims,
internal states, etc.). In addition, regularities in the speech samples are

formally represented by a variety of means—namely, by mathematical-statistical formulae and by sociolinguistic rules. Taken together, the studies represent the "building-block" strategies on which future research in this area will continue to draw, and hopefully develop.

Obviously, the strategies used to study the communication between therapist and client have not been devised with the principal intent of discovering regularities in speech and speech-related phenomena alone. The strategies have been applied in investigating topics of obvious significance for the conduct of psychotherapy, and for the understanding of normal and abnormal patterns of adjustment. To this end, emotional expression, interpersonal relatedness, ideational preoccupations, strategic interaction, and anxiety—to name only a few general categories of shared interest—have all been illuminated in the following pages. Keeping in mind the thankless relationship between the meticulousness of one's empirical scrutiny and the degrees of difficulty involved in systematization, the "tough-mindedness" of the selections should stand out quite clearly, especially when one considers the relatively short time which has elapsed since objective studies began. Hopefully, the degree of success achieved by these individual strategies of discovery will prompt integrational work in the future, helping to link, for example, emotional expression and interpersonal relatedness, psychotherapeutic techniques and strategic interaction, statistical-mathematical formulae and sociolinguistic rules. Such multidimensional focus will undoubtedly illuminate the complexities characteristic of language use in psychotherapy.

THE ORGANIZATION AND CONTENT OF THIS VOLUME

As suggested above, the following chapters present differing strategies of discovery. As a means to highlight these differences, and to underscore interchapter affinities, the studies in this volume have been grouped in terms of the kinds of categories they employ in coding specific speech or speech-related variables. In addition, in each of the first eight chapters, the authors have been asked to address the following three questions in the course of their presentation: (1) Why choose this particular system of analysis?; (2) how has it been employed in the past, and what can be its uses in the future?; and (3) what has it revealed? In addressing question one, the authors have presented the theoretical rationale and developmental histories of their systems. In addressing question two, each contributor has presented a detailed demonstration of how their system can be applied to the talk in psychotherapy. And lastly, in addressing question three, the contributors have reviewed their findings to date, and have suggested further applications for their systems.

Part I: The two chapters in Part I present schemes of analysis employing content categories. In Chapter 1 entitled "Content Category Analysis: The Measurement of the Magnitude of Psychological Dimensions in Psychotherapy," Louis A. Gottschalk presents a model of content analysis based on the construction and validation of formal scales of weighted content categories. He reports research results concerning such psychological states as anxiety, hostility, hope, personal disorganization, and achievement. In Chapter 2, entitled "Concept Analysis of Language in Psychotherapy," Julius Laffal presents a system of content analysis based on the development of a concept dictionary, which can be utilized to analyze lexical items in terms of their component semantic commonalities and differences. This approach to content analysis is illustrated in several case studies, one of which is the famous Schreber case, in which Freud attempted an analytic account of Schreber's psychosis and religious delusions—an account which gave rise to the familiar linking of homosexuality and projection in paranoia.

Part II: The two chapters in Part II present schemes of analysis employing what have been termed intersubjective categories, that is, categories such as self-disclosure, interpretation, giving direction, and so on, which are descriptive of syntactically implied and other interpersonal relationships between a communicator and a recipient. In the third chapter, entitled "Snyder's Classification System for Therapeutic Interviews", William U. Snyder presents his pioneering system of intersubjective categories, used to describe both therapeutic techniques and the relationships between therapist intersubjective category usage and client responses. In the fourth chapter, entitled "Verbal Response Modes as Intersubjective Categories," William B. Stiles presents a system of intersubjective categories generated by the use of formal principles of classification. The taxonomy of verbal response modes, which can be used to classify both the form and intent of client or therapist utterances, has been utilized in the study of technique usage among competing schools of psychotherapy, and in extensive empirical investigations of doctor–patient interviews.

Part III: The two chapters in Part III present schemes of analysis employing what have been termed extralinguistic categories—categories used to code such speech-associated phenomena as pauses, interruptions, dysfluencies, and the temporal patterning of dialogue. In chapter 5, entitled, "A Speech Interaction System," Joseph D. Matarazzo, Donald J. Kiesler, and Arthur N. Wiens present an extra linguistic category scheme used to explore the durations of communicative activity, silence, and simultaneous talk (i.e., interruptions) in therapeutic and analog experimental encounters. In addition to presenting the results of extensive experimental and naturalistic research, an objective application of the speech interaction system to the problem of empathy in interview situations is reviewed. In chapter 6 entitled "Everyday Disturbances of Speech," George F. Mahl presents a system of speech-disturbance categories (e.g., repetitions, stuttering, tongue slips, and so on) found to be a valid instrument in the investigation of anxiety and conflict in a wide variety of contexts.

Part IV: The two chapters in Part IV present comparatively recent additions to the literature concerned with psychotherapeutic talk, and both draw heavily on traditions of language analysis developed within linguistics or philosophy of language. In chapter 7, entitled "The Analysis of Natural Language in Psychological Treatment," Michael J. Patton and Naomi M. Meara present a system of analysis, based on a conception of case grammar (see Chafe, 1970; Cook, 1979), which analyzes verbs into category types—for instance, "process verbs define a causal relation, without specification of an agent, in which something is happening to a person or thing (see Chapter 7, p. 284)." With such a system of verb types and the case role designations for relevant noun phrases, Patton and Meara present research results concerning convergence and tracking in psychotherapy sessions. In chapter 8, entitled "Ethnography and the Vicissitudes of Talk in Psychotherapy," Roy D. Pea and Robert L. Russell illustrate and critically review ethnographically inspired microanalytic systems applied in the investigation of psychotherapeutic talk. With special emphasis on Comprehensive Discourse Analysis, developed by William Labov and David Fanshel (1977), Pea and Russell develop an initial exposition of this style of analysis, emphasizing its roots in ordinary language philosophy, interpretive sociology, and the new ethnography of speaking.

In the ninth and concluding chapter, Robert L. Russell attempts to raise several key issues with which analyses of talk in psychotherapy will have to wrestle in pushing toward further success. The brief discussion centers on the important role of developmentalism, sociological variables, and new data-analytic techniques in future studies of psychotherapeutic talk.

CONCLUDING COMMENT

Innumerable facets can be singled out of the complex interpersonal activity we call psychotherapy, and the selection of some small fraction of them for critical study is itself a difficult methodological and theoretical decision. However, it seems evident that if psychotherapy is to be understood, then, at the very minimum, the talk which to a large degree constitutes the therapeutic encounter must be carefully analyzed. The following studies illustrate where we stand in putting together the basic building blocks for the empirical investigation of what client and therapist "do" and accomplish on an utterance-by-utterance basis. Taken singly or as a group, the studies will necessarily appear less than conclusive, not only because we are still in the infancy of this tradition of research, but because the talk between therapist and client represents only one facet of the psychotherapeutic process. If this volume helps to motivate and orient future studies, while informing prospective investigators about the different strategies available, then its purpose will have been fulfilled.

REFERENCES

Auld, F., Jr. & Murray, E. J. (1955). Content analysis studies of psychotherapy. *Psychological Bulletin, 52*, 377–395.
Breuer, J. (1981). Case 1: Fraulein Anna O. In J. Breuer & S. Freud, *Studies on hysteria* (J. Strachey, Ed. & Trans.), pp. 21–47. New York: Basic Books. (Originally published in 1893).
Breuer, J. & Freud, S. (1981). *Studies on hysteria* (J. Strachey, Ed. & Trans.) New York: Basic Books. Originally published in 1893).
Brill, A. A. (1972). *Basic principles of psycho-analysis.* New York: Washington Square Press.
Chafe, W. S. (1970). *Meaning and structure in language.* Chicago: University of Chicago Press.
Cook, W. A. (1979). *Core grammar: development of the matrix model* (1970–1978). Washington, D.C.: Georgetown University Press.
Forrester, J. (1980). *Language and the origins of psychoanalysis.* New York: Columbia University Press.
Frank, J. (1961). On the history of the objective investigation of the process of psychotherapy. *Journal of Psychology, 15*, 89–95.
Kiesler, D. J. (1966). Some myths of psychotherapy research and the search for a paradigm. *Psychological Bulletin, 65*, 110–136.
Kiesler, D. J. (1973). *The process of psychotherapy.* Chicago: Aldine Publishing Company.
Labov, W. & Fanshel, D. (1977). *Therapeutic discourse: psychotherapy as conversation.* New York: Academic Press.
MacCabe, C. (1981). *The talking cure: essays in psychoanalysis.* New York: St. Martin's Press.
Marsden, G. (1965). Content analysis studies of therapeutic interviews: 1954 to 1964. *Psychological Bulletin, 63*, 298–321.
Marsden, G. (1971). Content analysis studies of psychotherapy: 1954–1968. In A. E. Bergin & S. L. Garfield (Eds.), *Handbook of psychotherapy and behavior change.* New York: Wiley.
Rogers, C. R. (1942). The use of electrically recorded interviews in improving psychotherapeutic techniques. *American Journal of Orthopsychiatry, 12*, 429–434.
Russell, R. L. (1986). The inadvisability of admixing psychoanalysis with other forms of psychotherapy. *Journal of Contemporary Psychotherapy, 16*, 76–86.
Russell, R. L. & Stiles, W. B. (1979). Categories for classifying language in psychotherapy. *Psychological Bulletin, 86*, 404–419.

Smith, J. H. (Ed.). (1978). *Psychoanalysis and language: Psychiatry and the humanities* (Volume 3). New Haven and London: Yale University Press.

Stiles, W. B. (1979). Verbal response modes and psychotherapeutic technique. *Psychiatry, 42*, 49–62.

Strupp, H. H. (1973). Foreword. In D. J. Kiesler (Ed.), *The process of psychotherapy.* Chicago: Aldine Publishing Company.

I
Content-Category Strategies

1

Content-Category Analysis

The Measurement of the Magnitude of
Psychological Dimensions in Psychotherapy

Louis A. Gottschalk

The general problem with which the content-analysis procedure developed by Gottschalk and his associates deals is the accurate measurement of psychological states or traits, a problem of equal consequence to psychiatrists, psychologists, behavioral and social scientists.

The measurement method chosen utilizes a function that is uniquely human, namely speech and its content (or its semantic aspect). Small samples of speech, as brief as two or five minutes, have been found sufficient to provide objective measures of various psychological dimensions with the use of this method. The development of the method has involved a long series of steps. It has required that the psychological dimension selected for measurement, for example, anxiety or hostility, be carefully defined; that a unit of communication, the grammatical clause, be specified; and that the content, or lexical cues, from which a receiver of the verbal message infers the occurrence of the psychological state, be spelled out. Furthermore, it is necessary that the linguistic cues conveying intensity, principally syntactical in nature, also be specified; that differential weights, signifying relative intensity, be assigned to semantic and linguistic cues whenever appro-

With the permission of the publisher parts of this chapter have been adapted from a previous publication of the author: "Some Psychoanalytic Research into the Communication of Meaning through Language: The Quality and Magnitude of Psychological States." *British Journal of Medical Psychology*, 1971, 44, 131–147.

LOUIS A. GOTTSCHALK • Department of Psychiatry and Human Behavior, College of Medicine, University of California at Irvine, Irvine, CA 92717.

priate; and that a systematic means of correcting for the number of words spoken per unit time be determined, so that one individual can be compared to others, or to himself on different occasions, with respect to the magnitude of a particular psychological state as derived from the content of verbal behavior. The method also requires that a formal scale of weighted content categories be specified for each psychological dimension to be measured; that research technicians be trained to apply these scales to typescripts of human speech (much as biochemical technicians are trained to run various complex chemical determinations by following prescribed procedures); and that the interscorer reliability of two trained content technicians using the same scale be .85 or above (a modest but respectable level of consensus in the psychological sciences for these kinds of measurements). Moreover, a set of construct validation studies, including the use of four kinds of criterion measures—psychological, psychophysiological, psychopharmacological, and psychobiochemical—have had to be carried out to establish exactly what this content-analysis procedure is measuring. On the basis of these construct-validation studies, changes have been in the content categories and their associated weights in each specific scale, in the direction of maximizing the correlations between the content-analysis scores with these various criterion measures.

Construct validation is a step-by-step process that requires repeated reexamination and retesting, in new situations, of the constructs being evaluated. After initial validation studies were completed for verbal behavior measures of the psychological constructs of anxiety, hostility out, hostility in, ambivalent hostility, and social alienation-personal disorganization (the schizophrenic syndrome), a large variety of additional investigations were carried out using these verbal behavior measures. These have provided considerable data on the ways in which such verbal behavior scores relate to other relevant measurable phenomena. These data afford growing evidence as to how the constructs examined by these verbal-behavior measures "fit" with other empirical data (Gottschalk, Gleser, Daniels, & Block, 1958; Gottschalk, Gleser, Springer, Kaplan, Shanon, & Ross, 1960; Gottschalk, Gleser, Magliocco, & D'Zmura, 1961; Gottschalk, Springer, & Gleser, 1961; Gottschalk, Gleser, & Springer, 1963; Gottschalk & Gleser, 1964; Gleser, Gottschalk, & Springer, 1961).

The formulation of these psychological states has been deeply influenced by the position that they have biological roots. Both the definition of each separate state and the selection of the specific verbal-content items used as cues for inferring each state were influenced by the decision that whatever psychological state was measured by this content-analysis approach should, whenever possible, be associated with some biological characteristic of the individual, in addition to some psychological aspect or some social situation. Hence, not only psychological, but also physiological, biochemical, and pharmacological studies have all provided further construct validation.

The details of these steps, including many reliability and validity studies and the specific investigations pinning down each point, have been published over the past 30 years (Gottschalk & Hambidge, 1955; Gottschalk & Gleser, 1969; Gottschalk, Winget, & Gleser, 1969; Gottschalk, 1979a). Content-analysis scales applicable to speech have been developed for objectively and precisely measuring anxiety, hostility (in or out), the capacity for human relations, social alienation-personal disorganization (schizophrenia), cognitive impairment, achievement strivings, dependency, dependency frustration, hope, and health-sickness.

EMPIRICALLY DERIVED STEPS FOR MEASURING THE MAGNITUDE OF PSYCHOLOGICAL STATES

1. Research has demonstrated that the relative magnitude of a psychological state can be validly estimated from the typescript of 2–5 minutes of speech of an individual, using solely content variables, and not including any paralanguage variables. In other words, the major part of the variance in an immediate psychological state of an individual can be accounted for by variations in the content of the verbal communications (Gottschalk, Gleser, Magliocco, & D'Zmura, 1961; Gottschalk, Springer, & Gleser, 1961; Gottschalk, Gleser, & Springer, 1963; Gottschalk, Mayerson, & Gottlieb, 1967; Gleser et al., 1961; Gottschalk & Gleser, 1969; Gottschalk & Kaplan, 1958).

2. On the basis of verbal content alone, the type and magnitude of any one psychological state at any one period of time are directly proportional to three primary factors: (a) the frequency of occurrence of categories of thematic statements; (b) the degree to which the verbal expression directly represents, or is pertinent to, the psychological activation of the specific state (e.g., to say that one is killing or injuring another person or wants to do so is regarded as a more direct representation of hostile aggression than to say that one simply disapproves of another person); and (c) the degree of personal involvement attributed by the speaker to the emotionally relevant idea, feeling, action, or event.

3. The degree of direct representation can be represented mathematically by a weighting factor. Higher weights have tended to be assigned to scorable verbal statements which communicate feelings that, by influence, are more likely to be strongly experienced by the speaker. Completely unconscious or repressed feelings of any kind are not, by

this method of weighting, considered to signify states of high magnitude, but rather are cut to amount to zero or no feelings. This numerical weight, which is assigned to each thematic category, designates roughly the relative probability that the thematic category is associated with the psychological state. Initially, weights have been assigned deductively on the basis of common sense (as in the Example 2 above) or from clinical judgment (as in 4 below). Subsequently, the weights have been modified and revised whenever further empirical evidence has been sufficient to warrant such a change (Gottschalk, Gleser, Magliocco, & D'Zmura, 1961; Gottschalk, Gleser, & Springer, 1963; Gottschalk & Gleser, 1964).

4. The occurrence of suppressed and repressed feelings can be inferred from the content of verbal behavior by noting the appearance of a variety of defensive and adaptive mechanisms. The assumption is that the verbal content of spontaneous speech, like dream content, contains the workings of primary- and secondary-process thinking, though speech presumably employs different proportions of these kinds of thinking than the dream. Thus, the immediate magnitude of a psychological state is considered to be approximately the same, whether the affectively toned verbal thematic reference is expressed in the past tense, present tense, or future tense, as an intention, as a conditional probability, or as a wish. Some of the defensive and adaptive mechanisms signaling the presence of suppressed and repressed feelings in language are: (a) the psychological state, or its associated ideation or behavior, are attributed to other human beings; (b) the psychological state, or its associated ideation or behavior, are said to occur in sub-human animals or in inanimate objects; (c) the psychological state and its equivalents are repudiated or denied; and (4) the psychological state and its equivalents are acknowledged, but reported to be present in attenuated form.

5. The product of the frequency of use of relevant categories of verbal statements and the numerical weights assigned to each thematic category provides an ordinal measure of the magnitude of the psychological state. That is, the greater the speaker's specific feeling state over a given unit of time, the more verbal references will be made, per 100 words, to experiences or events classified into verbal categories relevant to the specific psychological state. Thus, multiplying the weight for the category by the number of references in the verbal sample classified in that category, and then summing all the content categories pertinent to the specified state, provides an ordinal index of the intensity of the psychological state.

6. Individuals differ considerably in the rate of speech, and the same individual may vary in rate of speech from one unit of time to

another. Since numerical indices of the magnitude of emotion can vary with the number of words spoken per unit time, the numerical score derived from one verbal sample may be compared to the score derived from another, composed of a different number of words, only by using some correction factor expressing the score of the feeling state of the speakers in terms of a common denominator, for example, the score per 100 words.

Initially, this correction was made by dividing the total raw score by the number of words spoken, and multiplying by 100. It was decided later that the most satisfactory and simplest way to take into consideration rate of speech for the measurement of affects is by adding 0.5 to the raw score, multiplying by 100, and dividing by the number of words spoken. This method avoids the discontinuity occurring whenever no scorable items have occurred in some verbal samples. It also provides a uniform transformation over all samples and, with rare exceptions, reduces the correlation between the score of the psychological state and the number of words essentially to zero.

A further transformation is made to obtain the final score when measuring affects, namely, using the square root of the corrected score. This transformation is intended to reduce the skewness of the score distribution, thus making the measure more amenable to parametric statistical treatment. This square-root transformation tends to make the ordinal scale approximate the characteristics of an interval scale.

To illustrate the findings of this method of measuring the intensity of any psychological state, applications will be drawn from one of the simplest content-analysis scales, the anxiety scale:

SCHEDULE 1
Anxiety Scale*

1. Death anxiety—references to death, dying, threat of death, or anxiety about death, experienced by or occurring to:
   a. self (3)
   b. animate others (2)
   c. inanimate objects destroyed (1)
   d. denial of death anxiety (1)
2. Mutiliation (castration) anxiety—references to injury, tissue, or physical damage, or anxiety about injury or threat of such, experienced by or occurring to:
   a. self (3)
   b. animate others (2)
   c. inanimate objects (1)
   d. denial (1)
3. Separation anxiety—references to desertion, abandonment, loneliness, ostracism, loss

*Numbers in parentheses are the weights.

of support, falling, loss of love or love object, or threat of such, experienced by or
occurring to:
   a. self (3)
   b. animate others (2)
   c. inanimate objects (1)
   d. denial (1)
4. Guilt anxiety—references to adverse criticism, abuse, condemnation, moral disapproval, guilt, or threat of such, experienced by:
   a. self (3)
   b. animate others (2)
   c. denial (1)
5. Shame anxiety—references to ridicule, inadequacy, shame, embarrassment, humiliation, over-exposure of deficiencies or private details, or threat of such, experienced by:
   a. self (3)
   b. animate others (2)
   c. denial (1)
6. Diffuse or nonspecific anxiety—references by word or in phrases to anxiety and/or fear,
   without distinguishing type or source of anxiety:
   a. self (3)
   b. animate others (2)
   c. denial (1)

   The type of anxiety that this scale attempts to measure is what
might be termed "free" anxiety (in contrast to "bound" anxiety), which
manifests itself in conversion and hypochondriacal symptoms, in com-
pulsions, in doing and undoing, in withdrawal from human relationships, and so forth. It is likely that some aspects of bound anxiety
are registered by this scale, particularly by means of those content items
in the scale which involve the psychological mechanisms of displace-
ment and denial. This bound anxiety is preconscious, is relatively readily accessible to consciousness, and is capable—along with grossly conscious anxiety feelings—of activating autonomic nervous system and
central nervous system signs of arousal. There is evidence, in fact, that
these anxiety scores reflect not only the subjective awareness of anxiety
from the conscious and the preconscious level, but also the level of
relevant autonomic arousal and the level of relevant postural and kinesic
activity.
   Anxiety has been classified, on the basis of clinical experience, into
six subtypes: death, mutilation, separation, guilt, shame, and diffuse or
nonspecific anxiety (see Schedule 1). It is true that the nature and
sources of anxiety may be classified in other ways. Furthermore, it is
acknowledged that the content categories used are not always discrete
and unique, but this circumstance is consistent with the impression that
people may be experiencing different kinds of anxiety simultaneously.
This procedure does not differentiate between fear and anxiety, since it

is impossible to make this distinction on the basis of such short samples of verbal content alone.

In the classification of death anxiety, only those items dealing directly with death and destruction have been included. Mutilation fear and anxiety, as the term has been conceptualized, is synonymous with castration anxiety, and the descriptive items on the anxiety scale pertaining to this type are derived from psychoanalytic psychology (Freud, 1926; May, 1950). The concept of separation anxiety and the descriptive items designating what references in speech are to be counted under this heading have also been derived from psychoanalytic psychology, and specifically from Bowlby (1960) and others. In the descriptive items differentiating between shame and guilt anxiety the work of Piers and Singer (1953) has been used.

Actually, the categories for the anxiety scale were selected by listening to many people who were considered to be anxious and not anxious, and noting that these categories of anxiety were both relatively frequently present and readily identifiable. Further crystallization of the ideas for the descriptive features of the content items under each category heading came from listening to tape-recordings of hypnotically induced anxiety states.[1] In these tape-recordings, student nurses told stories in reaction to the same Thematic Apperception Test cards while in a hypnotic trance, before and after it was suggested that they were very anxious. The categories and descriptive details in Schedule 1 give the content items which were eventually selected.

The weights for each subcategory were assigned on the basis of the principles discussed above, namely, on the basis of the degree of personal involvement and direct representation. These weights are, of course, approximations. The square-root transformation of these anxiety scores in various validation studies appears to provide a scaling of anxiety by this verbal-behavior approach that has some earmarks of an interval instead of an ordinal scale. For example, when parametric as well as nonparametric statistics are used in evaluating the relationship of our anxiety measures to other psychological, physiological, biochemical, and pharmacological variables, a comparison of the statistical indices usually shows negligible differences. An example of a coded and scored speech sample follows. This and most of the speech samples used in the illustrative findings were obtained by telling subjects that we were doing studies of speaking and conversational habits, and getting them to talk into a tape-recorder for 5 minutes about any interesting or dramatic

---

[1]These tape-recordings were lent to L. A. Gottschalk by Levitt, Persky, and Brady, who made them in connection with an investigation of anxiety (1964).

personal life experience (Gottschalk & Hambidge, 1955; Gottschalk, 1968; Gottschalk & Gleser, 1969).

Example 1 illustrates the technique of scoring just those clauses which have scorable anxiety items, with appropriate symbols designating each category in the anxiety scale (Schedule 1). The numbers in parentheses indicate the weights assigned to each scorable content item. The diagonal marks indicate grammatical clauses. (A detailed description and discussion of scoring procedures, with many examples, is given by Gottschalk, Winget & Gleser, 1969.)

EXAMPLE 1

Verbal Sample No. 1 Coded for Anxiety

Name of subject:
(Male medical
in-patient)

Total words: 188
Correction factor: 0.5319

Well, here I am again doing this. / If I knew
$5a3$

something to talk about / I could / I could / I could
tell it better. / I don't know / whether this goes
over to the Board of Directors or what / but I
$5a3$

do / the best I know for a poor uneducated old
man. / Everything I know about myself / I like to
$5a3$ $4a3$

keep to myself. / Well, maybe the law is trying to
$4d1$

find out about me. / I was never arrested before
$4a3$

in my life. / I'd like to get arrested sometimes /
$4a3$

just to see how it feels to go to jail. / I guess / I
$5a3$ $5a3$

sound / like I'm off my rocker. / But what little I
$5a3$

know, / why it ain't hardly worth the telling. /
That nurse, she came to get more blood this
afternoon. / I just held out my arm / she jabbed
$2a3$ $2a3$

me with a needle. / Seems like / I'll run out of
$2a3$ $2a3$

blood. / I won't have any left. / Been jabbed so
$2a3$

much now, / I got a black and blue spot in my
$4a3$

arm. / I don't know / what'll happen to me / after
$3a3$

I make these complaints. / So they might discharge me / even if I am sick. /

Tabulation of Verbal Sample No. 1 Coded for Anxiety

Correction Factor (C.F.) = 0.5319

Subcategory	Total weight	Raw score
Death		
	0	—
Mutilation		
$2a3 \times 5$	15	7.98
Separation		
$3a3 \times 1$	3	1.60
Guil		
$4a3 \times 4$	13	6.91
$4d1 \times 1$		
Shame		
$5a3 \times 6$	18	9.57
Diffuse		
	0	—
Total	49	26.06

$26.06 \times \tfrac{1}{2}\text{C.F.} = 26.33$
Square root = 5.13

In this speech sample, the rationale for the scoring is as follows: "If I knew something to talk about" is scored 5a3, to signify shame anxiety (self) because this statement fits the category—"references to ridicule, inadequacy, shame, embarrassment, humiliation . . . or threat of such experienced by self." The same reasoning applies to the verbal statements: "the best I know for a *poor uneducated* old man," "like I'm off my rocker," "what little I know," "it ain't hardly worth telling."

"I'd like to get arrested sometimes" is scored 4a3, as *guilt anxiety*, because the speaker is making a "reference to adverse criticism, abuse, condemnation, moral disapproval, guilt or threat of such experienced by the self."

"She jabbed me with a needle" is classified 2a3, as *mutilation anxiety*, because it fits this content category.

SCORING FOR CONTENT CATEGORIES

The content-analysis technician applying this procedure to type-scripts of tape-recorded speech has not had to worry about approaching the work of content analysis through prolonged familiarization with, and training in, one theoretical orientation or another. Rather, the technician follows a strictly empirical approach, scoring the occurrence of any content or themes in each grammatical clause of speech according to a "cookbook"; namely, sets of various, well-delineated language categories making up each of the separate verbal-behavior scales. A manual (Gottschalk, Winget, & Gleser, 1969) is available that indicates what verbal categories should be looked for, and how much the occurrence of each one is to be weighted. Following initial coding of content in this way, the technician then follows prescribed mathematical calculations leading up to a final score for the magnitude of any one psychological state or another.

MATERIAL TO WHICH CONTENT ANALYSIS MAY BE APPLIED

This content-analysis procedure can be and has been applied to interview material, psychotherapeutic, diagnostic, or otherwise. The content-analysis scales can be applied to different kinds of language materials, obtained in a variety of situations, in both spoken and written form. Most of the reliability and validity studies have been done on small samples of speech, 2 to 5 minutes in duration, obtained in response to standard instructions. The typed data can be broken down into equal temporal units (for example, 2 to 5 minute segments). Or the units can be based on the number of words spoken by one or both participants (or more, if they are present); for example, consecutive 500-word sequences of the speaker can be coded for content. Depending on the purpose or research design of the study, these content-analysis scales have also been applied to dreams, projective test data (specifically, tape-recordings of Thematic Apperception Test responses), written verbal samples, and even to literature, letters, public speeches, and any other type of language material.

ANXIETY SCALE: NORMATIVE STUDIES[2]

The overall percentile anxiety scores for several nonpsychiatric patient samples combined ($N = 282$)[3] and also for 107 psychiatric outpatients and for 107 psychiatric inpatients, are shown in Table 1 (Gotts-

---

[2]The square-root score, corrected for discontinuity at zero, is the score used for norms and for all statistical comparisons.

[3]The samples used were the Kroger sample ($n = 94$), undergraduate college students ($n = 87$), psychiatric residency applicants ($n = 22$), Veterans Administration Hospital medical in-patients ($n = 29$), and private hospital medical in-patients ($n = 50$).

TABLE 1
Percentile Scores for the Total Anxiety Scale
in Three Groups

	Nonpsychiatric employees, students, medical in-patients ($N = 282$)	Psychiatric out-patients ($N = 107$)	Psychiatric in-patients ($N = 107$)
95	2.65	3.40	3.25
90	2.40	3.20	2.77
85	2.20	3.02	2.52
80	2.05	2.83	2.35
75	1.90	2.50	2.20
70	1.78	2.27	2.07
60	1.58	1.97	1.80
50	1.45	1.78	1.60
40	1.28	1.59	1.41
30	1.10	1.40	1.22
25	0.98	1.31	1.10
20	0.85	1.22	0.98
15	0.68	1.13	0.83
10	0.53	1.02	0.70
5	0.35	0.82	0.50
Mean	1.46	1.92	1.68
SD	0.71	0.82	0.81

chalk & Gleser, 1969). From these distributions, and from a validity study, it has been found that a score of 2.2 indicates moderate anxiety, while a score of 3.0 or more is indicative of the presence of pathological anxiety. Thus, the illustration above depicts a speech sample from a speaker suffering from a high level of anxiety.

ANXIETY AND INTELLIGENCE

A statistical test of the verbal-anxiety scores for 90 individuals employed at the same company (Kroger) revealed no difference between males and females in average anxiety, but a significant negative trend in anxiety with IQ level ($p < .05$), the lowest IQ group having the highest anxiety score ($r = -.28$). These data are shown in Figure 1. This difference is probably not due to IQ and/or education *per se;* rather, speaking extemporaneously involves a task for which individuals of lower IQ sometimes feel inadequate.

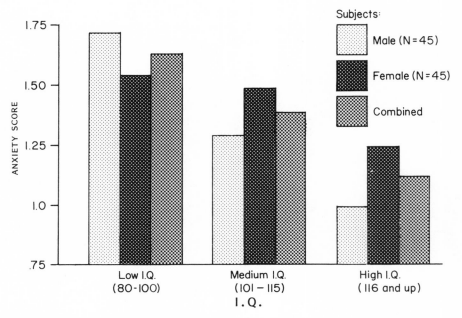

FIGURE 1. I.Q. and anxiety scores for males and females.

ANXIETY AND SEX DIFFERENCES

Although no significant sex difference has been found for overall anxiety in our sample of nonpsychiatric subjects, some interesting differences have occurred in the type of anxiety expressed, as indicated by the separate category scores for anxiety. When these were analyzed separately, again using the square-root transformation, it was found that females had significantly lower average scores than males in the categories for "death" and "mutilation" anxiety, and significantly higher average scores on "shame" anxiety. In fact, for females, shame anxiety was by far the most important category scored; whereas for the males, death, mutilation, and shame were scored with about equal average frequency.

Sex differences in anxiety subscale scores were reexamined, using the total normative sample of 173 males and 109 females. For the larger sample, the females had significantly higher mean scores on separation and shame anxiety, and significantly lower scores on death anxiety (see Figure 2). Using the median test, the difference in medians for shame and separation anxiety are significant, the median for females being higher. However, males have considerably higher scores in death anx-

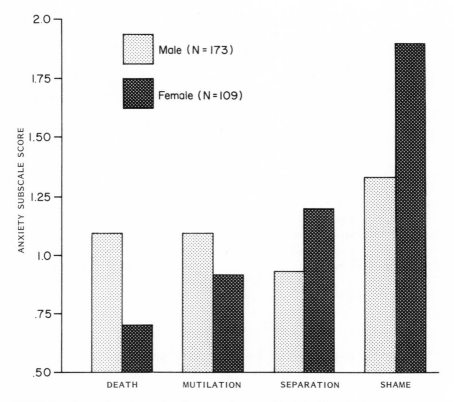

FIGURE 2. Sex and anxiety subscale scores (nonpsychiatric subjects).

iety, so that the difference is significant ($p < .05$) at the 75th percentile. There is also a tendency for the males to have higher mutilation anxiety.

Sex differences in the subscales were also examined in samples of 107 psychiatric outpatients and 107 psychiatric inpatients. For outpatients, the females again had significantly higher mean scores on separation and shame anxiety. The females were also significantly higher on diffuse anxiety. In the median test, the sexes differed significantly only on shame and diffuse anxiety. There were no significant differences between the sexes in the inpatient sample.

ANXIETY AND AGE

The relationship between age and anxiety has been examined in several samples of adults. There is no evidence of a linear relationship, correlations in all samples yielding nonsignificant coefficients. If there is a trend in anxiety with age, it is probably of a curvilinear form, increasing up to some age and then decreasing. However, the variance in anxiety scores accounted for by age of the subject would at most be quite small.

One subscale of anxiety, however, evidently increases consistently with age. In three separate samples we have found correlations of .25, .24 and .28 between age and death anxiety. Such a relationship makes considerable sense, since death appears increasingly important and threatening as one grows older. It is interesting that such a trend can be found in our data, inasmuch as death anxiety is one of the more infrequently scored subcategories of the total anxiety scale. Some additional evidence that the death anxiety score relates to the increased risk of dying is provided by the study of Miller (1965), who—using our content analysis method—found significantly higher scores on death, separation, shame, and diffuse-anxiety scores in a group of medical outpatients who had suffered, but recovered from, a myocardial infarction, as compared to such scores from a group of outpatients with other medical diseases.

INTERCORRELATIONS AMONG THE ANXIETY SUBSCALES

The intercorrelations among the anxiety subscales were examined in three separate samples of individuals. For the most part, these subscales tend to be uncorrelated, and hence may be assumed to measure independent psychological components of anxiety.

In the light of classical psychometric theory, one might question whether it is meaningful to combine such noncorrelated scores into a single score, let alone to speak of the resulting scale as measuring a single construct, anxiety. However, it has not been assumed that scores on the separate subscales represent the same dimension or kind of anxiety, but rather that they are interchangeable with regard to the intensity of anxiety. It thus might be noted that this total anxiety score can be conceptualized as the resulting magnitude of anxiety—that is, the square root of the sum of squares of the intensities on the separate subscales. The direction of this result, which would depend on the relative magnitude of the separate subscores, has, so far, been ignored. The physiological and biochemical concomitants of immediate anxiety relate to the overall intensity, rather than to the kind of anxiety, that a person is experiencing.

OTHER RELATIONSHIPS AMONG VERBAL THEMATIC CONTENT SCORES

Relationships between Measures of Anxiety and Hostility (Gottschalk & Gleser, 1969)

Correlations of the total anxiety scores and the anxiety subscale scores with the several hostility measures for two samples of people are presented in Table 2. It may be noted that total anxiety is only moderately correlated with total hostility out, hostility in, and ambivalent hostility[4] in the sample of employed personnel. The total anxiety score is somewhat more highly correlated with hostility in, and with ambivalent hostility, in the sample of psychiatric outpatients. Although the correlation between anxiety and total hostility out is about the same in the two samples, it stems from a correlation between anxiety and covert hostility[5] in the sample of employed personnel, whereas the higher correlation is between anxiety and overt hostility[6] in the patient group.

Looking at the subscales, it appears that at least part of this shift may be due to the fact that guilt anxiety is positively correlated with overt hostility in the patient group, but not in the group as employed personnel. Furthermore, shame anxiety is significantly negatively correlated with covert hostility in the patient sample. In this regard, it is interesting to note that shame is significantly correlated with hostility inward in both samples, whereas guilt is highly correlated with hostility out in both samples.

SOME EXAMPLES OF APPLICATIONS OF THE ANXIETY SCALE

A method of measuring the magnitude of any psychological state from small samples of speech would not be worth the trouble of formulating its underlying principles, or testing its reliability and validity, if it did not have applications well beyond its psychoanalytic precursors and its theoretical and empirical origins. This method of measuring psychological states from the content analysis of short samples of speech has scientific applications which justify the time and work that have

[4]Ambivalent hostility: derived from verbal communications suggesting destructive and critical thoughts or actions of others to the self.
[5]Overt hostility outward: derived from verbal communications about the self being hostile to others.
[6]Covert hostility outward: derived from verbal communications about others being hostile to others.

TABLE 2

Correlations between Anxiety Subscales and Hostility Scales Derived from Verbal Samples[a]

Anxiety subscales	Number of words	Hostility in	Ambivalent hostility	Total hostility out	Overt hostility out	Covert hostility out
(a) Employed personnel (n = 94)						
Death	0.06	−0.01	**0.28**	0.23	−0.10	**0.35**
Mutilation	−0.01	0.08	0.18	**0.46**	0.04	**0.55**
Separation	0.12	0.16	0.18	0.15	0.16	0.06
Guilt	0.22	−0.09	0.05	**0.26**	−0.15	**0.38**
Shame	**−0.31**	**0.43**	0.02	−0.09	0.15	−0.13
Diffuse	0.16	−0.03	0.07	0.18	0.16	0.11
Total anxiety scale	−0.18	**0.35**	**0.34**	**0.39**	0.10	**0.46**
(b) Psychiatric out-patients (n = 50)						
Death	0.28	−0.10	0.16	**0.36**	0.08	**0.38**
Mutilation	0.19	−0.28	−0.02	0.11	−0.24	**0.32**
Separation	0.29	**0.36**	**0.41**	0.06	0.07	−0.04
Guilt	0.05	**0.37**	**0.46**	**0.56**	**0.30**	**0.43**
Shame	−0.23	**0.43**	0.02	−0.10	0.21	**−0.32**
Diffuse	0.06	**0.54**	**0.38**	0.07	0.16	−0.13
Total anxiety scale	−0.06	**0.64**	**0.55**	**0.35**	**0.32**	0.13

[a]Higher correlations are given in bold type for emphasis.

been invested in its development. Numerous applications are outside the psychotherapeutic situation. Taking the very simplest content-analysis scale as a prototype, namely, the anxiety scale, let several studies be briefly cited which illustrate some uses of the method. (Up to now such studies would have been impossible because of the lack of just such a measurement procedure and technique).

Correlations between Anxiety Scores and Skin Temperature Changes

A group of 12 high school boys, 16 to 17 years old, gave four verbal samples (in response to standard instructions to talk about any interesting or dramatic life experiences) on each of two separate occasions, while continuous measurements of skin temperature were being taken (Gottlieb, Gleser, & Gottschalk, 1967). The first 5-minute verbal sample was taken prior to hypnotizing the subject, whereas the subsequent three samples were obtained while the subject was in a hypnotic state. The anxiety scores from six verbal samples obtained under hypnosis were correlated with the decrease in skin temperature occurring during the giving of the verbal sample for each student separately, using a rank-order correlation. Ten of the 12 correlations were positive ($p < .04$), yielding an average intrasubject correlation of .31.

In another study, examining the correlations between 5-minute sequences of two psychotherapeutic interviews and skin temperature (Gottschalk, Springer, & Gleser, 1961), a significant correlation was found between the anxiety scored in each 5-minute interval and the decrease in skin temperature from the beginning to the end of each 5-minute interval (Gottschalk & Gleser, 1969.)

Anxiety Scores from Dreams and Inhibition of Penile Erection with Rapid Eye Movement Sleep

Karacan, Goodenough, Shapiro, & Starker (1966) studied the relationships of penile erections during episodes of rapid eye movement (REM) sleep to the anxiety scores derived, by this method, from the tape-recorded dreams reported upon awakening from such periods of sleep. A statistically significant association was found between anxiety scores from such dreams and the lack of penile erections.

Studies of Relationships of Emotions to Plasma Lipids

A natural history study (Gottschalk, Cleghorn, Gleser, & Iacono, 1965) disclosed different relationships between several types of emotions and blood lipids in a group of 24 men who had fasted 10–12 hours.

Findings were cross-validated in a study of a second group of 20 men. Anxiety scores had a significant positive correlation with plasma-free fatty acids (FFA) in both groups—a sign of catecholamine (adrenergic) secretion in individuals fasting for this period of time—, whereas three types of hostility indices had essentially zero correlation with FFA. In reaction to venipuncture and free associating for 5 minutes, more anxious men tended to have higher FFA levels and sharper rises in FFA than nonanxious men. There was evidence for positive correlations between triglyceride levels and both anxiety and hostility inward scores, as well as for total hostility outward scores and levels of blood cholesterol. In contrast to studies where higher levels of emotional arousal have often been involved, and no differential relationship has been found between blood lipid levels and the kind of emotions one is experiencing, plasma lipid levels in this study were found related differently to anxiety than to hostility at relatively low levels of acute arousal.

Anxiety Levels in Dreams: Relation to Changes in Plasma-Free Fatty Acids

Blood samples for determination of plasma-free fatty acids were obtained throughout the night, by means of an indwelling venous catheter. The first blood sample was drawn at the onset of rapid eye movements, and a second after 15 minutes of these eye movements. Subjects were then awakened and asked to relate their dreams; a third sample was drawn 15–25 minutes later. Anxiety scores derived from 20 dreams of nine subjects had significant positive correlations with changes in free fatty acids occurring during the 15 minutes of REM sleep. (No statistically significant relation was found between anxiety and the changes in free fatty acids occurring from the time just before awakening to 15–25 minutes later.) These findings indicate that anxiety aroused in dreams triggers the release of certain catecholamines into the cardiovascular circulation, and these catecholamines mobilize proportional amounts of free fatty acids from body fat (Gottschalk, Cleghorn, *et al.*, 1965; Gottschalk, Stone, Gleser, & Iacono, 1966).

COMPUTER PROGRAMMING OF CONTENT ANALYSIS

One of the problems in a content-analysis system of the kind described here is the training time required to obtain high reliability of coding content according to any one scale; another problem is the time required to accurately score typescripts of interviews. Different content-analysis scales require different amounts of time to score—which includes coding content, tallying scores, and calculating raw and corrected scores. The total time range for these operations is from 10 to 60 minutes per 5-minute speech sample per scale.

In collaboration with J. S. Brown and C. Hausmann, Computer Sciences Division, University of California at Irvine, and with the technical assistance of M. Syben from my laboratory, some definite progress has been made toward developing a completely automated system for analyzing the content of natural language according to our hostility-outward scale (Gottschalk, Hausmann, & Brown, 1975). A parsing program was first developed, adapted in part from the LISP program (Lunar System, NASA). This computer program is capable of parsing natural language in a highly accurate fashion, far beyond the precision currently necessary for the level of detail and comprehension of the computerized content-analysis procedure developed at this moment. In this computer system, the denotation of hostility outward is assessed only from verbs. The specification of the agent that initiates or carries out the hostility and the object on whom the hostile action is focused require specifying the subject of the verb (a noun, pronoun, or phrase) and the direct or indirect object, and these operations are also carried out by the computer program. Admittedly, considerable meaning is lost by ignoring hostile content conveyed in adverbs, adjectives, or certain types of noun or pronoun referents. But the computer program has proved capable of correctly scoring 70 out of a series of 100 clauses scorable for hostility outward, and taken from the *Manual* for scoring these hostility scales (Gottschalk, Winget, & Gleser, 1969). Also, a nonparametric correlation of .91 was obtained between hostility-outward scores derived from six 5-minute speech samples (totaling around 3,000 words) scored by hand (i.e., by trained content-analysis technicians), compared to scores obtained from this computer program.

Another computer software program for scoring anxiety using the Gottschalk–Gleser Anxiety scale (1969) was developed and tested on 25 5-minute speech samples (Gottschalk & Bechtel, 1982). Like the computer program for scoring the Gottschalk–Gleser Hostility Outward scale, it utilized a PDP-10 mainframe and LISP software (Meehan, 1978). A Pearson product moment correlation of .85 was found between human and computer scoring, which is quite acceptable in view of the fact that training for reliability of human scores by this method call for a .85 level of inter- and intra- scorer reliability.

At the present time, Gottschalk and Bechtel are in the process of developing software for computer scoring of verbal samples applicable to the IBM Personal Computer.

PSYCHOPHARMACOLOGICAL STUDIES EMPLOYING
CONTENT ANALYSIS

In our drug society, a serious investigator in psychotherapy research, whether doing outcome or process research, cannot ignore the fact that about 65% of patients, whether they come to a Mental Health Outpatient Clinic or a General Medical Clinic, are taking some kind of psychoactive drug, either by prescription, or via the sharing of drugs from relatives or friends, or from an over-the-counter source (Gottschalk, Bates, Waskow, Katz, & Olsson, 1971). This percentage does not include such psychoactive agents as alcohol, coffee, and tobacco. Controlled studies, using this content-analysis method with a sizable number of commonly used psychoactive drugs, have demonstrated that these medicaments significantly alter an individual's psychological state. As such, the open or covert use of such psychoactive drugs may confound the researcher of psychotherapy, who may be involved in noting and measuring changes in the same psychologic continua that are influenced by pharmacologic agents. What follows are some examples of the many content-analysis studies Gottschalk and his coworkers have undertaken that indicate these psychopharmacologic influences.

1. Twenty dermatological inpatients (10 men and 10 women) were given 16 to 24 mg a day of perphenazine by mouth for one week, alternating with a placebo for one week, using a double-blind, crossover design (Gottschalk *et al.*, 1960). Analysis of the content of 5-minute speech samples obtained from these patients showed a reduction of hostility outward scores with perphenazine in 16 of the 20 patients (p < .01) and a decrease in anxiety scores among those patients who had elevated predrug anxiety scores.

2. Forty-six juvenile delinquent, 160 to 17-year-old boys were administered 20 mg of chlordiazepoxide or a placebo. Using the content analysis of 5-minute verbal samples, significant decreases were found in anxiety, ambivalent hostility, and overt hostility outward, 40 to 120 minutes after ingesting the chlordiazepoxide (Gleser *et al.*, 1961).

3. A significant increase occurred in anxiety and overt hostility outward scores, derived from verbal samples in nondepressed outpatients receiving the antidepressant drug imipramine, as compared to a placebo (Gottschalk, Gleser, Wylie, & Kaplan, 1965).

4. An oral dose of 15 mg of dextroamphetamine, as compared to a placebo or 25 mg of chlorpromazine, in a group of 33 incarcerated criminals at Patuxent Institution, Baltimore, significantly increased achievement-strivings scores derived from 5-minute speech samples (Gottschalk, Bates, Fox, & James, 1971).

5. Content analysis of speech of individuals administered either

psychotomimetric drugs (LSD-25, Ditran, or psilocybin) or a placebo showed that people receiving psychotomimetric drugs do not have higher average anxiety or hostility scores, but do have significantly higher content-analysis scores on a Cognitive and Intellectual Impairment Scale, than when they receive a placebo (Gottschalk & Gleser, 1969).

6. The relationship of plasma drug level and clinical response was studied in a double-blind, drug–placebo, crossover study, in which the antianxiety effects of a single oral dose of chlordiazepoxide (25 mg) on 18 chronically anxious, paid volunteers were observed. Though the subjects had the same oral drug dose, their plasma levels of chlordiazepoxide ranged from 0.26 to 1.63 µg/ml; and only those 11 subjects whose plasma chlordiazepoxide levels exceeded 0.70 µg/ml had a statistically significant decrease in anxiety scores, as measured from 5-minute speech samples (Gottschalk *et al.*, 1973).

7. Six former street addicts, incarcerated in Vacaville Institution, California, were administered 100 mg of meperidine (Demerol) by mouth, and another six received the same dose intramuscularly. Significant decreases in anxiety and hostility scores occurred, one hour post-drug, in both groups of subjects as derived from verbal samples (Elliott, Gottschalk, & Uliana, 1974). A significant correlation occurred between plasma meperidine concentrations and decrease in anxiety scores.

8. A group of 12 male college students gave 5-minute speech samples, after 12 to 14 hours of fasting, following ingestion of either a placebo or propranolol (40 mg), the latter being a beta adrenergic blocking agent. Resting anxiety scores were significantly lower ($p < .05$) when the subjects were on propranolol, but there was no difference, under the drug or placebo condition, in the magnitude of anxiety aroused in reaction to a stress interview. These findings, plus, in this specific study, heart rate and plasma-free fatty acid reduction, suggest that propranolol reduces anxiety primarily by reducing the afferent feedback to the central nervous system of autonomic nervous system correlates of anxiety (Gottschalk, Stone, & Gleser, 1974).

THE USE OF THIS CONTENT ANALYSIS METHOD IN PSYCHOTHERAPY RESEARCH

One of the shortcomings of any content-analysis procedure is that it discards data that might be of considerable value to the psychotherapist in a global approach to his roles. A content-analysis method cannot supplant the broad perspectives of a psychotherapist, nor his ability to synthesize many different points-of-view in listening and reacting to a community of forces. The value of a content analysis method in psychotherapy research lies more in its capacity to give objective assessments about the magnitude of specific psychological states. As such, high level measurement precision is reached, while global interrelationships may be lost. Such precise and accurate assessments of specific psychological dimensions may have considerable usefulness, for example, in the prediction of treatment outcome, whether one is interested in psychotherapy or in any other kind of treatment or change agent.

PREDICTION OF TREATMENT OUTCOME

These content-analysis scales have been used with encouraging success in a wide variety of studies on prediction of therapeutic outcome.

1. In a Brief Psychotherapy Clinic at the Cincinnati General Hospital, 5-minute speech samples were obtained from 22 clinic patients before assignment for psychotherapy (Gottschalk, Mayerson, & Gottlieb, 1967). A tape-recorded standardized interview was used to rate psychiatric change (the Psychiatric Morbidity Scale, Gottschalk et al., 1967, Gottschalk, Fox, & Bates, 1973) in terms of functional adaption, along four dimensions: psychological, interpersonal, vocational, and somatic. Pretreatment human-relations scores derived from spoken verbal samples correlated with posttreatment Psychiatric Morbidity Scale scores ($r = .66, N = 22, p < .01$). Also, scores from the pretreatment social alienation-personal disorganization scores correlated with posttreatment Psychiatric Morbidity Scale scores 7–10 weeks later ($r = .39, N = 22, p < .05$). In other words, pretreatment social alienation-personal disorganization scores predicted unfavorable therapeutic outcome, and pretreatment human-relations scores predicted favorable outcome, in this study.

2. A similar investigation of outcome in a Crisis Intervention Clinic at the Orange County Medical Center in Orange, California (Gottschalk, Noble, Stolzoff, Bates, Cable, Uliana, Birch, & Fleming, 1973) indicated that pretreatment human-relations scores predicted ($r = -.26, p < .05, N = 35$) favorable outcome assessed by a Psychiatric Morbidity Scale 7 to 10 weeks later. In this study, a randomly selected Waiting List group was asked to wait six weeks for treatment, instead of receiving it immediately. With these waiting list patients, pretreatment human-relations scores and hope scores correlated poorly with treatment-outcome, Psychiatric Morbidity Scale scores ($r = -.18$ and $r = .17$ respectively), that is, in the expected direction, but nonsignificantly; this contrasts to the results obtained with patients treated immediately (Gottschalk et al., 1973). Pretreatment hope scores correlated significantly ($p < .05$) with improvement in social alienation-personal disorganization scores for

those patients in an Actual Treatment Group, and these same hope scores correlated significantly positively ($p < .01$) with getting worse in human relations scores for those patients in a Waiting List Group. Two studies have indicated a high negative intercorrelation ($r = -.37$, $N = 22$; $r = -.58$, $N = 109$, $p < .001$) between social alienation-personal disorganization scores and human relations scores (Gottschalk & Gleser, 1969). Human relations scores and hope scores, as might be expected, are highly positively correlated (Gottschalk, 1974a); for example, in an adult group of 54, $r = .68$, ($p < .005$) and in a group of 109 school children, $r = .51$, ($p < .001$).

3. Social alienation-personal disorganization scores were predictors of a favorable response to a major tranquilizer (thioridazine) among 75 chronic schizophrenic patients at Longview State Hospital, Cincinnati, Ohio. Patients with pretreatment social alienation-personal disorganization scores greater than 2.0 were highly responsive to the administration (improvement) or withdrawal (worsening) of this tranquilizer (Gottschalk, Gleser, Cleghorn, Stone, & Winget, 1970). Patients with social alienation-personal disorganization scores less than 2.0 were relatively unresponsive to the administration or withdrawal of this major tranquilizer.

4. A recent study of the relationship of psychoactive drug blood levels to clinical response has revealed that when a single standard oral dose of thioridazine (4 mg/kg) was administered to 25 patients with acute schizophrenia at the Orange County Medical Center, predrug social alienation-personal disorganization scores were predictive of postdrug indices of plasma thioridazine concentration, such as the thioridazine half-life ($r = .44$, $p < .03$) and area-under-the-curve of decreasing drug levels with time ($r = .43$, $p < .03$). Moreover, the degree of improvement among these schizophrenic patients over the first 48 hours postdrug, in terms of factor scores from the Overall Gorham Brief Psychiatric Rating Scale, the Hamilton Depression Rating Scale, and the Wittenborn Rating Scale, was highly positively correlated with these indices of plasma thioridazine concentration, as well as with the predrug treatment social alienation-personal disorganization scores (Gottschalk, Biener, Noble, Birch, Wilbert, & Heiser, 1975).

5. Pretreatment human relations scores ($r = .40$, $p < .05$) and hope scores ($r = .38$, $p < .05$) were predictive of survival time of patients ($N = 16$) with metastatic cancer receiving partial or total body irradiation from radioactive cobalt (Gottschalk, Kunkel, Wohl, Saenger, & Winget, 1969). Further studies with 20 or more such cancer patients replicated the positive correlational trends observed in the initial study (Gottschalk, 1974a).

6. Hope scores were derived from 5-minute speech samples ob-

tained from psychiatric patients coming to the emergency room of a general hospital in Pittsburgh, Pennsylvania. These scores significantly predicted those patients who would seriously follow up with treatment recommendations (Perley, Winget, & Placci, 1971).

7. Anxiety scores were derived from reports of dreams given by women in the third trimester of pregnancy attending an outpatient ob-gyn clinic at the Cincinnati General Hospital. The absence of anxiety in these dreams was highly predictive of women who would undergo prolonged labor during childbirth (Winget & Kapp, 1972). From these early studies, one can see that various psychological dimensions, derived from the content analysis of language behavior, are predictive of a number of biological as well as psychosocial processes.

8. Viney, Clarke, Bunn, & Teak (1983) found that psychotherapy with a group ($N = 223$) of medical inpatients, in comparison with a group of medically hospitalized patients who did not receive psychotherapy, led to a significant decrease in anxiety, as measured by the Gottschalk–Gleser Anxiety scale, and an increase in self-esteem and positive feelings, that persisted for at least 15 months after the psychotherapy. Female patients proved more responsive to psychotherapy than male patients. While the psychotherapy had little impact on the physical status of the patients while they were in the hospital, for patients with more serious medical problems, psychotherapy was found to lead to less need for medication and quicker recovery. Patients who received psychotherapy had less costly consultations and fewer hospitalization costs during the 15-month follow-up period.

It is an intention, using a fuller range of the Gottschalk–Gleser and similar content-analysis scales, to explore the predictive value of combinations of these content-analysis scores for more complex outcomes. For example, what children or adults are likely to evidence continuing sociopathic or criminal behavior? Which individuals are most readily psychoanalyzable, if analyzability can be described in objective and operational terms?

STUDIES OF THE PSYCHOTHERAPEUTIC PROCESS

There have been several studies involving the use of these content-analysis scales in studying various aspects of the process of psychotherapy.

1. In one study (Gottschalk, 1974b), during the psychoanalysis of a male patient, the therapist studied what the patient was saying before, during, and after he fingered his lips, mouth, or nose. Transcripts of 14 psychoanalytic sessions, tape-recorded over a one-year period, were

divided into the smallest possible communication units (the grammatical clause). Two content-analysis technicians independently scored the typescript of each clause, according to an object–relations scale for references to females (F), males (M), sexually unspecified humans (O), and inanimate objects (I), and for positive valence (+), neutral (=), and negative feelings (−) toward any objects. Each clause was then scored for the accompanying hand position: hand touching mouth or lips (I), hand on face but not touching lips (II), and hands away from face (III). Eight hundred and thirty-six statements were scored along the three dimensions: object relations, valence, and hand position during utterance. Significantly more references were made to females while the hand was touching the mouth or lips than when not, and there were relatively more positive statements when fingering the lips or mouth than when not doing so. This investigation was seen as demonstrating that kinesic activity during psychotherapy definitely influences, or is associated with, differences in the content of thought as reflected in speech.

2. Freedman, Blass, Rifkin, & Quitkin (1973) examined the relationship between kinesic behavior, defined by a scoring system of object- and body-focused hand movements, and the direction of aggression as measured by the Gottschalk–Gleser hostility scales. Motor behavior and concomitant speech samples were scored from videotaped interview segments of 24 college students. Intercorrelational analysis revealed that object-focused movements were related to overt hostility ($r = .49$) and that body-focused movements were related to covert hostility ($r = .53$) and, specifically, to hand-to-hand motions ($r = .52$). These findings were interpreted as revealing the differential role of object- and body-focused movements in the encoding of affect.

3. During two psychotherapeutic sessions, each 5-minute segment of a patients' verbal interactions was scored for anxiety according to the Gottschalk–Gleser anxiety scale, and the change in skin temperature before and after each 5-minute segment was noted. A significant correlation ($p < .02$) was found between the anxiety score from each 5-minute speech interval and a decrease in skin temperature (Gottschalk, Springer, & Gleser, 1961). This was one finding that substantiated the hypothesis that the anxiety measured by the Gottschalk–Gleser Anxiety Scale was associated with the release of adrenergic chemical substances in the body (Gottschalk, Stone, Gleser, & Iacono, 1966).

4. From simultaneously tape-recorded interviews and electroencephalograms of a twenty year old male patient, high amplitude bursts of paroxysmal electroencephalographic activity were found to be preceded by higher anxiety ($p < .05$) and hostility inward ($p < .05$), derived from the content analysis of 30-word segments of speech occurring just

before a paroxysmal EEG burst, than from a 30-word speech sample not followed by such abnormal electroencephalographic activity (Gottschalk, 1972; Luborsky, Docherty, Todd, Kanpp, Mirsky, & Gottschalk, 1975). This study is a contribution to the understanding of psychological trigger mechanisms in some epileptic seizures.

5. Changes in anxiety, hostility outwards, and social alienation-personal disorganization, as well as other psychological states, were scored from successive 5-minute segments of two psychotherapeutic interviews, using the Gottschalk–Gleser scales (Gottschalk *et al.*, 1961b). The interrelationships of these changes across psychological states were examined, as were the psychological responses to the psychotherapist's interventions. This study represents one of the first investigations measuring sequential changes in affects and other psychological states during the psychotherapeutic process.

6. Schöfer, Balck, and Koch (1979), in applying the Gottschalk–Gleser method to psychotherapy research, have proposed defining "natural" summarizing units appropriate to the quality of the psychotherapeutic dialogue. They suggested three kinds of summarizing units: (a) the individual sentence; (b) the individual statement; (c) the individual session. They demonstrated that the analysis of representative sections from a psychotherapeutic session could provide indices typifying the whole psychotherapy. For example, by scoring the first, the last, and the longest speech samples of an hour, scores representative of the total hour were obtained. If this could be generalized to other psychotherapeutic session, the time involved in scoring could be greatly decreased.

In another study cited by these investigators (Schöfer, Balck, & Koch, 1979, pp. 857–870) a session score was obtained by combining all statements from one patient having more than 90 words from 17 transcribed psychotherapeutic hours. All affects scored in the course of the therapy had a tendency to decrease. All affect scores were combined into a "total affect" score, and the 9th and 14th hours were noted to be prominent because of their relatively high scores. In both these sessions, the patient relapsed into reporting her chief complaint, strong itching of the skin. Immediately after both of these hours the therapist expressed his skepticism in regard to a successful outcome of the therapy. In each of the following sessions, the 10th and 15th, the therapist's skepticism turned to optimism, while the patient's affectivity greatly decreased.

7. Witkin, Lewis, & Weil (1968) were the first group of investigators to demonstrate that shame anxiety, as measured by the Gottschalk–Gleser Anxiety Scale, was more likely to be prominent in less differentiated (field-dependent) patients and that guilt anxiety was more prominent in differentiated (field-independent) patients. These authors also

report interesting interactions between the therapist's cognitive style, that is, whether the therapist was field-dependent or independent, and the patient's anxiety during the psychotherapeutic process.

8. Lewis (1979) has illustrated how she has used the Gottschalk–Gleser method of analyzing content to examine the role of shame and guilt in neurosis, and to explore sex differences in superego style. She demonstrated an affinity between *shame*, field-dependence, depression, and hysteria, and between *guilt*, field-independence, paranoia, and obsessive-compulsive neurosis.

Lewis (1971, 1979) has also written extensively about how guilt-ridden, as compared to shame-ridden, individuals are psychodynamically organized, especially with respect to their aggression and hostility. To independently verify her clinical differentiations of guilt and shame, as well as the relationship of these affects to various kinds of hostile affects, she sent segments of the typescripts of tape-recorded psychotherapeutic interviews for independent and blind scoring of anxiety and hostility by content analysis. According to the Gottschalk–Gleser scales, content analysis showed that guilt-anxiety scores correlated significantly and positively with hostility outward scores in the same speech samples, and shame anxiety scores correlated significantly and positively with hostility-inward scores (Gottschalk & Gleser, 1969). Of further interest in these elaborate psychotherapy studies is the finding that patients with high guilt-anxiety content-analysis scores tend to be perceptually and cognitively organized in the direction of field independence, as assessed by the Rod-and-Frame Test (Witkin, 1949), and that patients who have high shame-anxiety content-analysis scores are field dependent. These affective perceptual-cognitive orientations definitely influence the course of psychotherapy and the nature of the psychotherapeutic interventions necessary to effect therapeutic change.

CONTENT-ANALYSIS STUDIES OF INTERVIEWER–INTERVIEWEE INTERACTION

Several studies have been carried out exploring interviewer effects on interviewee anxiety and hostility. These studies suggest that different response patterns of interviewees can be obtained with different interviewers. The importance of such studies for psychotherapy is that they provide some experimental means of demonstrating exactly how either countertransference or conscious attitudes of the psychotherapist are capable of influencing the responses of a patient. The effects of countertransference on the patient are already familiar to psychotherapists, but the more subtle mechanisms of the communication of such emotional states are not completely understood, and the extent of such effects in extrapsychotherapeutic situations is not realized.

1. Two male interviewers each obtained two 5-minute verbal samples from eight normal, employed subjects (Gottschalk, 1971). The first of these two verbal samples was elicited by using a so-called "visual" method of induction (Gottschalk & Hambidge, 1955), which involved giving each subject a series of Thematic Apperception Test (TAT) cards (7 GF, 13 MF, 2 BM, 3 BM) and asking the subject to tell stories about the pictures for 5 minutes. The second verbal sample was elicited by using a standard "verbal" method of induction in which the subjects were asked to speak for 5 minutes about any interesting or dramatic life experiences.

The order of obtaining the verbal samples by each interviewer was balanced. That is, one interviewer elicited verbal samples first from four of the subjects, and the other interviewer elicited verbal samples first from the other four subjects. Anxiety and hostility outward scores were determined from the speech samples by a technician unfamiliar with this study. The effects of interviewer, method of induction of speech ("visual" or "verbal"), order, and their interactions on affect scores were statistically computed (by analysis of variance). The results of this study are illustrated in Figure 3.

Anxiety scores were significantly lower ($p < .005$) when obtained by interviewer A than by interviewer B. This difference was consistent over both methods of obtaining verbal samples. No differences in hostility outward scores were noted with respect to which interviewer obtained the verbal samples.

2. The opportunity to look further at the effect of the sex of personality or sex of the interviewer on the content of verbal samples was afforded by a study of 170 freshman college students, participating in preacademic orientation exercises (Gottschalk & Gleser, 1969). These subjects, who were paid $1.00 each to volunteer their services, all gave 5-minute verbal samples on the same day, in response to standard instructions to one of four interviewers, two male and two female. The assignment of interviewer was unsystematic. When the verbal samples were sorted, it was found that one interviewer had seen only ten subjects of each sex. Thus, an equal number of each sex was randomly selected from the verbal samples of the other three interviewers. These 80 verbal samples were scored for anxiety and hostility. Differences in these scores attributable to the sex or personality of the interviewer were sought statistically, using a mixed-model, nested analysis of variance.

The average anxiety scores for male and female subjects classified according to the interviewer are shown in Figure 4. From the analysis of variance of these data it was determined that the sex of the interviewer

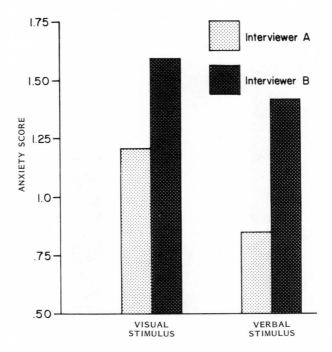

FIGURE 3. Effect of two different interviewers on anxiety scores from eight subjects.

per se had no effect on anxiety scores, but that some interviewers, regardless of their sex, obtained higher anxiety scores on the average than did others ($F = 3.60$; $p < .05$). Furthermore, some interviewers consistently obtained higher anxiety scores from female subjects, whereas for other interviewers, the higher scores were obtained with male interviewees.

The findings with respect to hostility-inward scores were similar to those for anxiety, as indicated in Figure 5. However, for this variable, the interviewer effect (for a given sex) reached a higher level of significance than for anxiety.

The hostility-outward scores, averaged according to interviewer and sex of subject, are shown in Figure 6. Again the sex of the interviewer had no significant effect on scores, but certain interviewers, regardless of sex, differed significantly in the amount of hostility outward they elicited from both male and female subjects.

Ambivalent hostility scores (derived from references to critical or destructive thoughts, or to actions of others towards self), unlike those of the other three affects, showed a definite (interaction) effect of sex of

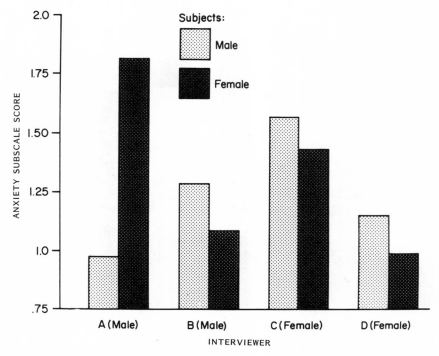

FIGURE 4. Anxiety scores for male and female subjects (in groups of 10) interviewed by different interviewers.

interviewer with sex of interviewee ($p < .001$). Female subjects responded with higher ambivalent hostility scores when interviewed by males than when interviewed by females. Male subjects, on the other hand, had higher ambivalent hostility scores when interviewed by females than when interviewed by males (see Figure 7).

An interesting feature of these findings was that the higher hostility scores were elicited by a male and a female interviewer who were in the throes of divorce proceedings, and these interviewers evoked especially high hostility scores from interviewees of the opposite sex. These interviewers were unaware of any specific feelings or behavior on their part that might have been provocative. If either of them had been psychoanalysts, which they were not, they would hopefully have recognized any subtle reactions to their interviewees, helping us understand why their interviewees responded in such a fashion to them. But how these attitudes are communicated needs to be ascertained more precisely. Videotaping such an interview might provide some answers.

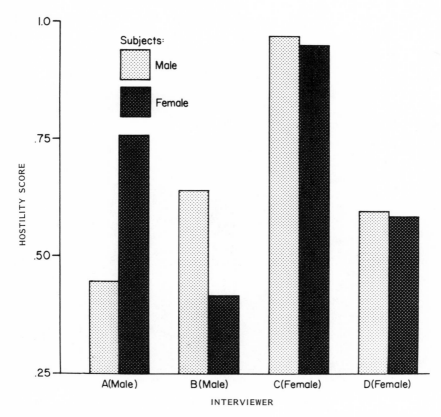

FIGURE 5. Hostility inward scores for male and female subjects (in groups of 10) interviewed by different interviewers.

3. Other experimental studies of the effects of the interviewer on the interviewer have been reported by Gottschalk and Gleser (1969). One of these examined the effect of personality or sex of the interviewer on sexual references, self-references, and affect scores (p. 261 f.). Another examined whether an interviewer can deliberately influence the frequency of the verbal response of the speaker without the speaker's awareness (p. 273 f.). Both of the studies illustrated the potentialities of interpersonal, interactional investigations using content analyses.

4. Schöfer, Koch, and Balck (1979) have examined the relationship of hostile and anxious affects, as measured by the Gottschalk–Gleser content-analysis method, to sex of the interviewee, sex of the interviewer, socioeconomic class, and age, in a German-speaking population of subjects.

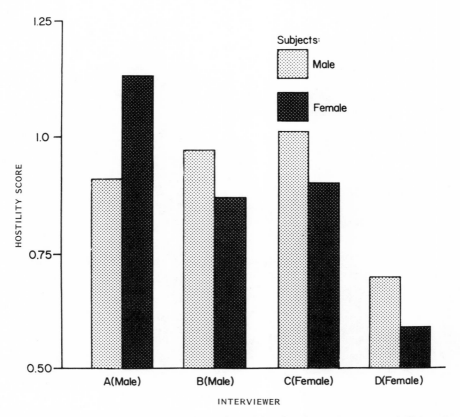

FIGURE 6. Hostility outward scores for male and female subjects (in groups of 10) interviewed by different interviewers.

In a pilot study, Schöfer (1977) showed that the scores themselves, as well as the intercorrelations of the hostility and anxiety scores of a subsample ($N = 200$) of a larger sample were very similar to the normative scores (Kroger sample) published by Gottschalk and Gleser (1969). This finding illustrates the cross-ethnic and cross-language applicability and generalizability of this method.

This careful study revealed that social class is definitely related to the magnitude of affect expression, and that the lower social class in West Germany has significantly higher affect scores than the upper social class. This investigation, moreover, unearthed interviewer–interviewee interactional effects not previously explored by American behavioral scientists.

5. Lolas and von Rad (1982) studied alexithymia characteristics in psychosomatic and psychoneurotic patients, examining the first 30 min-

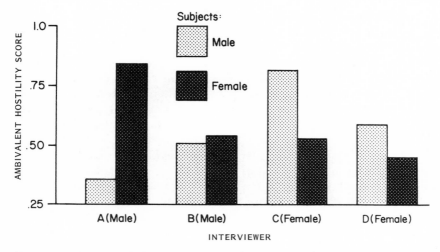

FIGURE 7. Ambivalent hostility scores for male and female subjects (in groups of 10) interviewed by different interviewers.

utes of an interview obtained from tape recordings. Both the interviewers' and patients' utterances were content-analyzed for anxiety, by means of the Electronic Verbal Analysis System (Grünzig, Holzcheck, & Kächele, 1976) implemented at the Telefunken TR 40 computer at the university of Ulm. Interviewers showed a tendency to produce more words in the separation-anxiety category ($p < .01$) when talking with psychoneurotic patients, who emitted more shame anxiety ($p < .05$) when compared with psychosomatic patients.

These psychotherapy studies provide only a brief example of the range and kinds of applications of these content-analysis scales to psychotherapy research. With appropriate research goals and research design, the applications of these measurement tools are limited only by the ingenuity and innovativeness of the serious investigator.

The usefulness of these content-analysis scales in following psychotherapeutic interaction has hardly been touched on thus far. A few studies have looked into interactional approaches (Gottschalk, Springer, & Gleser, 1961; Witkin, Lewis, & Weil, 1968; Schöfer et al, 1979; Lolas & von Rad, 1982). But none has applied content analysis to the extent that it can and should be used. One of the main reasons for this situation is that construct-validation studies have had higher priority. Secondly, other applications, for example, to prediction of outcome, psychopharmacology, and psychophysiology, have somehow taken precedence. Interactional studies could objectively examine whether certain types of comments by the psychotherapist are more likely to produce one effect or another. There is a belief among psychodynamically oriented therapists, for example, that a direct interpretation of the presence of a client's unconscious urge or affect will lead to its inhibition, whereas pointing out irrational bases for inhibiting such an urge or affect will enhance its expression. Content analysis of the kind described here could easily objectively test such a hypothesis or many others. Such research might be time-consuming, but the results could help move psychotherapy research into a position where it would become less of an art and more of a science.

Recently Viney (1983) in Australia has provided an excellent review and appraisal of the assesment of psychological states through content analysis of verbal communication. The review not only provides information about available content-analysis scales, but also provides and suggests applications in personality, developmental psychology, and social psychology, as well as in clinical, community, and health psychology.

A SUMMARY OF OTHER GOTTSCHALK–GLESER CONTENT SCALES APPLICABLE TO PSYCHOTHERAPY RESEARCH

There are many other Gottschalk–Gleser content-analysis scales besides the Anxiety scale that can be applied to psychotherapy research. Although there is not space available here to review in detail the reliability and validity studies on which these scales are based, this information is available in other publications (Gottschalk & Gleser, 1969; Gottschalk, 1979a). But there is space to summarize what these scales were designed to measure, to give references to pertinent investigations involving these scales, and to provide a description of the verbal categories employed in each scale. In addition, it is relevant to mention that these scales have undergone separate reliability and validity studies in connection with their applicability to children ranging in age from 6 to 16 (Gottschalk, 1976; Gottschalk & Uliana, 1979; Gottschalk et al., 1979; Gleser, Winget, Seligman, & Rauh, 1979; Winget, Seligman, Rauh, & Gleser, 1979).

Hostility Scales

The Hostility scales were designed to measure three types of hostility of a transient, rather than sustained, affect. The Hostility Directed Outward scale measures the intensity of adversely critical, angry, assaultive, asocial impulses and drives towards objects outside oneself. The Hostility Directed Inward scale measures degrees of self-hate and self-criticism and, to some extent, feelings of anxious depression and masochism. The Ambivalent Hostility scale, though derived from verbal communications suggesting destructive and critical thoughts or actions of others to the self, also measures, not only some aspects of hostility directed inward, but at the same time some features of hostility directed outward. All three hostility scales assign higher weights to scorable verbal statements communicating hostility that, by inference, is more likely to be strongly experienced by the speaker; on the other hand, completely repressed hostility is not scored.

Reliability and validity studies of hostility scales are numerous, and have been published elsehwere (Gottschalk & Gleser, 1969; Gottschalk, 1979a).

SCHEDULE 2

Hostility Directed Outward Scale: Destructive, Injurious, Critical Thoughts
and Actions Directed to Others

I. Hostility Outward—Overt
    Thematic Categories

a 3* Self killing, fighting, injuring other individuals or threatening to do so.

b 3 Self robbing or abandoning other individuals, causing suffering or anguish to others, or threatening to do so.

c 3 Self adversely criticizing, depreciating, blaming, expressing anger or dislike of other human beings.

a 2 Self killing, injuring or destroying domestic animals, pets, or threatening to do so.

b 2 Self abandoning, robbing, domestic animals, pets, or threatening to do so.

c 2 Self criticizing or depreciating others in a vague or mild manner.

d 2 Self depriving or disappointing other human beings.

II. Hostility Outward—Covert
     Thematic Categories

a 3* Others (human) killing, fighting, injuring other individuals or threatening to do so.

b 3 Other (human) robbing, abandoning, causing suffering or anguish to other individuals or threatening to do so.

c 3 Others adversely criticizing, depreciating, blaming, expressing anger, dislike of other human beings.

a 2 Other (human) killing, injuring, or destroying domestic animals, pets, or threatening to do so.

b 2 Others (human) abandoning, robbing, domestic animals, pets, or threatening to do so.

c 2 Others (human) criticizing or depreciating other individuals in a vague or mild manner.

d 2 Others (human) depriving or disappointing other human beings.

e 2 Others (human or domestic animals) dying or killed violently in death-dealing situation or threatening with such.

*The number serves to give the weight, as well as to identify the category. The letter also helps identify the category.

SCHEDULE 2 (*Continued*)

I.   Hostility Outward—Overt
       Thematic Categories

a 1 Self killing, injuring,
       destroying, robbing wild life,
       flora, inanimate objects or
       threatening to do so.

b 1 Self adversely criticizing,
       depreciating, blaming,
       expressing anger or dislike of
       subhumans, inanimate objects,
       places, sittuations.

c 1 Self using hostile words,
       cursing, mention of anger or
       rage without referent.

II. Hostility Outward—Covert
       Thematic Categories

f 2 Bodies (human or domestic
       animals) mutilated,
       depreciated, defiled.

a 1 Wild life, flora, inanimate
       objects, injured, broken,
       robbed, destroyed or
       threatened with such (with or
       without mention of agent).

b 1 Others (human) adversely
       criticizing, depreciating,
       expressing anger or dislike of
       subhumans, inanimate objects,
       places, situations.

c 1 Others angry, cursing,
       without reference to cause or
       direction of anger. Also
       instruments of destruction not
       used threateningly.

d 1 Others (human, domestic,
       animals) injured, robbed,
       dead, abandoned, or
       threatened with such, from
       any source including
       subhuman and inanimate
       objects, situations (storms,
       floods, etc.).

e 1 Subhumans killing, fighting,
       injuring, robbing, destroying
       each other, or threatening to
       do so.

f 1 Denial of anger, dislike,
       hatred, cruelty, and intent to
       harm.

SCHEDULE 3

Hostility Directed Inward Scale: Self-Destructive, Self-Critical Thoughts and Actions

I Hostility Inward

Thematic Categories

a 4* References to self (speaker) attempting or threatening to kill self, with or without
       conscious intent.
b 4 References to self wanting to die, needing or deserving to die.
a 3 References to self injuring, mutilating, disfiguring self, or threats to do so, with or
       without conscious intent.

*The number serves to give the weight, as well as to identify the category. The letter also helps identify
  the category.

SCHEDULE 3 (*Continued*)

Thematic Categories

b 3   Self blaming, expressing anger or hatred to self, considering self worthless or of no value, causing oneself grief or trouble, or threatening to do so.

c 3   References to feelings of discouragement, giving up hope, despairing, feeling grieved or depressed, having no purpose in life.

a 2   References to self needing or deserving punishment, paying for one's sins, needing to atone or do penance.

b 2   Self adversely criticizing, depreciating self; references to regretting, being sorry or ashamed for what one says or does; references to self mistaken or in error.

c 2   References to feeling of deprivation, disappointment, lonesomeness.

a 1   References to feeling disappointed in self; unable to meet expectations of self or others.

b 1   Denial of anger, dislike, hatred, blame, destructive impulses from self to self.

c 1   References to feeling painfully driven or obliged to meet one's own expectations and standards.

SCHEDULE 4

Ambivalent Hostility Scale: Destructive, Injurious, Critical Thoughts and Actions of Others to Self

II Ambivalent Hostility

Thematic Categories

a 3*   Others (human) killing or threatening to kill self.

b 3   Others (human) physically injuring, mutilating, disfiguring self, or threatening to do so.

c 3   Others (human) adversely criticizing, blaming, expressing anger or dislike toward self, or threatening to do so.

d 3   Others (human) abandoning, robbing self, causing suffering, anguish, or threatening to do so.

a 2   Others (human) depriving, disappointing, misunderstanding self or threatening to do so.

b 2   Self threatened with death from subhuman or inanimate object, or death-dealing situation.

a 1   Others (subhuman, inanimate, *or situation*) injuring, abandoning, robbing self, causing suffering, anguish.

b 1   Denial of blame.

*The number serves to give the weight as well as to identify the category. The letter also helps identify the category.

Social Alienation and Personal Disorganization Scale

The Social Alienation and Personal Disorganization scale was, originally, designed to measure the relative degree of personal disorganization, social alienation, and isolation of schizophrenic patients. The common denominators of the schizophrenic syndrome are considered to be disturbances in the coherence and logicality of thinking processes and disturbances in human relationships, especially in the form of withdrawal, avoidance, and antagonism. Another principal characteristic of this concept of the schizophrenic syndrome is that it is a phenomenon quantitatively describable, that is, that there are relative degrees of severity of schizophrenia and that, in some schizophrenic individuals, the severity can fluctuate considerably from day to day. This concept of the schizophrenic syndrome, in fact, holds that these principal and characteristic features of schizophrenia—social alienation and personal disorganization—are present to varying extents in nonschizophrenic individuals, but not in such a continuous and/or extreme fashion.

Reliability and validity studies of these social-alienation and personal-disorganization scales are intensive and have been published elsewhere (Gottschalk & Gleser, 1969; Gottschalk, 1979a).

SCHEDULE 5

Content-Analysis Scale of (Schizophrenic) Social Alienation
and Personal Disorganization

Scores (Weights)		Categories & Scoring Symbols:
Modified*	Original+	
		I. Interpersonal references (including fauna and flora).
		A. To thoughts, feelings, or reported actions of avoidance, leaving, deserting, spurning, not understanding of others.
0	+1	1. Self avoiding others
+1	+1	2. Others avoiding self.
		B. To unfriendly, hostile, destructive thoughts, feelings, or actions.
+1	+1	1. Self unfriendly to others.
+½	+1	2. Others unfriendly to self.
		C. To congenial and constructive thoughts, feelings, or actions.
−2	−1	1. Others helping, being friendly towards others.
−2	−1	2. Self helping, being friendly towards others.
		3. Others helping, being friendly towards self.
		D. To others (including fauna, flora, things, and places).
0	+1	1. Bad, dangerous, low value or worth, strange, ill, malfunctioning.
−1	−½	2. Intact, satisfied, healthy, well.
		II. Intrapersonal references
		A. To disorientation-orientation, past present, or future. (Do not include all references to time, place, or person, but only those in which it is

*The number serves to give the weight as well as to identify the category. The letter also helps identify the category.

SCHEDULE 5 (*Continued*)

Scores (Weights)		
Modified*	Original+	Categories & Scoring Symbols:

Modified*	Original+	Categories & Scoring Symbols
		reasonably clear the subject is trying to orient himself, or is expressing disorientation with respect to these. Also, do not score more than one item per clause under this category.)
+2	+1	1. Indicating disorientation for time, place, or person, or other distortion reality.
0	−½	2. Indicating orientation in time, place, person.
0	+½	3. Indicating attempts to identify time, place, or person, without clearly revealing orientation or disorientation.
		III. A. Signs of disorganization.
+1	+1	1. Remarks or words that are not understandable or inaudible.
0	+1	2. Incomplete sentences, clauses, phrases; blocking.
+2	+1	3. Obviously erroneous or fallacious remarks or conclusions; illogical or bizarre statements.
		B. Repetition of ideas in sequence.
0	+½	1. Words separated only by a word (excluding instances due to grammatical and syntactic convention, where words are repeated, e.g., "as far as," "by and by," and so forth. Also, excluding instances where such words as "I" and "the" are spearated by a word).
+1	+1	2. Phrases, clauses (separated only by a phrase or clause).
		New Items
+1	0	IV. A. Questions directed to the interviewer.
+½	0	B. Other references to the interviewer.
+1	0	V. Religious and biblical references.
		B. To self
0	+1	1a. Physical illness, malfunctioning (references to illness or symptoms due primarily to cellular or tissue damage).
+1	+1	1b. Psychological malfunctioning (references to illness or symptoms due primarily to emotions or psychological reactions not secondary to cellular or tissue damage).
0	+1	1c. Malfunctioning of indeterminate origin (references to illness or symptoms not definitely attributable either to emotions or cellular damage).
−2	−½	2. Getting better.
−1	−1	3a. Intact, satisfied, healthy, well; definite positive affect or valence indicated.

(*continued*)

SCHEDULE 5 (*Continued*)

Scores (Weights)

Categories & Scoring Symbols:

Modified*	Original+		
−1	−1	3b.	Intact, satisfied, healthy, well; flat, factual, or neutral attitudes expressed.
+⅟₁	+½	4.7	Not being prepared or able to produce, perform, act, not knowing, not sure.
+½	+1	5.	To being controlled, feeling controlled, wanting control, asking for control or permission, being obliged or having to do, think or experience something.
+3	−½	C.	Denial of feelings, attitudes, or mental state of the self.
		D.	To food.
0	+1	1.	Bad, dangerous, unpleasant, or otherwise negative; interferences or delays in eating; too much and wish to have less; too little and wish to have more.
0	−½	2.	Good or neutral.
		E.	To weather
−1	−½	1.	Bad, dangerous, unpleasant or otherwise negative (not sunny, not clear, uncomfortable, etc.)
−1	−1	2.	Good, pleasant or neutral.
		F.	To sleep
0	+1	1.	Bad, dangerous, unpleasant or otherwise negative; too much; too little.
0	−½	2.	Good, pleasant or neutral.

Human Relations Scale

The Human Relation scale provides a quantitative estimate of an individual's degree of interest in and capacity for constructive, mutually productive, or satisfying human relationships.

Details of initial and further validation studies of the Human Relations Scale scores are available. (Gottschalk, 1968; Gottschalk & Gleser, 1969, pp. 225–228).

SCHEDULE 6

Score each clause of the verbal sample with one of the code symbols preceding the following thematic categories, whenever the content of the clause denotes similar or equivalent content to any of these thematic categories. Many clauses may not contain themes that are similar to these categories and hence can be left unscored.

Scoring weights are given in the left-hand margin beside each category. Total words of the verbal sample should be counted and used as a correction factor to arrive at a final score. Where it is possible to score a clause under two different categories, choose scoring

SCHEDULE 6 (*Continued*)

which is weighted minus rather than plus, and give the lowest rating toward the negative pole, that is, give priority to pathology. Give only one score per clause.

Weight		Content Categories & Scoring symbols
	A1.	References to giving to, supporting, helping, or protecting others.
+2		a. Self to others—specific
+1		a'. Self to others—references in which the giving etc. is inferential or the object is unspecified.
+1		b. Others giving to others or others receiving from and being taken care of by others.
	A2.	References to warm, loving, congenial human relations or human relations in which a desire to be closer is expressed. The reference should be specific rather than inferred. Do not score such key words as marriage or friends in this category unless there is additional evidence of congeniality. Rather, score in B2, below.
+2		a. Involving self or self and others
+1		b. Involving others
	A3.	Concern for other people; references to missing others when they are away. References should be to specific others only.
+1		a. Self about others
+1		b. Others about self
+½		c. Others about others
	A4.	Praise or approval of others indicating more than neutral relations (see B2 below) but not conveying as much positive feeling or warmth as A2, above.
+1		a. Self to others
+1		b. Others to self
+½		c. Others to others
	B1.	References to manipulative relationships with other human beings. The reference should involve demanding someone do something largely in the service of one's own needs (exploitive), or deliberately making someone feel shame or guilt, e.g., by putting emphasis on how one is made to suffer.
−½		a. Self manipulating others
−1		b. Others manipulating self
−½		c. Others manipulating others
	B2.	Neutral: nonevaluative references to any kinds of human relations which specify the person(s) interacted with, but which do not specify the nature of the deeper involvement and which are not classified elsewhere. All references to self and others (e.g., we drove, we reached, we thought, etc.) not scorable elsewhere are coded B2a.
+¼		a. Self or self and others
+¼		b. Others
−½	B3.	Neutral: nonevaluative references to any kinds of human relations, which are generalized, ambiguous as to person(s) interacted with and impersonal.
	C1.	Expulsive: references to competitive, hostile, depreciating, and smearing attitudes, impulses, actions.
−½		a. Self to others

(*continued*)

SCHEDULE 6 (*Continued*)

Weight		Content Categories & Scoring symbols
−1		b. Others to self
−½		c. Others to others
	C2.	Retentive: references to withholding affection, interest, approval, or attention from people; references to disapproval.
−1		a. Self from others
−1		b. Others from self
−½		c. Others from others
	C3.	Distancing: references in which people are alienated, drawn apart, kept at a distance from one another.
−1		a. Focus on self
−½		b. Focus on others
	D1.	Optimism: references to self receiving from, getting from, being taken care of, by other people in gratifying and positive way; interest in other people based on what they can do for oneself; asking others for help, emphasis on the self as the recipient of nurturance and sustenance.
+2		a. Self receiving from others
	D2.	Pessimism: references to frustration in being taken care of or to poor or inadequate protection, support or care.
−½		a. Self
−½		b. Others
	D3.	Separation: any reference to separation, loss, death, not scored elsewhere.
−1		a. Self
−½		b. Others
	D4.	References to eating or to food in connection with others.
+½		(1) Positive valence
		a. Self
		b. Others
+½		(2) Neutral valence
		a. Self
		b. Others
		(3) Negative valence
−1		a. Self
−½		b. Others
0	D5.	References to difficulty talking, to not knowing what to say, to being at a loss for words with interviewer or others.
	D6.	Direct interaction with interviewer.
+½		a. Asking questions of interviewer when standardized verbal sample instructions have been used.
+½		b. Other direct references: "you know," or statements addressing interviewer directly by name or as "you."
−2	E1.	References to lack of humans or subhumans in the environment. The references must contain evidence of lack of interest in or need for human or subhuman objects.
−1	E2.	References to eating, food, drinking, meals, etc. out of the context of other people. Code both self and others.
−1	E3.	References to bathing alone (no other people in view) or to undifferentiated or amorphous substances or surroundings involving no discernible human beings.

Achievement Strivings Scale

The scale-measuring magnitudes of achievement strivings employs content categories pertaining to achievement strivings, and not to those involving frustration. The content categories are broken down into typically *vocational* (Categories I and II) and *avocational* (Categories V and VI) pursuits. Category III focuses on the sense of commitment or sense of obligation to responsible or constructive social and personal behavior, or to a feeling of obligation to perform well or to succeed in a task. Category IV focuses on inner or external deterrents towards achieving or succeeding.

Preliminary validation studies of this scale are available. (Gottschalk & Gleser, 1969, pp. 237–243).

SCHEDULE 7

Achievement Strivings Scale

Score all codable clauses. Distinguish between references to the self or others by adding the following notation: (*a*) self or self and others; (*b*) others.

I. Vocational, occupational, educational references, including naming and identification.

II. Other constructive activities where emphasis is on work or labor rather than play. Emphasis may be in form of overcoming hardships, obstacles, problems, toward reaching a goal. Exclude all sports and entertainment activities.
   A. Domestic activities: moving; buying or selling major items; decorating, painting, cleaning, cooking, doing chores.
   B. Activities that require some effort or perseverance to carry out or activities done with speed or accuracy, activities involving trying new experiences as in eating new food or travelling to new places (score no more than three in succession of references to travelling to new places). Score references to learning new information or habits, needing to satisfy curiosity, or attempting to unlearn undesirable attitudes or behavior.

III. References to commitment or sense of obligation to responsible or constructive social and personal behavior; to obligation to perform well or succeed in a task; to commitment to a task and to carrying it out or completing it. References to inculcation by others or self of sense of responsibility for one's actions or for welfare of others; responsibility for leadership; evidence of positive superego or ego ideal; evidence of high standards or standards that are hard to live up to (score these even when reference is to fears of not achieving, e.g., "I felt terrible about doing so badly on the test").

IV. Deterrents
   A. External dangers or problems or fear of loss of control or limit-setting on part of others. References to lack of control by others; references to errors or misjudgments by others that might injure the self.
   B. Internal obstacles: references to difficulties in setting limits on oneself or problems

(continued)

SCHEDULE 7 (*Continued*)

in disciplining the self; references to errors or misjudgments by self that might harm the self.
C. Interpersonal: arguments or troubles getting along with others; problems in interpersonal relations, such as inability to make friends.

V. Sports (note that some sports, such as swimming, may be A, B, or C, depending on context).
    A. Spectator.
    B. Team or organized.
    C. Solitary or small group.

VI. Entertainment.
    A. Spectator.
    B. Amateur.
    C. Professional.

Hope Scale

The Hope scale was designed to measure the intensity of the optimism that a "favorable outcome" is likely to occur, not only in one's personal earthly activities, but also in cosmic phenomena, and even in spiritual or imaginary events. The "favorable outcome" is intended to denote one which might lead to human survival, the preservation or enhancement of health, the welfare or constructive achievement of the self or any part of mankind.

Construct-validation data, as well as other relevant material on the Hope Scale, are available elsewhere (Gottschalk, 1974a).

SCHEDULE 8

"Hope" Scale

Weights	Content Categories & Scoring Symbols
+1	H 1. References to self or others getting or receiving help, advice, support, sustenance, confidence, esteem (*a*) from others; (*b*) from self.
+1	H 2. References to feelings of optimism about the present or future (*a*) others; (*b*) self.
+1	H 3. References to being or wanting to be or seeking to be the recipient of good fortune, good luck, God's favor or blessing (*a*) others; (*b*) self.
+1	H 4. References to any kinds of hopes that lead to a constructive outcome, to survival, to longevity, to smooth-going interper-

SCHEDULE 8 (*Continued*)

Weights		Content Categories & Scoring symbols
		sonal relationships (this category can be scored only if the word "hope" or "wish" or a close synonym is used).
−1	H 5.	References to not being or not wanting to be or not seeking to be the recipient of good fortune, good luck, God's favor or blessing.
−1	H 6.	References to self or others not getting or receiving help, advice, support, sustenance, confidence, esteem (*a*) from others; (*b*) from self.
−1	H 7.	References to feelings of hopelessness, losing hope, despair, lack of confidence, lack of ambition, lack of interest; feelings of pessimism, discouragement (*a*) others; (*b*) self.

Cognitive and Intellectual Impairment Scale

The Cognitive and Intellectual Impairment scale was designed to measure transient and reversible changes in cognitive and intellectual function as well as irreversible changes, all due principally to brain dysfunction, and minimally to transient emotional changes in the individual.

Preliminary validation studies on this scale have been published elsewhere (Gottschalk & Gleser, pp. 229–236). Further validation studies on this scale, and on other cognitive impairment scales which can be derived from this scale, have been reported (Gottschalk, 1978, pp. 311–330; Gottschalk, 1979a, pp. 9–40; Gottschalk, Eckardt, Pautler, Wolf, & Terman, 1983; Gottschalk, Eckhardt, Hoigaard-Martin, Gilbert, Wolf, & Johnson, 1983; Gottschalk, Hoigaard, Eckhardt, Gilbert, & Wolf, 1983).

SCHEDULE 9

Cognitive and Intellectual Impairment Scale

Weights			Content Categories and Scoring Symbols
	I.		Interpersonal References (including fauna and flora).
		B.	To unfriendly, hostile, destructive thoughts, feelings, or actions.
−½			1. Self unfriendly to others.
		C.	To congenial and constructive thoughts, feelings, or actions.
−½			1. Others helping, being friendly toward others.
−½			2. Self helping, being friendly toward others.
−½			3. Others helping, being friendly toward self.
	II.		Intrapersonal References.
+3		A.	To disorientation-orientation, past, present or future (do not

(*continued*)

SCHEDULE 9 *(Continued)*

| Weight | | | Content Categories & Scoring symbols |

Weight			
			include all references to time, place, or person, but only those in which it is reasonably clear the subject is trying to orient himself or is expressing disorientation with respect to these; also, do not score more than one item per clause under this category).
		B.	To self.
−½			1. Injured, ailing, deprived, malfunctioning, getting worse, bad, dangerous, low value or worth, strange.
+¼			3. Intact, satisfied, healthy, well.
+1			5. To being controlled, feeling controlled, wanting control, asking for control or permission, being obliged or having to do, think, or experience something.
+1		C.	Denial of feelings, attitudes, or mental state of the self.
		D.	To food.
−1			2. Good or neutral.
	III.		Miscellaneous.
		A.	Signs of disorganization.
+1			2. Incomplete sentences, clauses, phrases; blocking.
		B.	Repetition of ideas in sequence.
+1			2. Phrases, clauses (separated only by a phrase or clause).
+½	IV.	A.	Questions Directed to the Interviewer.

"Derived" Cognitive Impairment Scores from Speech Samples on Halstead–Reitan and Other Neuropsychological Measures. The so-called "derived" scores of cognitive impairment include some 18 different neuro-psychological test scores constituting the Halstead–Reitan neuropsychological test battery. These scores were derived, on an actuarial basis, from a sample of 116 chronic alcoholic patients who were administered all of these neuropsychological tests, and also were asked to give a 5-minute-speech sample. All 33 form and/or content verbal categories in the Social Alienation-Personal Disorganization scale were correlated with all the neuropsychological subtest scores. Verbal categories correlating at a $p < .05$ or better were combined in a multiple regression formula, which was capable of predicting, at a highly significant level, each neuropsychological subtest score (Gottschalk, Eckardt & Feldman, 1979, 1983a). Both linear and quadratic multiple regression formulas were developed, and the best formula has been selected to provide these "derived" scores (Gottschalk, Eckardt & Feldman, 1979; 1983a). Cut-off scores are available to indicate levels of probable impairment of brain function. (See Table 3).

THE MEASUREMENT OF PSYCHOLOGICAL STATES VERSUS TRAITS FROM SPEECH SAMPLES

Previous reports (Gottschalk & Gleser, 1969; Gottschalk & Uliana, 1979) have investigated and described the extent to which these content-

TABLE 3
"Derived" Score from Gottschalk Cognitive Impairment Scales

"Derived" scores	Cut-off scores[a]
1. Tactual Performance Test (Total time)	>15.7 minutes
2. Tactual Performance Test (Memory)	≧ 5.0 figures
3. Tactual Performance Test (Location)	≧ 4.0 figures
4. Tapping	≦50.0 taps
5. Trails A	>40.0 seconds
6. Trails B	>92.0 seconds
7. Categories	>51.0 errors
8. Speech Perception	> 8.0 errors
9. Seashores	> 6.0 (ranked score)
10. Wisconsin Card Sorting	< 6.0 suggestive; 3 probable
11. Digit Symbol	<48.0 (raw score); 9[b]
12. Digit Span	<10.0 (raw score); 9[b]
13. Block Design	<29.0 (raw score); 9[b]
14. Object Assembly	<24.0 (raw score); 9[b]
15. Rod/Frame	> 2.0
16. Benton Visual Retention	Below "expected" score
17. Shipley-Hartford-Verbal	<25.0 (raw score)
18. Shipley-Hartford-Abstract	<10.0 (raw score)

[a]Scores in the range indicated suggest brain function impairment
[b](Scaled score equivalents)

analysis scales measure states and/or traits. In brief, the affect scales applied to a single 5-minute speech sample measure psychological states, that is, relatively short-lived, transient feelings. Affect scores derived from the average of three or more 5-minute verbal samples (produced at intervals of at least an hour apart) approximate trait measures, in the sense of providing a measure of the relatively unvarying central tendency of a psychological characteristic. Moreover, the standard deviation of these affect scores provides a useful descriptive parameter. A social alienation-personal disorganization score, obtained from a speech sample, is more like a trait measure than an affect score that is based on content analysis. For example, the coefficient of generalizability of a social alienation-personal disorganization score in one study was .77 for males and .71 for females, and this compares to coefficients of generalizability of .19 to .43 for a single anxiety score, and .00 to .68 for three types of hostility scores—hostility outward, ambivalent hostility, and inward hostility (Gottschalk & Gleser, 1969, pp. 62–67). Achievement strivings, hope, and human relations scores are thought to be more like a trait measure than a state measure (Gottschalk & Uliana,

1969). Cognitive impairment scores are stable and, hence, trait-like in permanent brain damage, but they fluctuate with transient disturbances of brain function.

The characteristics of these content analysis scores should be kept in mind in any clinical or research applications of these measures.

NORMATIVE SCORES

Percentiles—Children and Adults

The normative scores on these various psychological scales were derived from various, stratified samples of children and adults, the stratification being based on either grade level, age, and sex for children, and sex for adults. The normative scores for white children, ages 6–16, were based on a sample of 109 children from an Orange County, California school district (Gottschalk, 1976). The normative sample of black children was also based on a sample drawn from an Orange County school district, of a middle to lower middle class (Hollingshead, Classification II to III), and consisted of 276 children (Uliana, 1979). The normative sample of adults was based on various-sized adult samples of employed adults ($N = 58$–322) not seen in a psychiatric clinic or setting.

Hence, psychological scores in the 5th percentile or less, or the 95th percentile or more, are relatively deviant, and merit attention. The clinician, however, may well be interested in scores below the 20th percentile, or above the 80th percentile, of normative children or adults.

Profiles and T-scores—Children

The clinician will note that we have also prepared profiles whereby scores derived from 5-minute speech samples for 17 different content-analysis scales may be converted readily to T-scores, and compared to normative scores obtained on a sample of white children ($N = 109$, Gottschalk, 1976) and black children ($N = 276$, Uliana, 1979). A T-score of 70 or greater, or of 30 or less, would be equal to or greater than 2.00 standard deviations from the normative score, and can be considered significantly different at the .05 level of confidence on a one-tail test.

POSSIBLE USES AND APPLICATIONS OF THE 5-MINUTE SPEECH SAMPLE TEST

General Information

All the different scales can be derived from the same speech sample. Hence, any one or a number of scores from different scales can be

TABLE 4
Normative Scores for Adults

Percentile	Anxiety total (N = 282)	Hostility outward (N = 322)			Hostility inward (N = 322)	Ambivalent hostility (N = 322)
		Overt	Covert	Total		
95	2.65	1.45	1.52	1.95	1.26	1.45
90	2.40	1.21	1.30	1.67	1.00	1.20
85	2.20					
80	2.05	0.96	0.97	1.35	0.83	0.86
75	1.90					
70	1.78	0.83	0.83	1.17	0.69	0.67
60	1.58	0.70	0.68	1.04	0.59	0.58
50	1.45	0.62	0.58	0.91	0.52	0.49
40	1.28	0.54	0.49	0.78	0.44	0.40
30	1.10	0.46	0.42	0.63	0.36	0.35
25	0.98					
20	0.85	0.38	0.35	0.51	0.30	0.30
15	0.68					
10	0.53	0.30	0.28	0.40	0.25	0.25
5	0.35	0.25	0.24	0.30	0.22	0.22
Mean	1.46	0.69	0.70	0.96	0.59	0.61
SD	0.71	0.36	0.42	0.50	0.35	0.39

Normative scores on assorted psychological scales for adults

Percentile	Hope (N = 91)	Social alienation personal disorganization (N = 58)	Cognitive impairment (N = 58)
95	2.63	1.00	2.15
90	1.90	−0.10	1.85
85	1.55		
80	1.35		
75	1.19	−1.20	1.27
70	1.08		
60	0.81		
50	0.47	−2.90	0.43
40	0.32		
30	0.16		
25	0.00	−4.90	0.34
20	0.00		
15	0.00		
10	−0.16	−6.70	−1.28
5	−0.54	−7.50	−2.12
Mean	0.73		0.38
SD	1.03		
Median		−2.90	

TABLE 5
Normative Scores for Children

| Percentile | Anxiety total | Hostility outward | | | Hostility inward | Ambivalent hostility |
		Overt	Covert	Total		
95	3.51	1.69	1.77	2.23	1.95	1.50
90	3.31	1.34	1.47	1.83	1.50	1.28
85	3.01	1.25	1.31	1.67	1.10	1.01
80	2.80	1.03	1.19	1.57	0.93	0.82
75	2.55	0.94	1.09	1.48	0.82	0.72
70	2.48	0.88	0.94	1.38	0.79	0.71
60	2.26	0.75	0.81	1.20	0.65	0.61
50	1.99	0.64	0.74	1.04	0.56	0.55
40	1.74	0.56	0.64	0.88	0.48	0.48
30	1.55	0.49	0.55	0.74	0.40	0.41
25	1.35	0.47	0.51	0.67	0.37	0.38
20	1.19	0.42	0.43	0.61	0.35	0.37
15	1.04	0.39	0.37	0.55	0.31	0.35
10	0.86	0.35	0.33	0.51	0.28	0.32
5	0.65	0.32	0.30	0.41	0.26	0.30
Mean	2.04	0.79	0.85	1.14	0.73	0.67
SD	0.89	0.48	0.48	0.58	0.54	0.38

Normative scores of assorted psychological scales for white children
($N = 109$)

Percentile	Achievement strivings	Hope	Human relations	Social alienation-personal disorganization	Cognitive impairment
95	5.53	1.90	3.60	4.38	5.40
90	4.31	1.37	3.22	2.74	4.62
85	3.90	1.04	2.94	1.94	4.23
80	3.26	0.83	2.75	1.30	3.67
75	2.65	0.61	2.57	0.79	3.51
70	2.12	0.40	2.42	0.61	3.18
60	1.75	0.19	2.06	0.04	2.76
50	1.22	0.01	1.78	−0.52	2.27
40	0.95	−0.07	1.50	−1.27	1.93
30	−0.04	−0.38	1.13	−2.53	1.56
25	−0.25	−0.50	1.01	−2.86	1.37
20	−0.44	−0.67	0.82	−3.56	1.17
15	−0.84	−0.95	0.45	−4.90	0.89
10	−1.37	−1.38	0.11	−5.89	0.69
5	−1.99	−2.30	−0.39	−7.13	0.22
Mean	1.40	0.04	1.83	−1.14	2.50
SD	2.25	1.25	1.46	4.24	1.80

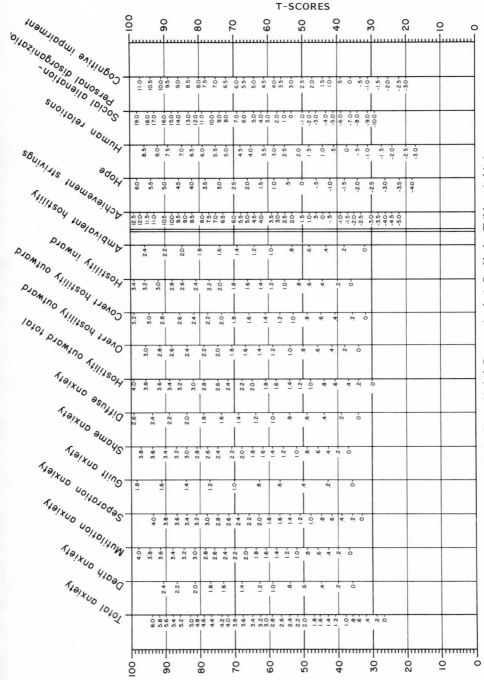

T-SCORES

FIGURE 8. Gottschalk–Gleser Verbal Content Analysis Profile for Children (white).

obtained from one sample, depending on what information one wants to learn. If possible, patients should be drug-free for 48 hours before giving a speech sample, since psychoactive drugs influence the scores.

Hope Scale. Higher scores predict more favorable outcomes with psychotherapy, crisis intervention, placebo, or the passage of time. How high the scores are for adults or children can be estimated from the percentiles or T-scores for these people.

The hope scores can, also, be used as a measure of change or of dependent variables (Gottschalk, 1975, 1976; Gottschalk, Uliana, & Hoigaard, 1979).

Social Alienation-Personal Disorganization (SA-PD) Scale. High Social Alienation-Personal Disorganization scale scores can predict unfavorable outcome with psychotherapy or crises intervention. Among schizophrenic patients, high Social Alienation-Personal Disorganization scores predict favorable responders to phenothiazine administration (Gottschalk, Gleser, Cleghorn, Stone, & Winget, 1970; Gottschalk *et al.*, 1979). These scores can be used as measures of change with drug therapy or psychotherapy among schizophrenic patients (Gottschalk, Mayerson, & Gottlieb, 1967; Gottschalk, Gleser, Cleghorn, Stone, & Winget, 1970; Gottschalk, Biener, Noble, Birch, Wilbert, & Heiser, 1975; Gottschalk, 1976; Gottschalk, Mennuti, & Cohen, 1979).

These scores are also useful as measures of general psychiatric morbidity among nonschizophrenic individuals, and among both children and adults (Gottschalk & Gleser, 1964; Gleser, Winget, & Seligman, 1979).

Criteria for distinguishing high and low social alienation-personal disorganization scores are available from percentile scores for normative adults and children, as well as from T-scores for white and black children.

Cognitive Impairment Scales. The Gottschalk-Gleser Cognitive Impairment scale provides rapidly accessible estimates of general cognitive impairment. It may be used as a quick-screening measure of cognitive impairment in children or adults, preliminary to the administration of other, more time-consuming and specific neuropsychological testing procedures. Or it may be used as the sole criteria, itself, of impairment of cognitive function.

The so-called "derived" measures of cognitive impairment are obtained from multiple regression formulas providing estimates of up to 18 neuropsychological test measures, including subtests of the Halstead–Reitan test battery (Gottschalk, Eckardt, & Feldman, 1979). These estimates correlate significantly with original neuropsychological test scores on a sample of 116 chronic alcoholic male patients (Gottschalk, Eckardt, & Feldman 1979, 1980).

What constitutes high scores on these measures of cognitive impairment is available from percentile scores and T-scores on normative children and adults, and cut-off scores suggestive of cognitive impairment for the "derived" measures.

Achievement Strivings Scale. These scores provide an estimate of the achievement orientation of any individual. Psychomotor-stimulant drugs, such as pipradrol (Gottschalk, Kapp, Ross, Kaplan, Silver, MacLeod, Kahn, Van Maanen, & Acheson, 1956) and amphetamine (Gottschalk, Gleser, Stone, & Kunkel, 1968, Gottschalk, Bates, Waskow, Katz, & Olsson, 1971) can significantly increase these scores.

Percentile scores and T-scores are available for the Achievement Strivings scale.

Human Relations Scale. This scale is useful for measuring various intensities of the orientation and drive for satisfying and constructive human relations. Its usefulness has not been extensively explored in predictive studies, but there is some evidence that high scores on this scale are correlated with favorable outcome in psychotherapy. (Gottschalk et al., 1967).

Percentile scores and T-scores from normative children and adults are available.

Anxiety and Hostility Scales. These scores are useful in any studies for which objective measures of these psychological states are needed. Such studies might include investigations of personality characteristics, psychotherapy, psychophysiology, neuropsychopharmacology, and so forth.

Normative percentile and T-scores are available. These scores are quite sensitive to the effects of psychoactive drugs.

REFERENCES

Bowlby, J. (1960). Separation anxiety. *International Journal of Psycho-Analysis, 41*, 89–113.

Elliott, H. W., Gottschalk, L. A., & Uliana, R. L. (1974). Relationship of plasma meperidine levels to changes in anxiety and hostility. *Comprehensive Psychiatry, 15*, 249–254.

Freedman, N., Blass, T., Rifkin, A., & Quitkin, F. (1973). Body movements and the verbal encoding of aggressive affect. *Journal of Abnormal and Social Psychology, 26*, 72–85.

Freud, S. (1905). Three essays on the theory of sexuality. III. Transformation of puberty. In J. Strachey (Ed.), *The standard edition of the complete psychological works of Sigmund Freud* (Vol. 20) London: Hogarth Press.

Freud, S. (1926). Inhibitions, symptoms and anxiety. In J. Strachey (Ed.), *The standard edition of the complete psychological works of Sigmund Freud* (Vol. 20). London: Hogarth Press.

Gleser, G. C., Gottschalk, L. A., & Springer, K. J. (1961). An anxiety scale applicable to verbal samples. *Archives of General Psychiatry, 5*, 593–605.

Gleser, G. C., Gottschalk, L. A., Fox, R., & Lippert, W. (1965). Immediate changes in affect with chlordiazepoxide in juvenile delinquent boys. *Archives of General Psychiatry, 13,* 291–295.

Gleser, G. C., Winget, C., & Seligman, R. (1979). Content scaling of affect in adolescent speech samples. *Journal of Youth and Adolescence, 8,* 283–297.

Gleser, G. C., Winget, C., Seligman, R., & Rauh, J. (1979). Evaluation of psychotherapy with adolescents using content analysis of verbal samples. In L. A. Gottschalk (Ed.), *The content analysis of verbal behavior: Further studies* (pp. 211–233). New York: Spectrum Publications.

Gottlieb, A., Gleser, G. C., & Gottschalk, L. A. (1967). Verbal and physiological responses to hypnotic suggestion of attitudes. *Psychosomatic Medicine, 24,* 172–183.

Gottschalk, L. A. (1968). Some applications of the psychoanalytic concept of object relatedness: Preliminary studies on a human relations content analysis scale applicable to verbal samples. *Comprehensive Psychiatry, 9,* 608–620.

Gottschalk, L. A. (1971). Some psychoanalytic research into the communication of meaning through language. *British Journal of Medical Psychology, 44,* 131–147.

Gottschalk, L. A. (1972). An objective method of measuring psychological states associated with changes in neural function. *Journal of Biological Psychiatry, 4,* 33–49.

Gottschalk, L. A. (1974a). A hope scale applicable to verbal samples. *Archives of General Psychiatry, 30,* 779–785.

Gottschalk, L. A. (1974b). The psychoanalytic study of hand–mouth approximations. In L. Goldberger & V. N. Rosen (Eds.), *Psychoanalysis and contemporary science* (Vol. 3, pp. 269–291). New York: International Universities Press.

Gottschalk, L. A. (1975). Drug effects and the assessment of affective states in man. In W. B. Essman & L. Valzelli (Eds.), *Current developments in psychopharmacology* (pp. 261–300). New York: Spectrum Publications.

Gottschalk, L. A. (1976). Children's speech as a source of data toward the measurement of psychological states. *Journal of Youth and Adolescence, 5,* 11–36.

Gottschalk, L. A. (1978). Cognitive defect in the schizophrenic syndrome as assessed by speech patterns. In G. Serban (Ed.), *Cognitive defects in the development of mental illness* (pp. 311–310). New York: Brunner/Mazel.

Gottschalk, L. A. (1979a). *The content analysis of verbal behavior: Further studies.* New York: Spectrum Publications.

Gottschalk, L. A. (1979b). A preliminary approach to the problems of relating the pharmacokinetics of phenothiazines to clinical response with schizophrenic patients. Prediction of placebo responders and responders to a single oral dose of a phenothiazine among acute schizophrenic patients. In L. A. Gottschalk (Ed.), *Pharmacokinetics of psychoactive drugs: Further studies* (Ch. 5, pp. 63–81). New York: Spectrum Publications.

Gottschalk, L. A., & Bechtel, R. J. (1982). The measurement of anxiety through the computer analysis of verbal samples. *Comprehensive Psychiatry, 23,* 364–369.

Gottschalk, L. A., & Gleser, G. C. (1964). Distinguishing characteristics of the verbal communications of schizophrenic patients. *Disorders of Communications,* Association for Research in Nervous and Mental Disorders (*A.R.N.M.D.*), 12, 100–113.

Gottschalk, L. A., & Gleser, G. C. (1969). *The measurement of psychological states through the content analysis of verbal behavior.* Berkeley: University of California Press.

Gottschalk, L. A., & Hambidge, G., Jr. (1955). Verbal behavior analysis: A systematic approach to the problem of quantifying psychological processes. *Journal Projective Techniques, 19,* 387–409.

Gottschalk, L. A., & Kaplan, S. M. (1958). A quantitative method of estimating variations in intensity of psychologic conflict or state. *Archives of Neurological Psychiatry, 79,* 688–696.

Gottschalk, L. A., & Kaplan, S. A. (1972). Chlordiazepoxide plasma levels and clinical responses. *Comprehensive Psychiatry, 13,* 519–528.

Gottschalk, L. A., & Uliana, R. L. (1979). Profiles of children's psychological states derived from the Gottschalk-Gleser content analysis of speech. *Journal of Youth and Adolescence, 8,* 269–282.

Gottschalk, L. A., Kapp, F. T., Ross, W. D., Kaplan, S. M., Silver, H., MacLeod, J. A., Kahn, J. B., Jr., Van Maanen, E. F., & Acheson, G. H. (1956). Explorations in testing drugs affecting physical and mental activity. Studies with a new drug of potential value in psychiatric illness. *Journal of the American Medical Association, 161,* 1038–1054.

Gottschalk, L. A., Gleser, G. C., Daniels, R. S., & Block, S. L. (1958). The speech patterns of schizophrenic patients: A method of assessing relative degree of personal disorganization and social alienation. *Journal of Nervous and Mental Disorders, 127,* 153–166.

Gottschalk, L. A., Gleser, G. C., Springer, K. J., Kaplan, S. M., Shanon, J., & Ross, W. D. (1960). Effects of perphenazine on verbal behavior patterns. *Archives of General Psychiatry, 2,* 632–639.

Gottschalk, L. A., Gleser, G. C., Magliocco, E. B., & D'Zmura, T. L. (1961). Further studies on the speech patterns of schizophrenic patients: Measuring interindividual differences in relative degree of personal disorganization and social alienation. *Journal of Nervous and Mental Disorders, 132,* 101–113.

Gottschalk, L. A., Springer, K. J., & Gleser, G. C. (1961). Experiments with a method of assessing the variations in intensity of certain psychological states during two psychotherapeutic interviews. In L. A. Gottschalk (Ed.), *Comparative psycholinguistic analysis of two psychotherapeutic interviews* (pp. 115–138). New York: International Universities Press.

Gottschalk, L. A., Gleser, G. C., & Springer, K. J. (1963). Three hostility scales applicable to verbal samples. *Archives of General Psychiatry, 9,* 254–279.

Gottschalk, L. A., Gleser, G. C., D'Zmura, T., & Hanenson, I. B. (1964). Some psychophysiological relationships in hypertensive women. The effect of hydrochlorothiazide on the relation of affect to blood pressure. *Psychosomatic Medicine, 26,* 610–617.

Gottschalk, L. A., Gleser, G. C., Wylie, H. W., & Kaplan, S. M. (1965). Effects of imipramine on anxiety and hostility levels derived from verbal communications. *Psychopharmacologia, 7,* 303–310.

Gottschalk, L. A., Cleghorn, J. M., Gleser, G. C., & Iacono, J. M. (1965). Studies of relationships of emotions to plasma lipids. *Psychosomatic Medicine, 27,* 102–111.

Gottschalk, L. A., Stone, W. N., Gleser, G. C., & Iacono, J. M. (1966). Anxiety levels in dreams: Relation to changes in plasma free fatty acids. *Science, 153,* 654–56.

Gottschalk, L. A., Mayerson, P., & Gottlieb, A. (1967). The prediction and evaluation of outcome in an emergency brief psychotherapy clinic. *Journal of Nervous and Mental Disorders, 144,* 77–96.

Gottschalk, L. A., Gleser, G. C., Stone, W. N., & Kunkel, R. L. (1968). Studies of psychoactive drugs effects on non-psychiatric patients. Measurement of affective and cognitive changes by content analysis of speech. In W. Evans & N. Kline (Eds.), *Psychopharmacology of the normal human.* Springfield, IL: Charles C Thomas.

Gottschalk, L. A., Winget, C. N., & Gleser, G. C. (1969). *Manual of instructions for using the Gottschalk-Gleser content analysis scales: Anxiety, hostility, and social alienation-personal disorganization.* Berkeley: University of California Press.

Gottschalk, L. A., Kunkel, R. L., Wohl, T., Saenger, E., & Winget, C. N. (1969). Total and half body irradiation. Effect on cognitive and emotional processes. *Archives of General Psychiatry, 21,* 574–580.

Gottschalk, L. A., Gleser, G. C., & Hanson, E. J. (1969). Positive and negative conditioning of self-references, 1963. In L. A. Gottschalk & G. C. Gleser (Eds.) *Measurement of psychological states through the content analysis of verbal behavior*. Berkeley: University of California Press.

Gottschalk, L. A., Gleser, G. C., Cleghorn, J. C., Stone, W. N., & Winget, C. N. (1970). Prediction of changes in severity of the schizophrenic syndrome with discontinuation and administration of phenothiazines in chronic schizophrenic patients: Language as a predictor and measure of change in schizophrenia. *Comprehensive Psychiatry, 11*, 123–140.

Gottschalk, L. A., Bates, D. E., Fox, R. A., & James, J. M. (1971). Patterns of psychoactive drug use found in samples from a mental health clinic and general medical clinic. *Archives of General Psychiatry, 25*, 395–397.

Gottschalk, L. A., Bates, D. E., Waskow, I. E., Katz, M. M., & Olsson, J. (1971). Effect of amphetamine or chlorpromazine on achievement strivings scores derived from content analysis of speech. *Comprehensive Psychiatry, 12*, 430–435.

Gottschalk, L. A., Noble, E. P., Stolzoff, G. E., Bates, D. E., Cable, C. G., Uliana, R. L., Birch, H., & Fleming, E. W. (1973). Relationships of chlordiazepoxide blood levels to psychological and biochemical responses. In S. Garattini, R. Mussini, & L. O. Randall (Eds.), *Benzodiazepines* (pp. 257–280), New York: Raven Press.

Gottschalk, L. A., Fox, R. A., & Bates, D. E. (1973). A study of prediction of outcome in a mental health crisis clinic. *American Journal of Psychiatry, 130*, 1107–1111.

Gottschalk, L. A., Brown, S. B., Bruney, E. H., Shumate, L. W., & Uliana, R. (1973c). An evaluation of a parents' group in a child-centered clinic. *Psychiatry, 36*, 157–171.

Gottschalk, L. A., Stone, W. N., & Gleser, G. C. (1974). Peripheral versus central mechanisms accounting for antianxiety effects of propranolol. *Psychosomatic Medicine, 36*, 47–56.

Gottschalk, L. A., Hausmann, C., & Brown, J. S. (1975). A computerized scoring system for use with content analysis scales. *Comprehensive Psychiatry, 16*, 77–90.

Gottschalk, L. A., Biener, R. A., Noble, E. P., Birch, H., Wilbert, D. E., & Heiser, J. F. (1975). Thioridazine plasma levels and clinical response. *Comprehensive Psychiatry, 16*, 323–337.

Gottschalk, L. A., Dinovo, E. C., Biener, R., Birch, H., Syben, M., & Noble, E. P. (1979). Plasma levels of mesoridazine and its metabolites and clinical response in acute schizophrenia after a single intramuscular drug dose. In L. A. Gottschalk (Ed.), *The content analysis of verbal behavior: Further studies*, (Ch. 26, pp. 471–490). New York: Spectrum Publications.

Gottschalk, L. A., Eckardt, M. J., & Feldman, D. J. (1979). Further validation studies of a cognitive-intellectual impairment scale applicable to verbal samples. In L. A. Gottschalk (Ed.) *The content analysis of verbal behavior: Further studies*, (Ch. 2, pp. 9–40). New York: Spectrum Publications.

Gottschalk, L. A., Mennuti, S. A., & Cohn, J. B. (1979). Thioridazine plasma levels and clinical response in five schizophrenic patients receiving daily oral medication: Correlations and the prediction of clinical responses. In L. A. Gottschalk (Ed.), *Pharmacokinetics of psychoactive drugs: Further studies*, (Ch. 6, pp. 83–95). New York: Spectrum Publications.

Gottschalk, L. A., Uliana, R. L., & Hoigaard, J. C. (1979). Preliminary validation of a set of content analysis scales applicable to verbal samples of psychological states in children. *Psychiatry Research, 1*, 71–82.

Gottschalk, L. A., Eckardt, M. J., Pautler, C. P., Wolf, R. J., & Terman, S. A. (1983). Cognitive impairment scales derived from verbal samples. *Comprehensive Psychiatry, 24*, 6–19.

Gottschalk, L. A., Eckardt, M. J., Hoigaard-Martin, J. C., Gilbert, R. L., Wolf, R. J. &

Johnson, W. (1983). Neuropsychological deficit in chronic alcoholism: Early detection and prediction by analysis of verbal samples. *Substance and Alcohol Actions/Misuse, 4,* 45–58.

Gottschalk, L. A., Hoigaard, J. C., Eckardt, M. J., Gilbert, R. L., & Wolf R. J. (1983). Cognitive impairment and other psychological scores, derived from the content analysis of speech, in detoxified male chronic alcoholics. *The American Journal of Drug and Alcohol Abuse, 9,* 447–460.

Gottschalk, L. A., Winget, C. N., Gleser, G. C., & Lolas, F. (1984). *Analisis de la conducta-verbal.* Santiago, Chile: Editorial Universitaria S.A.

Grünzig, H. J., Holzcheck, K., & Kächele, H. (1976). EVA-Ein Programmsystem zur Maschinellen. Inhaltsanalyse von Psychotherapie Protokallen. *Medinische Psychologie, 2,* 208–217.

Karacan, I., Goodenough, D. R., Shapiro, A., & Starker, S. (1966). Erection cycle during sleep in relation to dream anxiety. *Archives of General Psychiatry, 15,* 183–189.

Koch, U. & Schöfer, G. (Eds.). (1986). *Sprachinhaltnalyse in der psychosomatischen und psychiatrischen Forschung: Grundlagen und Anwendungstudien mit den Affektskalen von Gottschalk und Gleser.* Beltz Verlag: Weinheim.

Levitt, E. E., Persky, H., & Brady, J. P. (1964). *Hypnotic induction: A psychoendocrine investigation.* Springfield, IL: Charles C Thomas.

Lewis, H. B. (1971). *Shame and guilt in neurosis.* New York: International Universities Press.

Lewis, H. B. (1979). Using content analysis to explore shame and guilt in neurosis. In L. A. Gottschalk (Ed.), *The content analysis of verbal behavior: Further studies,* (Ch. 47, pp. 831–853). New York: Spectrum Publications.

Lolas, F. & von Rad, M. (1982). Psychosomatic disease and neurosis: A study of dyadic verbal behavior. *Comprehensive Psychiatry, 23,* 19–24.

Luborsky, L., Docherty, J., Todd, T., Knapp, P., Mirsky, A., & Gottschalk, L. A. (1975). A content analysis of psychological states prior to petit mal EEG paroxysms. *Journal of Nervous and Mental Disease, 160,* 282–298.

May, R. (1950). *The meaning of anxiety.* New York: Ronald Press.

Meehan, J. (1978). *The new UCI LISP manual.* Hillsdale, NJ: Erlbaum.

Miller, C. K. (1965). Psychological correlates of coronary artery disease. *Psychosomatic Medicine, 27,* 257–265.

Perley, J., Winget, C. N., & Placci, C. (1971). Hope and discomfort as factors influencing treatment continuation. *Comprehensive Psychiatry, 12,* 557–563.

Piers, G., & Singer, M. D. (1953). *Shame and guilt.* Springfield, IL: Charles C Thomas.

Schöfer, G. (1977). Das Gottschalk–Gleser-Verfahren: Eine Sprachinhaltsanalyse zur Erfassung and Quantifizierung von aggressiven und angstlichen Affecten 2. *Psychosomatische Medinishe Psychoanalysis, 23,* 1.

Schöfer, G. (Ed.) (1980). Sprachinhaltsanalyse Theorie und Technik. Studien zur Messung angstlicher und aggressiver Affekte. Weinnheim and Basel: Beltz Verlag.

Schöfer, G., Balck, F., & Koch, U. (1979). Possible applications of the Gottschalk-Gleser content analysis of speech in psychotherapy research. In L. A. Gottschalk (Ed.), *The content analysis of verbal behavior: Further studies,* (Ch. 48, pp. 857–870). New York: Spectrum Publications.

Schöfer, G., Koch, U., & Balck, F. (1979). The Gottschalk–Gleser content analysis of speech: A normative study (the relationship of hostile and anxious affects to sex, sex of the interviewer, socioeconomic class and age). In L. A. Gottschalk (Ed.), *The content analysis of verbal behavior: Further studies* (Ch. 4, pp. 97–118). New York: Spectrum Publications.

Uliana, R. L. (1979). Measurement of black children's affective states and the effect of interviewer's race on affective states as measured through language behavior. In L. A.

Gottschalk (Ed.), *The content analysis of verbal behavior: Further studies,* (pp. 173–209). New York: Spectrum Publications.

Viney, L. L. (1983). The assessment of psychological states through content analysis of verbal communications. *Psychological Bulletin, 44,* 542–563.

Viney, L. L., Clarke, A. M., Bunn, T. A., & Teak, H. Y. (1983). *Crisis counselling for ill or inured patients who are hospitalized.* A report to the Commonwealth Department of Health, Canberra, Australia (pp. 375), University of Wollongong.

Winget, C. N., & Gleser, G. C. (1971). Effect of total and half body radiation on patients with metastatic cancer. In E. L. Saenger (Ed.), *Metabolic changes in humans following total body radiation.* DASA 1848 Progress Report in Research Project DA-49-146-XZ-315, Defense Atomic Support Agency, Washington, D.C.

Winget, C. N., & Kapp, F. T. (1972). The relationship of the manifest content of dreams to duration of childbirth in primiparae. *Psychosomatic Medicine, 34,* 313–320.

Winget, C. N., Seligman, R., Rauh, J. L., & Gleser, G. C. (1979). Social alienation-personal disorganization assessment in disturbed and normal adolescents. *Journal of Nervous and Mental Disorders, 167,* 282–287.

Witkin, H. A. (1949). Perception of body position and of the position of the visual field. *Psychological Monograph, 63,* 1–46.

Witkin, H. A., Lewis, H. B., & Weil, E. (1968). Affective reactions and patient–therapist interactions among more differentiated and less differentiated patients early in therapy. *Journal of Nervous and Mental Disease, 146,* 193–208.

2

Concept Analysis of Language in Psychotherapy

Julius Laffal

INTRODUCTION

Explicitly or implicitly, psychotherapist and patient have agreed to a contractual relationship in which the therapist is to apply his skill to understanding and helping the patient. As a means of implementing this contract, the patient is to speak of himself, and the clinician is to question him, raise hypotheses about what he says or does, and offer interpretation and instruction. What the patient says is taken not only as information about particular subject matter, but as data about his way of viewing the world and about his difficulties. On the other hand, the clinician chooses his own contributions either to produce further clarification of the patient's statements or to facilitate changes in the patient's attitudes and behavior. The interaction between psychotherapist and patient is thus somewhat different from ordinary conversation (Streeck, 1980, p. 124).

The therapeutic relationship is an evolving one. Ultimately, for the therapist, a stable perception of the patient's personality and ideational organization will emerge, within which his communications and behaviors will be understood. Particularly for psychotherapy seeking to achieve basic changes in the individual's way of doing things, the therapist will gradually focus on themes that seem to be central to the individual's thinking, and will attempt to influence him through examination of these themes.

JULIUS LAFFAL • Department of Psychiatry, Yale University School of Medicine, New Haven, CT 06519.

It would be most desirable to be able to organize and study the information about a patient conveyed in his words in the course of psychotherapy. For the volume of such information, some form of psychologically valid summary is required, capable of tracking the themes revealed by the patient in his speech, and of highlighting changes and unusual material which might otherwise be lost in the sheer mass of data.

MEANING COMMONALITY OF WORDS AS A BASIS FOR LANGUAGE ANALYSIS

In what follows, I will describe a computer-based system for the analysis of conceptual content expressed in language, applicable to the spoken interaction in psychotherapy. The system deals with semantic content of words, but I will show how it might also be applied to sentence syntax, and to pragmatic aspects of the therapeutic interaction.[1]

That groups of words may have meanings in common is the key to a semantic description of language. Commonalities in meaning have been given such labels as *conceptual field* (Lyons, 1977, p. 253ff), *semantic marker* (Katz & Fodor, 1964, p. 496ff), and *semantic primitive* (Miller & Johnson-Laird, 1976, p. 326ff).

Katz and Fodor (1964) maintain that there are basic, unanalyzable meaning commonalities relating groups of language tokens. Ultimately, these commonalities depend on perceptual experiences. Pursuing this possibility, Miller and Johnson-Laird (1976) attempted a rigorous analysis of meanings based on spatial-perceptual primitives, but had to conclude that while some ideational commonalities lie in perceptual processes as such, most meaning relations are of a more complex, conceptual nature.

Rosch and Mervis (1975, p. 275) have suggested that natural semantic categories may be understood as networks of overlapping attributes: "members of a category come to be viewed as prototypical of the category as a whole in proportion to the extent to which they bear a family

---

[1]Semantics deals with the relations of signs to the objects, events, and abstractions which they denote (Morris, 1938, p. 99). Syntactics deals with relationships between signs, and by extension to relationships between objects, events, and abstractions denoted by signs. Pragmatics deals with the psychological, biological, and social aspects of the functioning of signs. Pragmatics includes the psychological states and intentions of speakers and listeners, social norms in speech, and the effects which speech may have on speakers. In the clinical situation, as Morris points out (p. 117), the same sign vehicle may be interpreted semantically as referring to its denotata, and pragmatically as revealing something about the patient.

resemblance to (have attributes which overlap those of) other members of the category." Such categories as "chair" and "car" are described as being at a basic level, since they contain the richest attribute information and form natural discontinuities with each other. At a higher level of abstraction are such concepts as "furniture" and "vehicle," in which the entries still have a family resemblance but share fewer attributes. In most discussions, it is the higher-level entities which are identified as the semantic commonalities of language, since categories at the more basic level are too numerous, and too restricted in conceptual content, to have practical value for revealing the semantic organization of vocabulary.

Miller and Johnson-Laird (1976, p. 329), in characterizing semantic commonalities, concern themselves with "the connections between words that meanings create." The goal of a semantic analysis, in their view, is to provide, not a complete definition of word meaning, but only enough of the meaning to identify the semantic components that serve to differentiate and relate words. The decomposition of a word into connective meanings (semantic commonalities) may therefore be described as a process of incomplete definition. If one seeks to substitute an incomplete semantic definition for the word it defines, the result may be quite different from the original. Thus, if "warm-blooded animal" is an incomplete definition of *elephant*, the sentence *Harold likes all elephants* will become, by substitution *Harold likes all warm-blooded animals*, which may or may not be true.

To what extent would a system of concepts based on semantic commonalities capture the meanings which may be carried by words in use? I will try to show that such a concept system can encompass major portions of the meanings of words in use, and accordingly can serve as an instrument for monitoring language and thought in psychotherapy. Below, some major sources of meaning of words in use are identified and discussed in terms of how they may relate to a concept system.

1. First, there is the explicit referential meaning of words. The standard dictionary definition approximates this meaning, which distinguishes the thing referred to from all other things. This is the richest meaning of a word, and the source of the greatest variation in meaning from word to word. But it is precisely this richness which prohibits use of referential meaning as a basis for analysis of meaning, and which makes it necessary to search for commonalities in meaning.

2. Words in use presumably evoke, at some level of awareness, the kinds of conceptual commonalities described by Miller and Johnson-Laird, and it is this second kind of meaning that a system for the conceptual categorization of words addresses most directly. Evidence for the

evocation of such ideational classes when specific word tokens occur is found especially in work on clustering in association and recall (Bousfield, Cohen, & Whitmarsh, 1958; Bousfield, Puff, & Cowan, 1964; Tulving, 1962; Cofer, 1965, 1968). Concepts do not deal with explicit references or with the unique meanings conveyed by dictionary definitions, nor do they show how words relate to each other syntactically. They deal only with the semantic fields or meaning commonalities relating individual word tokens to each other.

3. Syntactic meaning, a third type of meaning, provides such information as the way words modify and relate to each other, the roles which words have in sentences, and the mood, aspect, and tense of verbs. Later, I will discuss two components of syntax, word modification and case roles of words in sentences, and show how the first may be approximated by a concept analysis of texts surrounding key words, and how the second may be arrived at by adding case subscripts to designated words.

4. A fourth meaning may be called associative meaning, derived from the fact that separate objects and events consistently occur in close conjunction, in the real world or verbally, and are hence likely to be consciously evoked when related words occur. Idiosyncratic meanings, those peculiar to an individual for a given word, may be treated as instances of associative meaning. Idiosyncratic meanings are of particular importance in the language of psychologically disturbed individuals.

Associative meaning may relate words and things which are conceptually quite different. Thus, when presented as a stimulus in a word association task, the word *table* evokes the conceptually related words *chair* and *desk*, but also the conceptually unrelated word *food*, as well as other words having to do with eating (Russell & Jenkins, 1954). The basis of this associative relationship in the real world is readily apparent in the use of tables for eating. Individuals may also make idiosyncratic associations of this sort that are not so apparent in the real world.

Laffal (1960, 1963) has used the method of concept analysis to explore associated meanings. This approach depends on the assumption that words appearing in close textual association with key words under study represent the associative meanings which these key words have for the individual. An application of the method to the language of Daniel Paul Schreber, a German high court judge whose autobiography served as the basis for Freud's development of his theory of paranoia (1911), is described in the present paper.

5. A fifth meaning, metaphoric meaning, is in one sense a problem of undefined words. Where metaphoric meanings have become standardized, they are found as explicit submeanings in dictionary definitions. The *heart of the matter* is the crux of the matter, not a living organ.

Heart is so defined in the dictionary, and can be identified with other words having comparable meanings in a concept analysis. But in *her looks are petals,* a literal definition of *petal* as part of a flower, and a conceptual definition of it as vegetation, will miss the point. To make the formal conceptual analysis of nonstandard metaphors possible, it is necessary to add words which will convey the metaphoric meaning. Thus one might edit the sentence into: *her looks are petals, delicate, shy, colorful.* In texts involving little use of metaphoric language, this kind of attention might not be worthwhile. In poetry it would probably be essential. Once edited, the metaphor is available for concept analysis like other words.

6. A sixth meaning, contextual meaning, is that which stems from the interaction of sentences in context. Thus, in the exchange *A: Let's go to lunch; B: I am watching the birds,* B's negative response is given indirectly by the statement that he is engaged in a preferred activity. The fact that A has suggested going to lunch makes it possible to understand B's remark, which has nothing to do with eating, as saying *I prefer to skip lunch.* To become available for analysis, such implicit meanings must be inserted in the text by an editor in the same way that metaphoric meanings are added.

7. A seventh type of meaning, related to, but perhaps even more crucial than, contextual meaning, may be called interpersonal meaning. Interpersonal meaning derives from the interpersonal context, and the implicit intentions and reactions, of the participants in the verbal exchange. Particularly where the analyst values understanding of the interpersonal situation, as in psychotherapy, this type of meaning may be the most important part of the communication. One may describe the things and events referred to, display the concepts used, identify the meanings associated with grammatical form, show the associative environments of key words, interpret all the metaphors, and still miss the interpersonal thrust of a verbal exchange.

In the case of these interpersonal meanings, a second order of statements is called for, translating the implicit meanings into explicit ones. Thus *Mother asserts authority over son* may be the second order statement for *Go to your room!.* Once a gloss of this sort is added to a text to provide the understood meanings, the analysis problem is reduced to the standard one, in which all content is explicitly stated.

In effect, then, with the participation of an editor to fill out metaphoric and contextual meanings, and to make explicit the implicit interpersonal meanings in the verbal exchange, the range of meanings captured by a concept system abstracting semantic commonalities from words may incorporate major aspects of the actual meanings of words in use.

A CONCEPT SYSTEM

Development of the present concept system of word meanings for the analysis of texts has been detailed elsewhere (Laffal, 1973, 1979), but may be summarized here. The process began by grouping synonymous words. This creates a set of small groups of words bound by specific common meanings, but too large a set for practical use in reducing words to concepts. By making similarity of meaning a criterion of grouping, smaller groups can be joined, and the total number of groups of words reduced. Thus, while *chair, stool,* and *seat* form a loosely synonymous group, application of the criterion of similarity will draw into the same group such "seating" words as *bench, couch,* and *sofa*. Even so, the groupings remain too small in size and too numerous for application. If, now, relatedness of experience is taken as a broader basis for organizing words conceptually, such words as *chair, table, bureau,* and *bed* may be drawn together as referring to common household furnishings. This principle of relatedness is a crucial step, leading finally to a system with a manageable number of concepts, each with a sizable number of tokens.

As the system developed, there were realignments and restructurings of concept categories where border areas between concepts were seen to overlap, or where concepts became overly inclusive or too narrow. The core of the system is a concept dictionary translating each word of English into one or more of 116 concepts (up to the present the system has been limited to one or two concepts per word). Words of a text to be analyzed are matched against the dictionary, and a cumulative profile is obtained of references to the 116 concepts in the text. Such concept profiles may be used to compare texts from separate speakers, or from the same speaker over time, or to compare textual fragments surrounding separate key words for the same speaker. The concept dictionary has been incorporated in a computer system, analyzing text words and yielding a concept profile of the text. Table 1 gives the mnemonic names of the concept categories, and Table 2 shows the kinds of words identified with each concept category.

The concept system described has been employed in a number of studies (Laffal, 1960, 1961, 1963, 1965, 1967, 1968, 1969, 1979; Laffal & Feldman, 1962, 1963; Laffal, Monahan, & Richman, 1974; Watson & Laffal, 1963; Zakaras & Fine, 1979; Hyman, 1980). These studies dealt only with conceptual meanings of words in use (meaning 2). They did not systematically take into account meanings conveyed by syntax (meaning 3), nor did they deal systematically with nonstandard metaphoric meaning, sentence context meaning, or interpersonal pragmatics (meanings 5, 6, and 7). I will describe three of these studies to demon-

TABLE 1
Mnemonic Names of Concepts

AFAR	EASY	HEAT	MUCH	SIML
AGGR	EDUC	HOLW	MUSC	SIP
AGRE	EMPH	HOLY	MYTH	SOLE
AID	END	HOME	NEAR	SOMA
ANML	ERTH	HSCR[a]	NEW	SOME
ASTR	EVER	IDEA	NO	SUB
BACK	EVNT	IN	NSCR[a]	TALK
BAD	FABR	ION	NUMR	TIME
BGIN	FALS	JOIN	OPEN	TRIV
BLOK	FEM	KIN	OPPO	TRUE
BLUR	FLOW	LACK	OUT	UP
BODY	FOND	LARG	PANG	VAPR
BUG	FOOD	LAW	PAST	VARY
BULG	FOOL	LEAD	PATH	VEGT
CLEN	FORM	LITL	PLAC	VEHC
COLD	FORW	LIVE	PLAY	VIEW
COLR	FURN	MALE	POWR	WEA
COVR	GARB	MART	QUIK	WEAK
CRIM	GLAD	MECH	REST	WHOL
CRUX	GO	MEDC	SELF	WORK
DAMG	GOOD	MONY	SEP	WRIT
DEAD	GRUP	MOTV	SEX	YNG
DIRT	HAVE	MSMT	SHRP	
DOWN	HEAR	MTRL	SICK	

[a]HSCR ("Hand score") and NSCR ("No score") are not actually concepts.

strate the concept analysis method, and will then offer some suggestions and illustrations of how the other aspects of meaning may be incorporated in a concept analysis.

The Schreber Case: Concept Analysis of Key Words

The first study applying the concept-category system explored symbolism in the autobiography of the famous patient Daniel Paul Schreber (Laffal, 1960). Daniel Paul Schreber was a doctor of jurispridence and a prominent judge at the end of the last century, who, after becoming psychotic, published an account of his religious delusions (Schreber, 1955). Without having known Schreber personally, Freud (1911) undertook to trace the etiology of Schreber's delusions, and from the memoirs he formulated the now familiar paradigm of homosexuality and projection in paranoia. Macalpine and Hunter (1955), who published an English translation of Schreber's memoirs, disagreed with Freud's interpretation, maintaining that a wish for ambisexuality

TABLE 2
Concept Descriptions

AFAR.	The unusual, the unexpected, and the distant.
AGGR.	Disadvantages, detriment, dislike, and anger.
AGRE.	Cooperation, consent, approval, and agreement.
AID.	Help, advantage, and support.
ANML.	Animals other than insects. Fish are scored ANML FLOW; birds are scored ANML UP.
ASTR.	Astronomical bodies, space, astrology.
BACK.	Physical location or direction back or behind.
BAD.	Negative moral or ethical connotations.
BGIN.	Birth, creation, beginning.
BLOK.	Blocking, obstruction, confinement.
BLUR.	Obscurity and vagueness.
BODY.	External limbs and features of humans, animals, and plants.
BUG.	Insects and microscopic organisms.
BULG.	Fullness, mounds, and protrusions.
CLEN.	Cleanliness, grooming, and purification.
COLD.	Cold, winter, polar regions.
COLR.	Colors, including black and white.
COVR.	Being covered, secret or hidden.
CRIM.	Illicitness and lawbreaking.
CRUX.	Important, crucial, essential, or worthy.
DAMG.	Violence, harm, and danger.
DEAD.	Words relating to death.
DIRT.	Uncleanliness, filth, and deterioration.
DOWN.	Downward direction, below, under.
EASY.	Lightness, smoothness, and easiness.
EDUC.	Learning and teaching.
EMPH.	Emphasis, accentuation, and exclamation.
END.	Halting, finishing, and outcomes.
ERTH.	Earth, ground, and earth products.
EVER.	Constancy, habituation, duration.
EVNT.	Events, behavior, and circumstance.
FABR.	Fabrics and clothlike products.
FALS.	Deception, falseness, and affectation.
FEM.	Feminine references.
FLOW.	Water, bodies of water and related activities, liquidity.
FOND.	Loving, cherishing, and friendship.
FOOD.	Food and eating.
FOOL.	Foolishness and stupidity.
FORM.	Structures and configurations both of a concrete and abstract nature.
FORW.	Forward, front, and sequences.
FURN.	Furniture and household furnishings.
GARB.	Wearing apparel, sewing, clothing adornments.
GLAD.	Comfort, happiness, and humor.
GO.	Travel and movement.
GOOD.	Morality, propriety, goodness, and beauty.
GRUP.	Groups and bunches.

(continued)

TABLE 2 (*Continued*)

HAVE.	Having, holding, and possessing.
HEAR.	Sounds and noises.
HEAT.	Heat and warmth.
HOLW.	Containers, hollow objects.
HOLY.	Religion, religious activities, religious objects.
HOME.	Dwellings and enclosures within which men and animals live and work.
HSCR.	"Hand Score," indicating that an editor must substitute appropriate words.
IDEA.	Rational processes, thinking, and knowledge.
IN.	Inside, entering, being directed inward.
ION.	Electricity, atoms, and molecules.
JOIN.	Coming together and uniting.
KIN.	Kinship, marriage, family, and clan.
LACK.	Lack, absence, emptiness.
LARG.	Largeness, increase, weightiness.
LAW.	Law, law enforcement, and government.
LEAD	Authority, leading, and controlling.
LITL.	Smallness, brevity, diminution.
LIVE.	Mortality, living, and abiding.
MALE.	Maleness, and features and activities distinctively male.
MART.	Business, commerce, and trade.
MECH.	Machinery, instruments, and mechanical devices other than vehicles.
MEDC.	Medical matters, health, and cure.
MONY.	Money, buying, and selling.
MOTV.	Motivations, feeling states, wishes, and responsibilites.
MSMT.	Measurement and instruments of measurement.
MUCH.	Large amounts, abundance, plentifulness.
MUSC.	Music, musical instruments, musical sounds.
MYTH.	The supernatural, the mythical, and the unreal.
NEAR.	Near, native, and familiar.
NEW.	Newness, novelty, and the present.
NO.	Negation and denial.
NSCR.	"No Score" words which include articles, auxiliary verbs, and various function words.
NUMR.	Numbers and numerical operations.
OPEN.	Freedom, discovery, exposure, opening.
OPPO.	Dissimilarities, differences, and contests.
OUT.	Being outside, emanation, discharging.
PANG.	Upset feelings, including anxiety, fear, and guilt.
PAST.	References to the past and to age.
PATH.	Roads, passageways, directions.
PLAC.	Location, place, and place names.
PLAY.	Recreation and entertainment.
POWR.	Ability, achievement, strength, and bravery.
QUIK.	Speed, suddenness, and alertness.
REST.	Slowness, immobility, and resting.
SELF.	First person pronouns and references to the self.
SEP.	Separation and splitting apart.
SEX.	Words with sexual reference or implication.

(*continued*)

TABLE 2 (*Continued*)

SHRP.	Sharp edges, points, precision.
SICK.	Illness, infection, and malady.
SIML.	Similarity, equality, suitability.
SIP.	Drinking, sucking, and potables.
SOLE.	Singleness, uniqueness.
SOMA.	Bodily and vegetative processes and parts.
SOME.	Parts, segments, and bits.
SUB.	Subordination, dependence, and subjection.
TALK.	Language and vocal communication.
TIME.	Time and periods of time.
TRIV.	Triviality, vapidity, and valuelessness.
TRUE.	Truth, honesty, proof.
UP.	Being up and above, climbing, flight.
VAPR.	Vapors, gases, air, and mist.
VARY.	Alteration, deviation, instability, and transience.
VEGT.	Vegetation and plant products.
VEHC.	Vehicles, characteristic parts of vehicles, and conductors of vehicles.
VIEW.	Vision and light.
WEA.	Weather and climate.
WEAK.	Weakness, failure, inexpertness.
WHOL.	Totality, generality, universality.
WORK.	Work, tools, and related activities.
WRIT.	Written language, writing instruments, and documents.
YNG.	Immaturity, infancy, and youth.

and self-contained procreative powers was at the root of Schreber's illness. They pinpointed the difference between their view and Freud's by contesting Freud's interpretation that the sun symbolized "father" in Schreber's thinking. They contended, to the contrary, that the sun had feminine connotations for Schreber.

If Schreber used the same terms in writing of the sun as he did in writing of father figures, this could be taken as evidence that his associations for the two were alike and that, in effect, they had similar meaning for him, as Freud asserted. If, on the other hand, Schreber wrote about the sun the way he wrote about women, this could be taken as evidence for the Macalpine and Hunter view that the sun had important feminine meaning for Schreber. The problem posed was to compare the contexts of *sun* with those of masculine and feminine key words in Schreber's autobiography, in order to determine the relative similarity of the ideas associated with these key words to each other.

Unfortunately, the third chapter of Schreber's autobiography, which dealt intimately with members of his family, was deleted from the work by official censorship, so that there are practically no references to Schreber's father in the book. This makes a direct comparison of language related to Schreber's father with language related to the sun impossible. However, there are indirect ways of approaching the problem. It is clear in Freud's discussion that he believed God to be the father figure par excellence for Schreber. Macalpine and Hunter do not accept this connection and, consistently with their position about the sun, argue that Freud ignored the female significance of God as well. Some fairly definite predictions arise from these differences of view.

If Freud's contention that the sun and God were both father symbols for Schreber is correct, then there ought to be a similarity in the way Schreber wrote about both of these, and both ought to be more similar to the way Schreber wrote about male figures than to the way he wrote about female figures.

However, if the Macalpine and Hunter view is correct, then there ought to be a strong similarity between the way Schreber wrote about the sun and God; but how he wrote of both of these ought to be more similar to the way he wrote of females than to the way he wrote about males.

Freud held, in addition, that Dr. Flechsig, Schreber's physician, was the subject of the patient's homosexual longings, and that both God and Dr. Flechsig stood as dominant male figures in relation to Schreber. If Freud is correct, there ought to be a strong relationship in the way Schreber wrote about Dr. Flechsig and God, and both of these ought to be more strongly related to the way Schreber wrote about male references than the way he wrote about female references. Macalpine and Hunter are not specific in interpreting the symbolism of Dr. Flechsig in Schreber's psychology, but they also appear to suggest some element of identity with God.

Passages in the English translation of Schreber's autobiography that contained only one of the words *sun, God,* or *Flechsig,* or one male or female reference word (e.g., *man, woman*), were marked for transcription. A passage was defined as a sequence beginning three lines before a line containing a particular key word and ending three lines after the line containing the key word, with the proviso that the passage contain no other key word. A roughly equivalent number of such passages was taken out for each key word and consolidated into a single text for that word. It happens that the word *sun* occurs alone least often in the memoirs, and the total number of passages available for *sun* was used to determine the number of passages selected for each of the other key words. For all key words other than *sun* (for which no additional passages were available), an additional equivalent number of passages were taken out for reliability determinations.

In order to study reliability of concept profiles for those key words in which enough passages were available, the texts were randomly divided into two sets, each containing an equivalent number of lines in which the key word appeared, and an equivalent number of lines one, two and three lines above or below the key-word line. There were thus two texts each of words associated with *male, female, God,* and *Flechsig,* and one text of words associated with *sun.* All words in the key word texts were then handscored with the relevant concepts (the computerized system was not then in operation), and frequency profiles of concepts were prepared for all texts.

There were some concepts which rarely occurred in Schreber's writing, and some which occurred consistently and with great frequency. These concepts were taken to reflect Schreber's language style, applicable to all of his writing no matter what the subject, and were eliminated from the analysis, since they would have contributed only to a general increase in apparent similarity of all contexts, and obscured differences between the contexts associated with the key words. Further, the specific concepts under which *sun, God, Flechsig, male,* and *female* were scored were also eliminated from the comparisons, since selection of the critical passages had been based on the presence of one concept, and the absence of the others. The total number of concept categories was in this way reduced to 42, while the number of words remaining in the texts ranged from 192 to 258.

In Table 3 are shown the Pearson product–moment intercorrelations and reliabilities of the concept profiles. For the key word *sun,* no reliability was available.

To test the hypothesis that the way Schreber talked about God was more like the way he talked about male references than the way he talked about female references, the eight correlations involved (four for *God-male* and four for *God-female*) were compared with each other, making 16 comparisons. The *God-male* correlations were greater in 13 of the 16 comparisons.[2] Thus, the contexts of *God* in Schreber's autobiography were more like the contexts of *male* than of *female.* Similarly, the correlations of *Flechsig* and *male* were higher than those of *Flechsig* and *female* in 15 of the 16 comparisons.

With respect to the symbolism of the sun, Table 3 shows *female* and *sun* to be more highly related, on the average, than *male* and *sun.* Of the four direct comparisons between these correlations in Table 1, three show the *female-sun* correlation higher, and one shows the *male-sun* correlation higher. There is thus a tendency of the data to favor the Mac-

[2]An empirical test was made by computer on 2,500 sets of eight random numbers to determine how often by chance the members of one group of four numbers would be larger in various proportions than the members of another group of four numbers. The probability of obtaining a ratio of 13:3 was .15; the probability of a ratio of 14:2 was .11; the probability of a ratio 15:1 was .04; the probability of a 16:0 ratio was .02.

TABLE 3

**Pearson Product–Moment Correlations between Concept Profiles
of Key Words in Schreber's Autobiography[a]**

	Male profile		Female profile		God profile		Flechsig profile	
	1	2	1	2	1	2	1	2
Male								
Profile 1								
Profile 2	.706[b]							
Female								
Profile 1	.667	.561						
Profile 2	.457	.437	.566[b]					
God								
Profile 1	.226	.475	.166	.420				
Profile 2	.451	.534	.413	.352	.679[b]			
Flechsig								
Profile 1	.679	.645	.576	.504	.446	.598		
Profile 2	.556	.662	.516	.319	.552	.636	.737[b]	
Sun	.523	.330	.678	.356	.136	.444	.511	.397

[a]Source: Laffal (1960, p. 476).
[b]Reliabilities.

alpine and Hunter view that the sun is a feminine symbol in the memoirs.

The Schreber study illustrates the application of the concept-analysis system in the exploration of associative and idiosyncratic meaning (meaning 4). In this type of application, those parts of a text are selected which contain key words, the parts are merged to create a single text for each key word, and the concept profiles of these merged texts are compared with each other to determine the relative similarity of the key words. Hypotheses bearing on conceptual similarities and differences between key words are especially amenable to study using this approach. The key words may be drawn from a single speaker, from separate speakers, or from separate time periods.

Psychotherapy with a Disturbed Child: Qualitative Analysis of Concepts

The study by Zakaras and Fine (1979) is of interest in applying clinical interpretation to concept categories derived from therapeutic interviews between a therapist and a child. The patient was a 12-year-old boy, described as having a symbiotic psychosis. He was seen twice weekly for one-half hour in psychotherapy in a residential treatment center. Prior to admission to the center he was hallucinating, 40 pounds overweight, unaware of bodily boundaries, and unable to separate his identity from that of his mother. He had been attending school irregularly, tried to make friends by giving away toys, spoke in fantasy terms, and was unable to read above a second grade level. His score on the Wechsler Scale for Children was in the dull-normal range, although his school psychologist estimated that his potential was in the average range. The family was of Mexican-American descent, and the boy spoke fluent Spanish as well as English. After eight months of treatment the patient had improved, was discharged from the center, and was seen on an outpatient basis.

During treatment, each session had been tape-recorded for purposes of supervision. After the treatment, it was decided to examine the language interaction and language changes of patient and therapist, using the concept-analysis system described above. Six interviews out of the therapy series were selected for analysis: the 3rd, 15th, 27th, 39th, 58th, and 73rd. Complete transcripts of these interviews were made, keypunched onto IBM cards, and submitted to computer concept analysis. In the computer analysis, each text word is compared to a stored dictionary of words (25,000 at the time) with associated concepts, and the frequency of occurrence of each of the 116 concepts is cumulated in a profile. In preparing a text for concept analysis by computer, an editor substitutes relevant nouns for proper names and for pronouns, and adds a number subscript identifying the appropriate dictionary meaning in the case of homonyms. For example, *bear*(1) is scored ANML, *bear*(2) is scored HAVE, *bear*(3) is scored BGIN, and so forth. Words without numbers are matched against the first dictionary entry for that word, which will represent the most common meaning of the word.

In examining how the patient and the therapist used words in the category POWR, it was found that the therapist made frequent references to the abilities and strength of the patient, but few such references to himself. At the beginning of therapy the patient referred to the power and strength of others, but not of the therapist. Then, in the third session and continuing through the treatment, the patient began to refer to his own power, which the authors suggest indicates the patient's increased ego strength and self-confidence.

Turning to how the patient and the therapist used words in the concept JOIN, they found that the therapist employed unambiguous "union" words (*meet, together, connect*), whereas the patient's words in this concept included a large number with an additional BLOK or DAMG scoring (*knot, collide, tie*). Their interpretation of this finding is that, while the therapist was more inclined to discuss union itself, the patient had a marked ambivalence about union, seeing it as both gratifying and threatening.

The differences in the use of the concepts POWR and JOIN by therapist and patient were shown to be statistcally significant, but the authors also evaluated other, statistically nonsignificant differences in use of concepts. Thus, the therapist made more frequent use of the categories AGRE, TIME, SIML, OPPO, GOOD, BLUR, MOTV, PANG, and NO, while the patient favored the categories KIN, AID, GO, DAMG, MEDC, MALE, and BODY. By inspecting the contexts in which the words in these concept categories were used, the authors found that the therapist's reliance on AGRE reflected his conviction that ideas of cooperation, praise, and permissiveness were important to establish a trusting therapeutic relationship with the child. TIME reflected the therapist's personal style, his attempt to provide boundaries to the patient's confusion, and his desire to introduce consistency, regularity, and predictability. Equally, his use of the concept SIML, with words of sameness, consistency, and equality, reinforced the idea of structure, and was directed at reducing the patient's confusion. Nevertheless, while stressing sameness, the therapist also talked of differences (OPPO). The therapist's use of GOOD words came from a concern for morality and goodness as against evil and dishonesty, while BLUR words could be traced to a stylistic feature (*I guess, I wonder*) in the therapist's effort to relate to the patient.

The concepts MOTV and PANG were used more by the therapist than by the patient, suggesting that the therapist felt it important to discuss anxiety, fear, guilt, responsibility, and choice, while the patient had less interest in these areas.

The concept KIN was used with statistically significant greater frequency by the patient than by the therapist. This result had been predicted on the grounds that concepts reflecting union would be elevated in a childhood schizophrenic with symbiotic features. The patient's use of words in the AID category showed a need for nurturance and dependency, while the authors suggest that the therapist's greater use of the NO concept indicates that he responded to some of the patient's demands by refusals and limit-setting. GO, the movement category, mirrored the patient's concern with activity and movement, an aspect also shown in his speed and expressiveness of speech. The comparatively high frequency of DAMG words for the patient was taken to be a projection of feelings of harm, and to reflect a paranoid cognitive style. MEDC was viewed as reflecting the patient's concern for cure, and his attempts to conceptualize the psychotherapeutic activity.

Use of the concept MALE was of interest. Both patient and therapist talked more about FEM than MALE, but the patient used MALE much more than did the therapist. The authors take this to mean that the patient, who was entering puberty at the time of treatment, was more concerned with his own masculinity and his relationship with his father than the therapist perceived. The patient's use of the concept BODY may have been part of this same concern, as well as an effort to define his own physical boundaries.

The authors also took note of those concepts which were scarcely used by patient or therapist. Thus, the concept SUB drew few tokens, suggesting that obedience and subordination were not discussed in the therapy, a surprising fact in therapy with a child, where parental control might be assumed to be of importance. The authors suggest that the absence of such topics may have been partly due to the therapist's reluctance to see the inequality in the therapeutic relationship.

In assessing the concept-analysis system, the authors concluded that its major limitation was that, while it did an excellent job of determining important areas of conceptual content, it did not always evaluate the orientation and use of that content by the speaker. With respect to neglected topics, they found that the total content-analysis approach provided an otherwise lacking perspective: "For example, it brings to awareness which areas were talked about and which areas were ignored. In the present study, it suggests that the patient's relationship to father and issues of parental control were ignored and probably would have been important to discuss" (p. 450).

A result that surprised the authors was that, while their initial hypotheses called for significant differences in specific conceptual areas, therapist and schizophrenic patient turned out to be fundamentally similar in their use of concepts.

Perhaps this result should not have been surprising. Watson and Laffal (1963) had found that therapists, when they talked about their patients, tended to use substantially the same types of concepts that the patients had used. Laffal (1967) also found that in conversation, individual differences in speakers tend to be overridden by the subject matter discussed. To the extent that the therapist becomes an active participant in the verbal exchange, and the therapy begins to resemble ordinary conversation, the conceptual content of therapist and patient are likely to become increasingly similar. There may well be implications in this for treatment of schizophrenic patients, namely, that a more active role by the therapist could have a normalizing effect on the patient.

Concept Analysis of Thirty Interviews with a Schizophrenic Patient

The largest study using the concept analysis method has been an analysis of thirty therapeutic interviews with a schizophrenic patient (Laffal, 1979). The interviews were mostly of one hour length, but some were briefer. The total number of words in the thirty interviews, including the therapist's, was slightly over 93,000. Around 80% of this, an estimated 75,000 words, belonged to the patient, and it was this material that was analyzed.

The patient was a 28-year-old man born of parents of Irish descent. The father had graduated from an Ivy League college and held a supervisory position in a large firm. He was a mild, soft-spoken man who was baffled by his son's illness, but always made himself available to help, and came often to take his son out for visits. The mother was a large woman, and was felt by personnel who had seen her to be the dominant member of the family and a source of major difficulty for the patient. The patient was the youngest of three sons, and asserted that he had been born by Caesarian section, when in fact the mother reported a normal delivery. At the time of his birth, the mother had very much wanted a girl, and was disappointed at having a third boy. She found him not nearly as affectionate as the other children, feeling he was cold, withdrawn, and self-willed. The patient began school at the age of five. He made good grades, but missed nearly a year of high school at the age of fourteen because of a bicycle accident in which he sustained a skull fracture. He also lost time from school because of hay fever.

At the age of eighteen the patient was isolating himself in his room, refusing to go to school, and behaving in a negativistic manner. He graduated from high school at the age of twenty, worked briefly as a copy boy on a newspaper, then enlisted in the Army. He was in front line combat for several months, and was wounded in the chest. Subsequently he developed psychiatric problems, including auditory and visual hallucinations, and marked stereotypy in behavior and speech. He was easily distracted and constantly interrupted himself to comment on objects and noises. His language was pompous and aphoristic, and he was inclined to pun a great deal. Thus, when asked, "How are your spirits?" by an examining doctor, he responded, "I don't know, I don't drink." In the army hospital the patient was treated by insulin coma. He was twenty-three years old at the time of discharge from the army.

His adjustment at home was poor. He hounded and persecuted his mother, and finally, after a physical confrontation with her, he was brought to a psychiatric hospital. Three years after hospitalization he entered psychotherapy, the early part of which is analyzed below. The therapy itself lasted over seven years. During this period the patient went to a nearby community college, completing a two-year program in journalism. Ultimately—around ten years after the treatment reported here—he was able to leave the hospital and live on his own.

In preparation for the study, all of the patient's verbalizations in thirty tape-recorded interviews, drawn from the first year and a half of treatment, were cardpunched on IBM cards, with appropriate editing for proper names, pronouns, and common homonyms. Three analyses were undertaken: first, to determine, by means of contextual analysis of key words, what latent themes might underlie such words; second, to identify the major themes in the patient's total language; and third, to trace the rise and fall of themes over the course of the thirty interviews. The first analysis—of key words—was addressed especially to the hypothesis, based on clinical judgment, that the themes of *Language* and *Leadership*, were related respectively, at a latent level, to themes of *Mother* and *Father*.

A series of 23 key words which seemed clinically of importance to the patient, along with words which were sufficiently close to the key words to be considered references to the same conceptual content, were identified, and all usages of these words in the 30 interviews, along with their surrounding contexts, were collected for study. This was facilitated by the fact that an initial computer run of the 30 interviews produced an alphabetic listing of the text words, along with the lines in which each word occurred. A context was defined as that segment of the patient's language which incuded two lines of cardpunched text immediately preceding, and two lines immediately following, the line in which the key word occurred, without regard to sentence boundaries, but confined within a given remark by the patient. The key words and their related words are shown in Table 4. Texts surrounding each key word from throughout the thirty interviews were combined into a single text for that key word, as in the Schreber case study.

The texts were then subjected to computerized concept analysis (the dictionary now containing 42,000 entries), and a matrix of key-word concept-profile correlations was prepared and factor analyzed. An initial orthogonal factor analysis did not support the hypothesis of a relationship between *Language* and *Mother*, and between *Leadership* and *Father*, since it showed each of these four themes as dominant in a factor of its own.

The possibility was then raised that the hypothesized relationship lay at a level beyond that tapped by the first-order factor analysis, and might be revealed by a higher-order analysis. In order to do a second-order factor analysis, first-order factors must be allowed to correlate with each other. Oblique factor rotation provides for such correlation, where orthogonal analysis is predicated on independence of factors. The key word-profile correlations were therefore subjected to oblique factor analysis, the results of which are reported in Table 5.

The factor pattern, in the left hand part of the table, shows the factor grouping and the coordinates of each key word among the various factors, and gives a picture of the relative importance of key words in each factor. The factor structure, in the right hand part of the table, provides the correlations of the key words with the factors. At the bot-

TABLE 4
Key Words and Related Words[a]

1. *Authority*
2. *Book (author, write)*
3. *Brother (fraternal)*
4. *Child (baby, daughter, fetal, filial, kid, offspring, progeny, son)*
5. *Death (die, grave, homicide, kill, murder, suicide)*
6. *Deep (bottom, depth, down, subterranean, under)*
7. *English (Anglophobe, Anglo-Saxon, Great Britain)*
8. *Family (ancestor, generation, genetic, grandfather, marry, nephew, parent, progenitor, sister, uncle, wife)*
9. *Father (dad, paternal)*
10. *Female (girl, lady, woman)*
11. *Food (bread, cannibal, coffee, donut, drink, eat, feed, meat, restaurant, steak, tea)*
12. *God (deity)*
13. *Government*
14. *Language (grammar)*
15. *Lead*
16. *Learn (academy, college, mentor, pupil, school, student, study, taught, teacher, Yale)*
17. *Love*
18. *Male (boy, male, man, men, penis, phallic, virile)*
19. *Mother (ma, maternal)*
20. *President (White House)*
21. *Smoke (cigaret, tobacco)*
22. *Speak (talk)*
23. *Therapist (doctor, physician, psychiatrist, psychologist)*

[a]Source: Laffal (1979, p. 327).

tom of the table is shown the matrix of correlations between factors. In the original orthogonal factor analysis, the four factors were shown to account for 68.5% of the variance in the matrix of key word correlations.

Taking key words with coordinates of at least .50, those contributing to each factor, in order of importance, are:

Factor I. *Speak, English, Deep, Therapist, Death, Learn, Book, Male*
Factor II. *President, Government, Lead, Authority*
Factor III. *Mother, Female, God*
Factor IV. *Brother, Father, Family*

Some idea of the actual word content in the four factors may be garnered from the concepts which contribute most importantly to their factor scores. Concepts with the highest factor scores, in descending order, are shown below:

Factor I. GRUP, TALK, MALE, GO, HAVE, MOTV, OPPO, AID.

TABLE 5
Oblique Factor Analysis of Key Words[a]

		Factor pattern				Factor structure			
		I	II	III	IV	I	II	III	IV
1.	Authority	28	−62	03	−13	71	−83	44	−49
2.	Book	57	00	03	−01	58	−34	29	−31
3.	Brother	09	13	05	−95	53	−26	40	−97
4.	Child	36	−10	16	−42	71	−51	52	−70
5.	Death	60	−08	09	−08	73	−49	43	−45
6.	Deep	76	−09	06	03	82	−53	42	−41
7.	English	78	−02	−03	04	76	−44	32	−36
8.	Family	19	−09	22	−62	66	−49	58	−83
9.	Father	−15	−31	09	−88	53	−55	47	−94
10.	Female	05	−08	87	00	49	−44	92	−37
11.	Food	35	−06	34	−20	65	−46	60	−53
12.	God	11	−36	57	03	56	−63	74	−36
13.	Government	15	−81	01	−05	64	−92	41	−40
14.	Language	73	−13	07	07	80	−55	42	−38
15.	Lead	25	−73	−05	−07	68	−87	37	−42
16.	Learn	60	−11	−01	−21	76	−52	39	−55
17.	Love	42	−06	13	−02	52	−36	35	−31
18.	Male	53	−11	−04	−43	79	−54	40	−72
19.	Mother	00	17	92	−13	39	−23	90	−42
20.	President	−10	−102	01	−01	49	−97	36	−30
21.	Smoke	49	07	−11	−13	47	−21	14	−32
22.	Speak	90	−02	06	13	87	−52	43	−37
23.	Therapist	63	−05	10	02	69	−44	40	−36

	Correlations among factors			
	I	II	III	IV
I	1.00	−.58	.46	−.52
II		1.00	−.39	.33
III			1.00	−.38
IV				1.00

[a]Source: Laffal (1979, p. 333).

Factor II. LEAD, LAW, GRUP, TALK, MOTV, HAVE, OPPO, GO.

Factor III. AID, FEM, HOLY, KIN, LEAD, GRUP, TALK, JOIN.

Factor IV. MALE, KIN, LEAD, GO, HAVE, GRUP, NUMR, TALK.

Because of the dominance of group words (GRUP) and language words (TALK), the first factor may be labeled a *Group–Language* factor.

Because of the dominance of LEAD and LAW concepts—which are scored together for words relating to government—the second factor may be called a *Leadership* factor. The third factor may be called a *Mother* factor, while the fourth may be called a *Brother–Father* factor. Note that Factor II, the *Leadership* factor, has the concepts GRUP and TALK in common as very high frequency items with Factor I, the *Group–Language* factor, but the most heavily occurring concepts, LEAD and LAW, are unique to this *Leadership* factor. What this means is that when words relating to groups and language are the focus of discussion, words relating to government and leadership occur infrequently, while when words of government and leadership are being used primarily, words relating to groups and language still occur with moderate frequency. These two factors thus have a negative correlation, despite the fact that they have important elements in common.

Table 6 contains the second order orthogonal factor analysis of key words, based on the correlations of first-order factors at the bottom of Table 5. The analysis results in one second-order factor, shown in the left hand part of the table, which accounts for 46.0% of the variance in the matrix of first-order factor correlations. The table also shows, in the right hand part, an expanded two-factor analysis of the first-order correlations. The two-factor analysis accounts for 53.2% of the variance in the first-order matrix.

The one-factor result in Table 6 defines a single bipolar dimension on which both *Group–Language* and *Mother* load positively, and *Leadership* and *Brother–Father* load negatively. The hypothesis of a latent relationship between *Language* and *Mother*, and between *Leadership* and *Father*, is thus borne out at the higher level of analysis.

The two-factor expansion—Factors A and B in Table 6—adds further information about the patient's thinking. Factor A shows *Group–Language* and *leadership* as polar groupings, but Factor B also shows the *Brother–Father* factor, in its own right, to be negatively related to *Group-*

TABLE 6
Second Order Factor Analysis of Key Words[a]

	I	h^2	A	B	h^2
Group–Language Factor	86	74	61	54	67
Leadership Factor	−65	42	−74	−24	58
Mother Factor	58	33	39	41	32
Brother–Father Factor	−59	35	−23	−70	54
% Variance	46.0	46.0	28.1	25.1	53.2

[a]Source: Laffal (1979, p. 335).

Language. The *Group–Language* factor thus appears to anchor a central complex of ideas in the patient's thinking, against which other sets of ideas may clash. Figure 1 presents these relationships graphically, by plotting the first-order factors on the axes formed by the two second-order factors. It is not possible here to discuss this structure of themes as length, but it may be pointed out that the picture is not a simple Oedipal one. There is a single dominant thematic dimension—*Group–Language* versus *Leadership*—with *Mother* in the *Group-Language* end of the continuum; however, the *Brother–Father* factor, while distinctly related to the *Leadership* factor, appears to have some elements of uniqueness as well.

We turn now from the key-word analysis to concept analysis of the total language of the patient in the thirty interviews. The details of this analysis are available in Laffal (1979), and I will here concentrate on how the analysis highlights the character of particular interviews, and how it traces the ebb and flow in themes in the patient's language.

A factor analysis of the concept profiles of the thirty interviews, shown in Table 7, accounts for 72.4% of the variance in the matrix of correlations, and reveals four factors with category preeminence as follows:

Factor I. GRUP, TALK, AID, MOTV, LEAD, GO, OPPO, MEDC.

Factor II. MALE, KIN, GO, LEAD, GRUP, MOTV, TALK, HAVE.

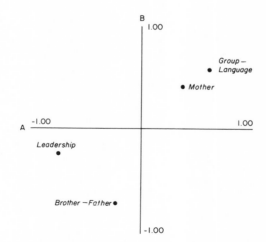

FIGURE 1. Plot of first-order factors on second-order factors: Laffal (1979, p. 336).

TABLE 7
Oblique Factor Analysis of Interviews

	Factor pattern				Factor structure			
Interview	I	II	III	IV	I	II	III	IV
1	92	−02	−12	−40	84	50	11	−32
2	62	37	−13	05	82	73	14	13
3	79	−07	10	30	80	49	31	37
4	64	25	01	20	82	67	26	28
5	89	03	00	05	91	60	25	13
6	91	03	−05	−10	91	59	20	−02
7	87	02	04	14	90	59	29	22
8	14	81	−13	−01	62	86	12	06
9	10	90	−20	−10	61	90	07	−03
10	72	18	−01	07	83	63	23	15
11	43	18	04	11	57	48	21	17
12	88	−05	00	03	85	51	23	10
13	78	12	−14	03	82	57	10	11
14	51	33	19	09	77	71	42	17
15	72	17	11	01	86	66	35	09
16	82	−04	17	11	85	54	39	19
17	85	06	05	−09	89	60	29	−01
18	99	−13	−09	01	89	47	14	08
19	52	19	09	−03	66	54	28	03
20	53	41	−06	05	77	73	20	12
21	02	02	69	01	22	22	70	04
22	60	00	01	51	66	43	20	56
23	63	23	23	−13	83	68	45	−05
24	68	12	31	−21	82	61	52	−13
25	03	71	31	−06	56	81	51	01
26	73	06	09	−44	76	52	29	−36
27	60	01	42	−07	71	50	59	00
28	03	55	20	21	45	64	36	27
29	35	51	−05	21	68	74	19	28
30	−08	85	15	−05	49	84	36	02

	Correlations among factors			
	I	II	III	IV
I	1.00	.63	.27	.09
II		1.00	.27	.08
III			1.00	.04
IV				1.00

[a]Source: Laffal (1979, p. 338).

Factor III. TIME, NUMR, GO, WRIT, DAMG, LEAD, PLAC, MEDC.

Factor IV. SICK, MEDC, GO, EMPH, TALK, AID, AGRE, BLUR.

Factor I is dominated by GRUP and TALK, which were also the two leading concepts in the *Group–Language* factor. The occurrence of LEAD and OPPO as prominent concepts in this factor suggests that the factor may to some extent represent the opposition *Group–Language* versus *Leadership*, which was found in the higher-order analysis of key words.

Factor II has substantially the same configuration of important concepts as the previously revealed *Brother–Father* factor.

Factors III and IV have dominant concepts not hitherto making significant contributions to any of the key-word factors. In Factor III, TIME and NUMR occurring together indicate reference to time of day and dates. This may therefore be labeled a *Time* factor. In Factor IV, the major themes appear to be illness, patients, and medical care (SICK, MEDC). This may be therefore labeled an *Illness* factor.

Factor III, the *Time* factor, has its major representation in Interview 21, as may be seen in the factor pattern of Table 7. Interview 21 was unique in that it was the shortest of all thirty interviews, and the last interview before a period of severe disturbance on the patient's part, lasting four months, in which further office interviews could not be held. Apparently, the interview was brief because the patient was already showing signs of disturbance. In it he spoke almost exclusively of days and dates, and it is for this reason that the concept analysis distinguishes the interview as being quite different from the others.

Only Interview 22 shows a coordinate above .50 in the factor pattern of Factor IV, the *Illness* factor. The central subject matter of this interview is the relationship between patients and doctors; however, it is also of note in marking the recovery of the patient from the long period of disturbance following Interview 21. Interview Factors III, *Time*, and IV, *Illness*, arise, it appears, from a disruption in the patient's mainstream thought processes, and together, they mark the beginning and the ending of the period of disruption. This suggests that while particular subject matter is of importance in itself, it may also be of significance in marking a deviation from the subject's expectable content. Only a large-scale analysis of the patient's language could have revealed such a phenomenon.

Finally, we examine how the major themes which were revealed in the key-word analysis distribute themselves throughout the thirty interviews. For this purpose, correlations between factor-score profiles of the key word factors (*Group–Language, Leadership, Brother–Father,* and *Mother*), and concept profiles of the interviews, were taken as indices of the importance of the themes in the interviews. These correlations were converted to standard scores, based on the mean correlation of each factor with all the interviews. The standard scores, shown in Figure 2 as bars for those correlations which exceed the mean, reveal the relative importance of the four themes in the various interviews, corrected for the mean level of production of each theme in all of the interviews.

The *Group–Language* factor, with a mean *r* of .73 and a standard deviation of .14, was a stable undercurrent throughout the interviews. The *Leadership* theme was most strongly represented in Interview 1, and subsequently received some emphasis in Interviews 6 and 19. *Brother– Father* was most marked in Interviews 8, 9, 25, and 30, while *Mother* was prominent only in Interview 2.

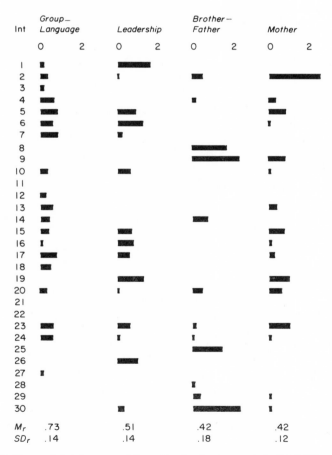

FIGURE 2. Theme–interview correlations (in standard scores): Laffal (1979, p. 343).

The pattern of relationships between themes and interviews in Figure 2 does not lend itself to simple description, and may best be characterized as portraying an ongoing interplay of themes. *Group–Language,* the generally prevailing motif, appears to become of less importance after Interview 22, the point at which an interlude of severe psychological disturbance for the patient ended. *Brother–Father* occupies two interviews in a major way in this postdisturbance sequence, suggesting that the patient was able then to drop his habitual talk, and to speak of more vital concerns. However, analysis of additional interviews over a more extended period of time would have been necessary to determine if this represented an enduring shift.

Extending the Analysis to Syntactics and Pragmatics in Psychotherapy

Having illustrated how the method of concept analysis deals with the semantic content of texts, we turn now to programmatic possibilities for extending the analysis to syntactic and pragmatic properties of a speaker's words.

Two major areas in which syntax adds meaning are in specification of the relationship between words and in grammatical case of words. According to Fillmore (1971, p. 374), relationships between most content words can be characterized by their use as predicates (assertions) and arguments (something about which assertions are made). Thus, in the phrase *tall man, tall* is the predicate and *man* is the argument. In *The boy runs swiftly, swiftly* is the predicate and *runs* the argument, while *runs swiftly* is the predicate of the argument *The boy.* Specification of predicates and arguments in the analysis of a text would show relationships between contents that a concept analysis does not provide.

However, since predication is a relationship between neighboring words, the same information can, to some extent, be developed by analysis of contents surrounding the key words to be studied. By such a context analysis one would know, for example, that for the key word *man,* words relating to *tall* appeared with a certain degree of frequency in the text; or for the key word *boy,* words such as *running* and *swift* tended to occur nearby. Thus, one could gather information that certain kinds of words appeared consistently in the environs of key words, even though one would not be able to specify the predicate nature of the contextual words.

Case is another source of meaning provided by syntax. In *Jim slapped John with a towel, Jim* is the agent who did the slapping and *John* is the person who received the action, while *towel* is the instrument of the action. A straightforward semantic concept analysis of separate word meanings does not specify the source of action, the recipient of action, or other roles in an action. The only way role relationships can be provided is by assigning cases based on the underlying sentence syntax. Case grammar, as proposed by Fillmore (1968, 1971), seems to hold promise here. Fillmore has outlined a set of cases identifying noun roles in sentences.[3] These include: the animate agent (A) identified by the verb action; the animate being experiencing or affected by the verb action (E); an object that moves or changes, or whose existence is in consideration by the verb action (O); a result (R) that comes into being as a consequence of the verb action; the instrument (I) by which the verb action is achieved; and a locative (L) that identifies a place marked by the verb action. Of these grammatical cases, our interest focuses on just two, of particular relevance to interpersonal pragmatics because they identify animate participants: Agent (A), the animate instigator of an action identified by a verb, and Experiencer (E), the being which experiences the effect of the action identified by the verb.

In a study of counseling, Bieber, Patton, and Fuhriman (1977) assigned Object, Experiencer, and Agentive cases based on type of verb used by client and therapist. They also employed a Benefactive case where the verb *to have* was used, while assigning Object case to stative (*to be*) verbs. In the example to follow, and for purposes of our psychological analysis, the only cases assigned are Agent and Experiencer. *A* may tell us something about active, self-generated moves by a person; *E* may tell us something about the extent to which a person is acted upon, or is a passive experiencer of actions identified by verbs. With respect to stative and benefactive verbs, their arguments are to be scored *A* or *E* as with other verbs, unless their meaning does not entail an action. Thus, *John is my brother* and *John has green eyes* are stative and benefactive sentences in which John is not scored *A*, because the verbs do not have the force of an action. In *John is angry* and *John is hurt*, John is identified as *A* in the first sentence and *E* in the second. In *John has a deep love for Joan*, John is *A* and Joan is *E*. The determining judgment of *A*, *E*, or no-case is based on whether the verb identifies an action with an instigator or an experiencer (not to be confused with traditional subject and object of the verb).

Furthermore, only indicative statements are subscripted for case. Sentences which demand that an action occur, or which raise possibilities and questions about an action, require careful consideration before applying case subscripts to the arguments of the verb whose action is in focus. Thus, in the following series of imperative, interrogative, subjunctive, optative, and indicative sentences, only the last

---

[3]Fillmore did not include nominal predicate sentences (of the N *be* N type) in his case system (1968, p. 84). For purposes of our psychological analysis, the types of sentences or clauses in which cases are assigned are further limited, as indicated, to indicative ones.

one—the indicative sentence—is subscribed for case: *Please leave! Is he leaving? He may leave. If only he would leave. He(A) is leaving.* Where a nonindicative sentence incorporates an indicative statement, case subscripts are applied in the indicative clause. Thus, *Did John throw the stone?* is an interrogative in which whether John did the act is in question, and John is therefore not subscripted. But, in *Why did John(A) throw the stone?* the action by John is presupposed, the inquiry being only about causes; therefore, John is identified as Agent.

How to include nonindicative statements in a case-grammar analysis for psychological purposes is a complex problem. I have no reasonable proposal for dealing with it at this point, and will confine my example to the use of case subscripts in indicative statements.

Adding case subscripts, as in *The man(A) is shouting,* amounts to the introduction of new contents, that is, *man* as agent of the *shouting.* If a text were edited in this manner, the subscripted words could be subjected to an analysis in their own right, to determine what persons and what concepts were assigned what case roles by each speaker. Thus, syntactic case-role information about animate beings could be incorporated in a concept analysis.

Of even greater psychotherapeutic interest is the question of how the implicit interpersonal and intrapsychic aspects of a communication, that is, the pragmatic aspects, might be managed.

Assume that *The man is shouting* is uttered in a context which indicates a possible attack. The statement might then have, as its pragmatic function, a message which might be expressed as *The man is warning us.*

If statements such as this last were appended to a text as pragmatic glosses, they themselves could be analyzed just as the content of the text is analyzed. How this may occur is illustrated below, in a segment from a tape recording of the beginning of a family therapy meeting.

A mother and an older daughter are in the family therapy meeting with a younger daughter, who is a patient in a psychiatric hospital, and a therapist. Mim is the older daughter, Vee is the younger daughter who is the patient. A brother, not present, is mentioned. Grammatical case, where applicable (i.e., occurring in indicative sentences or clauses) is shown in parentheses. Other parenthetical words are added to make understood words explicit (e.g., in sentence 17) or to provide some behavioral data (e.g., in sentence 5). Beside each remark are indicative, case-subscripted statements (1p, 2p, etc.), representing pragmatic interpretations by the therapist of the speaker's intentions or actions.

(1)	MIM: You look so skinny, kid.	(1p)	Mim(A) is concerned about Vee(E).
(2)	VEE: Well, they(A) keep me(E) jumping.	(2p)	Vee(A) is lighthearted. Others(A) dominate Vee(E).
(3)	MIM: Ah, they keep you jumping?	(3p)	Mim(E) is surprised.

(4)	VEE: Yes.	(4p)	Others(A) dominate Vee(E).
(5)	MIM: (laughs)	(5p)	Mim(E) is relieved.
(6)	MOTHER: Tell the truth, Vee.	(6p)	Mother(A) commands Vee(E). Mother(A) demands the truth. Vee(A) is untrustworthy.
(7)	VEE: Huh?	(7p)	Vee(E) is dismayed.
(8)	MOTHER: Tell the truth; you're(A) not eating.	(8p)	Mother(A) commands Vee(E). Mother(A) demands truth. Vee(A) is lying.
(9)	VEE: Oh!	(9p)	Vee(A) understands.
(10)	MOTHER: Are you?	(10p)	Mother(A) demands truth. Mother(A) commands Vee(E). Vee(A) is untrustworthy.
(11)	VEE: No.	(11p)	Vee(A) lied. Mother(A) has defeated Vee(E).
(12)	DR.: (to Mim) Have you not seen each other for some time?	(12p)	Dr.(A) changes topic. Dr.(A) protects Vee(E) from threatening mother(A), and encourages empathy between Mim(E) and Vee(E).
(13)	MIM: It's been since November. Ah, Thanksgiving. The last time I was home. Remember that, Vee? Remember Thanksgiving, you were home and I was home?	(13p)	Mim(A) encourages Vee(E) to remember.
(14)	VEE: Oh yeah.	(14p)	Vee(A) is unresponsive.
(15)	MIM: Do you come home?	(15p)	Mim(A) encourages Vee(E).
(16)	VEE: Yeah.	(16p)	Vee(A) is unresponsive.
(17)	MIM: You(A) did (come home), didn't you? Your next visit.	(17p)	Mim(E) is desperate. Mim(A) encourages Vee(E).
(18)	VEE: Yeah.	(18p)	Vee(A) is unresponsive.
(19)	MIM: (softly) What's the matter?	(19p)	Mim(A) is concerned about Vee(E).
(20)	VEE: Nothing. (Whispers).	(20p)	Vee(A) denies that she(E) is upset. Vee(A) confides in Mim(E).
(21)	MIM: Jimmy! No! Why do you(A) say that?	(21p)	Mim(E) is upset. Mim(A) denies something about Jimmy.
(22)	VEE: Oh, you(A) just scared me(E).	(22p)	Vee(A) blames Mim(E) for Mim(A) scaring Vee(E).
(23)	MIM: I scared you? How'd I(A) do that?	(23p)	Mim(E) is puzzled and guilty.
(24)	Well, you(A) said Jimmy was dead.	(24p)	Mim(A) is responsible, while Vee(E) is absolved, for saying Jimmy is dead.

Sentence 1 is taken as a descriptive statement without significant A or E component. The pragmatic feature of the sentence that appears to be of most importance is that the older sister, Mim, is expressing concern for the younger sister, Vee. This interpretation is shown in 1p. Sentence 2 is Vee's explanation of why she is so skinny: she (as Experiencer) is kept so active by others (as Agents) that she cannot put on weight. There is, at the same time, an element of lightheartedness in the phrase *keep me jumping*. These pragmatic aspects of the remark are represented in 2p. The syntactic and pragmatic analysis of the sample goes on in this manner.

How the semantic, syntactic, and pragmatic data may be organized is shown in Tables 8, 9, and 10. Table 8 provides a semantic concept distribution based on the words of each speaker. Table 9 displays those words which were subscripted for syntactic case. Table 10 summarizes the therapist's interpretations of the pragmatic functions of each speaker's remarks with respect to self and other speakers, linked to concepts.

TABLE 8
Concept Analysis of Family Interview

Concept	Speaker			
	Mim	Vee	Mother	Therapist
AGRE		4		
AID	2			
BACK	1			
BLUR	1			
BODY	1			
CRUX	1			
DEAD		1		
EMPH	3	5		
END	1			
EVER	1	1		
EVNT	1			
FOOD			1	
GO	3	1		
HOME	4			
IDEA	2			
JOIN	1			
LITL	1			
NEAR		1		
NO	2	2	1	1
PANG	2	1		
PAST	2			
QUIK	1	1		
SELF	4	2		
SOLE	4	2		2
SOMA			1	
SOME				1
TALK	1	1	2	
TIME	5			1
TRUE			2	
VIEW	1			1
YNG	1			

The data of Tables 8, 9, and 10 are open to interpretation. Table 8 represents the frequency of concepts for each speaker, hence may suggest each speaker's major preoccupations. One may look either at the categories which occur with highest frequency for a speaker, or at categories which occur only for that speaker. Mim and Vee, by virtue of the fact that they do most of the talking in the segment illustrated, have the broadest distribution of categories. Mim's major themes are TIME, HOME, SELF, and SOLE (self-reference). TIME appears to be largely a response to the therapist's inquiry about Vee and Mim seeing each other, while HOME reflects her sense of Vee's absence. Self-references may indicate some tendency to focus on herself, but this, of course, is a very small sample. Vee has a number of EMPH words—reflecting her use of interjections such as *well* and *oh*—and also a high AGRE score, reflecting her use of the affirmatives *Yes* and *Yeah* in response to questions. Vee also introduces the concept DEAD, which, because of its uniqueness, may say a great deal about her anxieties. The mother speaks of eating (FOOD, SOMA) and telling (TALK) the truth (TRUE), concerns which are directed at the younger daughter.

Table 9, which shows concepts as predicates whose arguments were case-conscripted personal references, provides information of a syntactic nature about how the speakers saw each other on the Agent—Experiencer dimension. It is of considerable interest here that Mim and Mother saw Vee, the patient, as an active Agent, in terms of the frequency with which they assigned her an *A* role (2A and 3A). However, for her part, Vee pictured herself as a passive Experiencer (4E), with others taking the Agent role.

Table 10, the summary of pragmatically oriented interpretations by the therapist about the therapeutic interaction, is most complex. It shows, for each speaker, a distribution of predicated concepts whose arguments are the various speakers, including self. Thus, as shown in column 1, the therapist believes Mim predicates of herself primarily an Experiencer role with considerable upset (PANG). Where she assumes the active Agent role (MOTV, AID), this appears to be in relationship to Vee, who is very much the target of her actions. Mim thus appears as a sensitive, anxious person who wants to help her sister.

According to the therapist, Vee assigns a mixed Agent–Experiencer role to Mim. While she accepts responsibility herself for some areas, as shown by the 4A MOTV score, it is clear that LEAD and POWR are attributed to others or to Mother as Agent, and she is the Experiencer of these predicates. Vee assumes the Agent role in the areas of AGGR, COVR, FALS, FOND, GLAD, IDEA, MOTV, NO, OPPO, SOMA, and TALK. There is in this some suggestion that aggression and negation, along with a range of other responses are, in the therapist's view, ac-

TABLE 9

Case-by-Concept Analysis of Family Interview[a]

Concept	Speaker											
	Mim				Vee				Mother			
	Mim	Vee	Mother	Others	Mim	Vee	Mother	Others	Mim	Vee	Mother	Others
EVER						E		A				
EVNT	A											
FOOD										A		
GO		A				E		A				
NO						E				A		
PANG					A	E						
QUIK						E		A				
SOMA												
TALK		A			A					A		
Sum A	1	2			2			3		3		
E						4						

[a] A = agent; E = experiencer.

TABLE 10
Pragmatics of Family Interview[a]

	Speaker									
	Mim					Vee				
Concept	Mim	Vee	Moth	Ther	Othr	Mim	Vee	Moth	Ther	Othr
AFAR	E									
AGGR						E	A			
AGRE							E			
AID	3A,E	3E								
BLUR	E									
COVR						E	A			
CRIM	E									
DAMG										
FALS							A			
FOND						E	A			
GLAD							A			
IDEA							A			
LEAD							2E			2A
MOTV	2A	2E				A,E	4A			
NO	A						A			
OPEN							E			
OPPO							3A			
PANG	2A,4E	2E				A	3E			
POWR							E	A		
SOMA							A			
TALK						A	A			
VARY										
WEAK							E	A		
Sum A	8					3	16	2		2
E	8	7				4	9			

[a]A = agent; E = experiencer.

	Speaker									
	Mother					Therapist				
Concept	Mim	Vee	Moth	Ther	Othr	Mim	Vee	Moth	Ther	Othr
AFAR										
AGGR		2A								
AGRE										
AID						E	2E		2A	
BLUR										
COVR										
CRIM										
DAMG								A		

(*continued*)

TABLE 10 (Continued)

	Speaker									
	Mim					Vee				
Concept	Mim	Vee	Moth	Ther	Othr	Mim	Vee	Moth	Ther	Othr
FALS		A								
FOND						E	E		A	
GLAD										
IDEA										
LEAD		3E	3A							
MOTV			3A							
NO										
OPEN										
OPPO										
PANG										
POWR										
SOMA										
TALK		A								
VARY									A	
WEAK		2A								
Sum A		6	6					1	4	
E		3				2	3			

tively available to her, despite her self-presentation as someone actively controlled by others.

Mother is quite active, as the therapist sees it, with respect to LEAD and MOTV (commanding and demanding), and she assigns Vee the subordinate E role with respect to LEAD. She is also inclined to see Vee as actively AGGR, FALS, and WEAK, that is, as deceptive and negativistic. On the other hand, the therapist assigns an active helping role (AID) to himself, with Vee the primary object of his ministrations, and he attributes an active DAMG role to Mother.

These comments are based on a small segment of an interview, and a limited number of pragmatic inferences about the speakers. As illustrations, however, they suggest how the concept-analysis method might be employed for systematizing large amounts of semantic, syntactic, and pragmatic material. It is a particular virtue of the system that separate individuals analyzing the same text may use ordinary language in noting their interpretations of speaker pragmatics, since the method reduces words to underlying concepts. This makes it possible to examine the reliability of, and the differences between, such pragmatic analyses, by comparing concept profiles derived from the separate analysts' statements.

SUMMARY AND CONCLUSIONS

This chapter describes a concept system for the analysis of semantic contents of language. Central to the system is a dictionary in which words are assigned one or more of 116 semantic concepts. Texts to be analyzed are compared word by word with the dictionary entries, and concepts are assigned to the text words. The cumulated concept profiles thus generated may be used to show similarities and differences between separate texts.

The syntactic cases of Agent and Experiencer may be applied by an editor to the sentences of a text, and the system is potentially able to incorporate this type of information, showing which persons in a text are assigned particular case roles with which concepts. Furthermore, if pragmatic interpretive statements, also showing case roles, are appended to the text, these statements can themselves be analyzed conceptually to reveal underlying ideational configurations in the interpretation of the text.

The work and the projections described in this presentation are based on a developing rather than a finished methodology. As one attempts to systematize language in order to abstract psychologically meaningful data, one has to sacrifice richness of meaning at every turn. Apparently—since studies with the method seem to have some face validity—the crudeness of the method has not negated its psychological relevance. Perhaps this is because, as has so often been pointed out, language is a robust instrument and what is lost in particular instances by narrowly limiting the meaning domains attributed to words is regained to some extent by cumulating large numbers of instances.

REFERENCES

Bieber, M. R., Patton, M. J., & Fuhriman, A. J. (1977). A metalanguage analysis of counselor and client verb usage in counseling. *Journal of Counseling Psychology, 24,* 264–271.

Bousfield, W. A., Cohen, B. H., & Whitmarsh, B. A. (1958). Associative clustering in the recall of words of different taxonomic frequencies of occurrences. *Psychological Reports, 4,* 39–44.

Bousfield, W. A., Puff, C. R., & Cowan, T. M. (1964). The development of constancies in sequential organization during repeated free recall. *Journal of Verbal Learning and Verbal Behavior, 6,* 489–495.

Cofer, C. N. (1965). On some factors in the organizational characteristics of free recall. *American Psychologist, 20,* 261–272.

Cofer, C. N. (1968). Associative overlap and category membership as variables in paired-associate learning. *Journal of Verbal Learning and Verbal Behavior, 7,* 230–235.

Fillmore, C. J. (1968). The case for case. In E. Bach & R. T. Harms (Eds.), *Universals in linguistic theory.* New York: Holt, Rinehart & Winston.

Fillmore, C. J. (1971). Types of lexical information. In D. D. Steinberg & L. A. Jakobovitz (Eds.), *Semantics: An interdisciplinary reader in philosophy, linguistics and psychology.* Cambridge: University of Cambridge Press.

Freud, S. (1953). Psychoanalytic notes upon an autobiographical account of a case of paranoia (1911). In J. Strachey (Ed.), *The standard edition of the complete psychological works of Sigmund Freud* (Vol. 13). London: Hogarth Press.

Hyman, B. (1980). "Intelligence" in early American psychology: From common parlance to psychological concept. *Dissertation Abstracts International, 42,* 335B.

Katz, J. & Fodor, J. A. (1964). The structure of a semantic theory. In J. A. Fodor & J. J. Katz (Eds.), *The structure of language.* Englewood Cliffs, NJ: Prentice-Hall.

Laffal, J. (1960). The contextual associates of sun and God in Schreber's autobiography. *Journal of Abnormal and Social Psychology, 61,* 474–479.

Laffal, J. (1961). Changes in the language of a schizophrenic patient during psychotherapy. *Journal of Abnormal and Social Psychology, 63,* 422–427.

Laffal, J. (1963). The use of contextual associates in the analysis of free speech. *Journal of General Psychology, 69,* 51–64.

Laffal, J. *Pathological and normal language.* New York: Atherton Press.

Laffal, J. (1967). Characteristics of the three person conversation. *Journal of Verbal Learning and Verbal Behavior, 6,* 555–559.

Laffal, J. (1968). An approach to the total content analysis of speech in psychotherapy. In J. M. Shlein (Ed.), *Research in psychotherapy* (Vol. 3). Washington, D.C.: American Psychological Association.

Laffal, J. (1969). Contextual similarities as a basis for inference. In G. Gerbner (Ed.), *The analysis of communication content.* New York: Wiley.

Laffal, J. (1973). *A concept dictionary of english.* New York: Halstead Press.

Laffal, J. (1979). *A source document in schizophrenia: Whoever had most fish would be lord and master.* Hope Valley, RI: Gallery Press.

Laffal, J. & Feldman, S. (1962). The structure of single word and continuous word associations. *Journal of Verbal Learning and Verbal Behavior, 1,* 54–61.

Laffal, J. & Feldman, S. (1963). The structure of free speech. *Journal of Verbal Learning and Verbal Behavior, 2,* 498–503.

Laffal, J., Monahan, J., & Richman, P. (1974). Communication of meaning in glossolalia. *Journal of Social Psychology, 92,* 277–291.

Lyons, J. (1977). *Semantics, Vol. I.* Cambridge: University of Cambridge Press.

Macalpine, I. & Hunter, R. A. (1955). Discussion of the Schreber Case. In D. P. Schreber, *Memoirs of my nervous illness.* Cambridge, MA: Robert Bentley.

Miller, G. A. & Johnson-Laird, P. N. (1976). *Language and perception.* Cambridge: Harvard University Press.

Morris, C. W. (1955). Foundations of the Theory of Signs. In O. Neurath, R. Carnap, & C. W. Morris (Eds.), *International Encyclopedia of Unified Science* (Vol. 1). Chicago: University of Chicago Press.

Rosch, E. & Mervis, B. (1975). Family resemblances: Studies in the internal structure of categories. *Cognitive Psychology, 7,* 573–605.

Russell, W. A. & Jenkins, J. J. (1954). *The complete Minnesota norms for responses to 100 words from the Kent–Rosanoff Association Test.* University of Minnesota Studies in the Role of Language in Behavior (Technical Report 11).

Schreber, D. P. (1955). *Memoirs of my nervous illness.* (Tr. by I. Macalpine & R. A. Hunter). Cambridge, MA: Robert Bentley.

Streeck, J. (1980). [Review of W. Labov & D. Fanshel, *Therapeutic discourse: Psychotherapy as conversation.*] *Language and Society, 9,* 117–126.

Tulving, E. (1962). Subjective organization in free recall of "unrelated" words. *Psychological Review, 69,* 344–354.

Watson, D. L. & Laffal, J. (1963). Sources of verbalizations of psychotherapists about patients. *Journal of General Psychology, 68,* 89–98.

Zakaras, M. E. & Fine, H. J. (1979). Schizophrenic language: an empiricized case study. *Psychotherapy: Theory, Research and Practice, 16,* 441–451.

II
Intersubjective Category Strategies

3

Snyder's Classification System for Therapeutic Interviews

William U. Snyder

THEORETICAL RATIONALE AND EVOLUTION

In 1943, I devised a system of categories, with later modifications, to be used for conducting research and training in psychotherapeutic interviewing and counseling. The two-way classification system includes categories primarily descriptive of the interaction between counselor or therapist verbal responses and the content and affect of client verbal responses. These systems have been used in many research projects since they were first developed. They are introduced below with brief descriptions, examples, and coding symbols. Some 1963 additions follow the presentation of the original systems.

CATEGORIES FOR THE SNYDER SYSTEM

Counselor Categories

Lead-Taking Categories. Those seeming to determine the direction of the interview, or indicating what the client should talk about.

- *XCS—Structuring.* Remarks defining the interview situation, or indicating purpose, such as telling "what we can do here." (Labeled XST later.)
- *XFT—Forcing the client to develop a topic.* Includes all efforts by a

---

WILLIAM U. SNYDER • Department of Psychology, Ohio University, Athens, OH 45701.

counselor to reject responsibility, for example, "What shall we talk about?"

- *XDQ—Direct questions.* Does not include interrogative statements, which are really reflections of feelings.
- *XND—Nondirective leads and questions.* Statements encouraging the client to state the problem further; for example, "Tell me more about it."

Nondirective Response-to-Feeling Categories. Those seeming to attempt to reflect or restate a feeling expressed by the client.

- *XSA—Simple acceptance.* "Yes," "M-hm."
- *XRC—Restatement of content or problem.* Simple repeating, although the wording need not be identical.
- *XCF—Clarification or recognition of feeling.* A statement by the counselor that puts the client's feeling in more recognizable form.

Semidirective Response-to-Feeling Category.

- *XIT—Interpretation.* The counselor points out patterns or relationships. This category includes statements of causation of behavior by the client.

Directive Counseling Categories. The counselor tries to change the client's expressed ideas.

- *XAE—Approval and encouragement.*
- *XIX—Giving information or explanation.*
- *XCA—Proposing client activity.* Later labeled *Calling Attention.* Enhancing client's awareness of a statement he has made.
- *XPS—Persuasion.*
- *XDC—Disapproval and criticism.*

Minor Categories. Those not related to the client's problems.

- *XEC—Ending the contact.*
- *XES—Ending the series.*
- *XFD—Friendly discussion.*
- *XUN—Unclassifiable.*

Client Content Categories

Problem Categories.

- *YSP—Statement of the problem (or symptoms).*

Simple Response Categories.

- *YAI—Asking for advice or information.*
- *YAQ—Answers to a question.*

- *YAC—Simple acceptance* or acquiescence to a clarification.
- *YRS—Rejection of a clarification or interpretation.*

Understanding or Action-taking Categories. Shows insight or discusses plans.

- *YUI—Understanding or insight.*
- *YDP—Discussion of plans,* decisions, or possible outcomes.

Minor Categories.

- *YEC—Ending of the contact.*
- *YES—Ending of the series.*
- *YNR—Not related to the problem.*
- *YFD—Friendly discussion.*
- *YUN—Unclassifiable.*

Client Feeling Categories

Positive Attitudes.

- *PAS—Positive attitudes toward the self.*
- *PAC—Positive attitudes toward the counselor or counseling.*
- *PAO—Positive attitudes toward others.*

Negative Attitudes.

- *NAS—Negative attitudes toward the self.*
- *NAC—Negative attitudes toward the counseling or counselor.*
- *NAO—Negative attitudes toward others.*

Ambivalent Attitudes.

- *AMS—Ambivalent attitudes toward the self.*
- *AMC—Ambivalent attitudes toward the counselor or counseling.*
- *AMO—Ambivalent attitudes toward others.*

NEW CATEGORIES ADDED IN 1963

Counselor Categories

Reflective or Reeducative Categories.

- *XAT—Attenuation.* "Well, perhaps I was wrong."
- *XAV—Advice.*
- *XEI—Education or Information.*

Relationship Category.

- *XRL—Relationship.* "Let's talk about our feelings for each other."

Supportive Categories.

- *XRS—Reassurance.*
- *XOH—Offers help.*
- *XAP—Approval.*

Redirective Categories.

- *XCH—Challenging.*
- *XWH—Withholding support.*

Categories for Different Types of Therapist Interpretations. (After Rausch & Bordin, 1957)

- XIT_4—Therapist connects two aspects of the contents of previous client statement.
- XIT_5—Therapist reformulates the behavior of the client during the interview in a way not explicitly recognized previously by the client.
- XIT_6—Therapist comments on the client's bodily or facial expressions as manifestations of the client's feelings.
- XIT_7—Therapist uses a preceding client statement to exemplify a process that has been building up during the interview and of which the client is seemingly unaware.
- XIT_8—Therapist speculates as to the possible childhood situation that may relate to current client feelings.
- XIT_9—Therapist deals with inferences about material completely removed from the client's awareness.

Categories for Client Need-Responses.

- Anx—Anxiety.
- Hos n—Hostility need.
- Hos p—Hostility pressure.
- Dep—Dependency need.
- Ego—Ego need.
- Nur—Nurturance need.
- Sex n—Sex need.
- Sex p—Sex pressure.
- Dom n—Dominance need.
- Dom p—Dominance pressure.
- Aff n—Affiliation need.
- Aff p—Affiliation pressure.
- Voc—Vocational concern.
- Mob—Mobility concern.
- Phy—Physical concern.

Categories for Client's Behavior in Therapy.

- Ins—Shows insight.
- Plans—Makes plans.
- Res—Shows resistance.
- Conf—Confirms an interpretation.
- Rel—Deals with the relationship.
- Ques—Asks a question.
- Drm—Reports a dream.
- Unc—Reveals unconscious material.

Categories of Sources of Client Affect.

* *Major Categories.*
* self—the client.
* par—client's parents.
* fa—father.
* auth—authority figure (other).
* mo—mother.
* sib—sister or brother.
* wife—client's wife.
* peers—associates.
* ther—the therapist.
* het—heterosexual love object.
* homo—homosexual love object.

* *Minor Categories.*
* masc—client's masculinity.
* enur—client's enuresis.
* phys—adequacy or physique.
* prof—professional adequacy.
* rival—admirer of spouse.
* matur—client's maturity.
* intel—client's intelligence.
* child—client's child.
* nur peo—nurturant people in general.
* anim—animals of the client
* relig—client's religion

As is evident, the overall original system incorporates 17 counselor categories, grouped under five main headings, 12 client (primarily content) categories grouped under four major headings, and nine client affect categories, grouped under three headings. The system was based on over 10,000 responses, which I personally coded. These were interactions occurring in 48 interviews with six clients, conducted by four therapists fairly experienced in doing nondirective or client centered psychotherapy. About two thirds of the interviews were either electrically recorded or secretly recorded by a stenographer listening over a sound system; the other interview reports were based on therapist's verbatim recall immediately after the interview.

RELIABILITY AND VALIDITY

Since approximately 10,000 responses were classified by the writer, the task was felt to be too large to request extensive cooperation by numerous other classifiers. For purposes of the reliability study, then, rechecks were made by me and one other person. One very significant question facing everyone who has attempted to objectify spoken or subjective statements has been the question of determining the boundaries of the units of material, that is, of "ideas." I felt that to include the question of reliability of breakdown *of units* would severely complicate the problem. I therefore concluded that the breaks between ideas should be arbitrarily decided by the classifier, in other words, that the reliability study would not be based on results obtained from unmodified data, without unit breaks already determined.

Two methods were used to show the reliability. The first was a recheck of my own classifications after an interval of more than a month, during which time numerous other interviews had been scored. Four interviews were rescored, two of them phonographic and two non-phonographic. Initial and terminal interviews were avoided, since it was felt that such interviews are more specialized in character, and therefore more consistently classified according to certain patterns. I was able to achieve a reliability ranging from .76 to .87 using this test–retest method. Corresponding chance-expectation scores would range from .06 to .33. Thus, it is evident that a high degree of reliability existed when checked by the test–retest method.

A further check of reliability was made by using a second classifier, who classified four other interviews previously classified by me. He had no previous experience in classifying interviews, and, after having carefully read the definitions of categories which I employed, read through only two interviews that I had previously classified. He was able to match my own scores with reliabilities ranging from .52 to .78. These compare with pure-chance expectations ranging from .06 to .33. Consequently, it may be said that the second classifier was able to match my scores with a reliability comparable to that found in the average standardized test. In view of the fact that he was not strongly indoctrinated in my scoring method, it is perhaps remarkable that he could achieve as similar scoring as he did.

In referring to the validity of a study, one is concerned with whether a measurement is really what it purports to be. It is difficult to show validity for the sort of material described above, except for face validity or consensual validity. This is demonstrated in the reliability scores reported above. That the second classifier was working on the basis of *a priori* definitions and achieved a highly similar scoring series, is strong evidence, I believe, of the presence of consensual or face validity.

ILLUSTRATION OF HOW THE SNYDER CODING SYSTEM WORKS

In order to illustrate how my Therapy Classification System works, I have included here a section of an interview from a case of a 22-year-old married graduate student whom I counseled in 1956.[1] The classifications

[1]This case was included in my book *Dependency in Psychotherapy*, New York: Macmillan & Co., 1963.

are given in the right margin of the page, with the 1943 classification coming first on each line. Therapist's statements are in italics. Following the excerpt, I give the rationale for scoring the selected categories.

(C) I've always felt socially inferior to my classmates because I   YSP; Anx—phys
was two years younger than most of them. I still cringe
when I remember how I was called "Fatso" because of my
somatotype. I also was called a fritterer, satisfied to have a
good time with no responsibilities.
(T) *Let's take the phrase "Fatso." Why does it bother you so?*   XDQ
(C) Well. I was somewhat heavy, and I was pretty touchy about   YSP; Anx—phys
that. Until I was fourteen, I was quite a butterball. Then I
went on a really strict diet. And as I started to grow tall, my
proportions improved. I'm sensitive about overweight, and
no matter how much I diet, I can't avoid some chubbiness.
Unfortunately, I like fattening foods, and when I'm depressed, I let go of my self-control and start guzzling a
milkshake. I don't know why I'm so sensitive about it.
(T) *Why do you think it bothers you, though? What elements of it*   XDQ
seemed derogatory?
(C) Well, to my way of thinking, anybody who is fat is not taking   YSP;YUI
care of himself. I probably equate fatness with general sloppiness. I'm trying to figure out why fatness would have
picked up such negative connotations for me. Probably because people use the concept in a derogatory manner.
(T) *I wonder if it's deeper than that. You said that fatness is parallel to*   XIT
sloppiness. Is it parallel to anything else?
(C) Yeah. It isn't masculine. The ideal man is the mesomorph.   YSP; Anx—phys
That's my ideal, too. I've always wanted to have muscles
and good build. Even now I'm quite embarrassed in a
bathing suit, although I'm not that fat, really.
(T) *You've always wanted to be an inverted triangle.* (Both laugh) *So*   XCF
the inference about overweight is that it isn't masculine. (Pause)   XIT
Which makes it what?
(C) Feminine. (Sighs) You caught me, didn't you. (Laughs)   YRL; Rel—ther
(T) *I had to beat you over the head with it.* (Both laugh)   XRL
(C) The next question is why I react so strenuously when I feel   YSP: Anx—masc
feminine. (Sighs) There're so many things that might be a
part of it. The male role in society, for one thing, is *the* role.
The man is important, and the woman is submissive. And
also in my own family situation: the male was the au-
thoritarian, the potent one. I wonder if also the fact that,
since my parents' divorce, for some time after that I lived
with my mother and might have been reacting against being
a "mamma's boy." People might have assumed that I was.
(Pause) It was much easier to identify with her, because she
was easier to get to.
    I wonder also if the homosexual behavior might have fit   YUI; Anx—masc
into it, too. I may equate homosexuality with being sort of
feminine, perhaps.
(T) *You mentioned three possible sources of anxiety about seeming*   XRC
feminine. One is the ego concern: the position of the male as

dominant in our society, and particularly in your family. And	
another was the possibility that you might be perceived as identify-	
ing with your mother. And third, you mentioned the possibility that	
people might think you were more homosexual. Perhaps you were a	XIT
little bit reaction-sensitive to this because of the incidents that had	
taken place, is that it?	
(C) Yeah. (Deep sigh)	YAC
(T) Does it bother you to think about it now?	XDQ
(C) Yeah.	YAC
(T) Why do you think that it does?	XDQ
(C) Because I don't think it's good. It's not healthy or well-	YSP; Anx—homo
adjusted behavior. Although there are supposedly well-ad-	
justed homosexuals.	
(T) But this didn't make you a homosexual, did it?	XRS
(C) No.	YAC
(T) But you still feel embarrassed to think about it, and talk about it.	XCF
(C) Yeah. (Deep sigh)	YAC
(T) That's a pretty deep sigh.	XIT_6
(C) (Client laughs) It's a very bothersome topic.	YSP; Anx—homo

All of the above category assignments were determined on the basis of (1) actual content expressed, (2) feelings implicit or expressed in the excerpt, and (3) the context in which these occurred. Thus, the rationale for scoring unit "1" in the category YSP; Anx–phys was that the client was telling about difficulties, he obviously felt distressed (a negative feeling), and the focus of his concern was his poor physique. In the initial study of the six psychotherapy cases, my scoring resulted in the distribution of category frequencies seen in Table 1.

USE OF THE SNYDER SYSTEM: A REVIEW OF SOME SIGNIFICANT STUDIES

The purpose of my original study, for which this system was devised, was to examine the nature of nondirective or client-centered psychotherapy. By analyzing the content of six representative therapy cases, I was able to demonstrate (1945) that (1) psychotherapy interviews are measurable data which can be labelled; (2) people who are trying to be client-centered are relatively successful in doing what they are attempting to do; (3) it was their nondirective techniques that were producing the more therapeutic outcomes, such as insight and discussion of plans; (4) the more nondirective procedures produced less resistance and hostility from the clients than do the directive techniques; (5) certain therapist trends existed; for example, interpretations, although not used a great deal, did tend to increase as the therapy progressed; and (6) the clients' discussion of plans for new behavior almost always followed their arrival at insights and understanding. These were just some of the 28 conclusions which were derived from the initial

TABLE 1
Therapists' responses

Code	Label	Percentages
XCF	Clarification of Feeling	31.6
XSA	Simple Acceptance	27.7
XIT	Interpretation	8.1
XDQ	Direct Question	5.7
XAE	Approval and Encouragement	4.7
XCS	Structuring	3.6
XND	Nondirective Lead	2.3
XPS	Persuasion	2.0
	Clients' responses	
YSP	Statement of the Problem	33.0
YUI	Understanding and Insight	29.8
YAC	Acquiescence to Counselor	17.9
YNR	Not Relevant to Problem	7.3
YAI	Asking for Information	4.1
YDP	Discussion of Plans	3.4
YRS	Rejection of Interpretation	3.2

study. Later, Seeman (1949) did a modified replication of the procedure I had used, and confirmed most of the results, except that he found the client-centered therapists, at that time, becoming even more nondirective; their interpretation, for instance, had fallen to almost a zero level.

Beginning in 1949, I directed three groups of integrated doctoral dissertations that made extensive use of my coding system. The first group contained nine students, and the second and third groups (1955 and 1957) each contained four. In each of these programs, the groups planned integrated studies, involving pools of clients and data that all the members of the group investigated, although each of the studies had independent hypotheses and results. Thus the research groups were able to study as many as 43 different clients, thereby greatly enlarging the useable subject pool. In the first group, eight of the studies employed my classification, and in the second and third groups all of the studies did so. (There were some slight modifications introduced in some studies, usually consisting of breaking down certain categories of client or therapist responses into several subcategories.) A brief summary of these findings reveals the marked diversity of studies which may emanate from use of my classification system.

Gillespie (1953) investigated resistance in therapy. He hypothesized that verbal signs of resistance are preceded by counselor "errors" such as statements that reflect unverbalized feelings, make inaccurate clarifications of feelings, or interpret the meaning of the client's remarks; that a high frequency of these signs of resistance is negatively correlated with the success of the therapy; and that it is positively correlated with the length of the treatment process. He found that the resistance category having the highest frequency was that of "resistance within the client," accounting for 60% of the total. The most frequently coded sign of resistance was "short answers." This correlated .58 with the total signs of resistance.

In studying the relationship between specific counselor categories and signs of resistance, Gillespie found that "persuasion" had the highest mean resistance per counselor statement, and "ending of the contact" had the lowest. There was a significant positive correlation between the *number* of counselor statements in each category and the amount of resistance following those statements, regardless of category.

Somewhat surprisingly, Gillespie also found that the *total* verbal signs of resistance occurred less often after the counselor "errors" mentioned above than after the nonerror categories. But, significantly, if the signs of resistance considered are those directed toward the therapist and the therapy, and not the ones "within" the client, these signs of resistance are, in fact, preceded by counselor-error categories more frequently than by nonerror responses.

Tucker (1953) developed a multiple criterion for successful outcome of therapy. The criterion was made up of a Client Rating Scale filled out at the conclusion of therapy, a Counselor Check List, filled out at the conclusion of therapy by both the counselor and an independent judge who had read the case, and a ratio between the positive and negative feelings found in the first and last interviews. Tucker found that the client's judgment of what happened in therapy may not necessarily coincide with the judgment of the therapist or of the independent judges. He concluded that caution needs to be employed in using excessively phenomenological measures of client change in therapy.

In another one of the studies, Aronson (1953) found no difference between counselors with regard to the success of their therapy based on Tucker's criteria, although they differed in degree of nondirectiveness. Since none of the counselors had a significantly larger proportion of their clients dropping out of therapy than did other counselors, it seems that the relative nondirectiveness of this group of counselors had little to do with whether clients remained in or left therapy. Aronson postulated that factors "within" the clients, such as strong anxiety, were of considerable significance in determining whether clients remained in the counseling.

Aronson's study of the counselors' personality characteristics, and of their relationship to the client's personality and interview behavior, indicated that the counselors were rated as differing significantly from each other in personality, and that their characteristics were positively correlated with a score of directiveness. The counselors who tended to be most consistently nondirective were those who most easily develop warm social and personal relationships, whose behavior was relatively consistent but flexible enough to meet changing situations, and whose display of emotion was more appropriate than was that of their colleagues; the more nondirective counselors were also the ones considered to be more easily upset, anxious, and submissive, and to be more dependent than their colleagues. Aronson also found that counselors who were ranked highest in intellectual curiosity, achievement, and exploratory interests relied less upon nondirective techniques in their therapy. But Aronson found that it was impossible to relate particular counselor personality characteristics to specific client behavior in therapy.

Page (1953) studied the ability to predict the outcome of therapy with measures of client verbalizations in initial therapy interviews. He postulated that the client whose language is characterized by productivity and variability will be more likely to work through his problems successfully than will be the client who is more restricted. He found a low positive relationship between the total number of words used and the Tucker multiple criterion of success, and a significant correlation between the measures of variability, except for the Type–Token ratio.

Roshal (1953) also made use of the Type–Token ratio (TTR), starting from the hypothesis that if a client goes from a less adjustive to a more adjustive condition, there will be an increase of TTR. She found that the mean gain in TTR is higher for the more improved cases (Tucker's multiple criterion) than for the less improved ones.

Blau (1953) attempted to compare more improved with less improved cases. He found that the total number of client responses in therapy bears no relation to the successful outcome of therapy. There were no significant differences between the two groups in their discussion of their problems during the initial phase of the therapy. The more improved group, however, differed significantly from the less improved group in having more statements indicating relief from symptoms and discussion of plans during the latter part of therapy.

Rakusin (1953) studied the concept of response variability as revealed in therapy and in the Rorschach. He found that the amounts of client insight, planning, and variability of approach to the problem would covary with reduction in discomfort and resolution of the problem. There was some indication that the number of responses to the Rorschach may be predictive of the amount of planning behavior during therapy.

Kahn (1953) investigated whether generality as a personality trait would consistently affect perceptions of therapy interviews and the Rorschach, but did not obtain any positive results. There are several possible reasons why Kahn and Rakusin did not obtain more positive findings. First, the client population was quite homogeneous. Second, we know that this client population was only mildly maladjusted. It may be that the Rorschach can be appropriately used for this purpose only with more maladjusted persons.

Much more material on the client–therapist relationship comes to us from our *Core Group II*, completed in 1956. This group of four integrated studies, conducted by Ashby, Ford, Guerney, and Guerney (1957), was designed to examine differences in the relationship formed between clients and their therapists during the process of two brief verbal psychotherapies. The effects of two independent variables were examined. The first was the verbal behavior of the therapist. Therapists were required to administer either a leading or a reflective type of psychotherapy, with a random assignment of clients to both treatment and therapist, by means of a table of random numbers. The same therapists administered both therapies, having been given special training in the differentiation of the two. Therapists were 10 advanced graduate students; clients were 40 individuals who came to the Psychological Clinic consecutively in a 4-month period. Most were young adults whose symptoms were primarily neurotic; twenty were assigned to each treatment.

The second independent variable consisted of a group of six scales of personality characteristics of the therapists: (a) ability to enter the phenomenological field of another; (b) sympathetic interest; (c) acceptance of others; (d) social stimulus value; (e) need for aggrandizing the self; and (f) aggressiveness. In general, these characteristics seemed to have little effect on the outcome of therapy, at least as they were able to be measured in the Core Group II studies.

The dependent variables included:

(1) Four measures of the relationship between client and therapist.
(2) Pretherapy measures of client's autonomy, succorance, deference, dominance, aggression, and cognitive ambiguity, based on Edwards' Personal Preference Schedule and Hathaway and McKinley's Minnesota Multiphasic Personality Inventory (MMPI).
(3) Six measures of client reactions in the therapy interviews: verbally-expressed dependency, guardedness, covert resistance, overt resistance, openness, and defensiveness.

Since these four studies were integrated, it is feasible to report their results jointly. Pretherapy defensiveness and aggressiveness of clients related differentially to the two therapy techniques and to the amount of verbal behavior of clients. Similarly, pretherapy need for deference and autonomy related to the subjective defensive reactions of clients in therapy. Clients who were more aggressive when they entered therapy tended to react more defensively in the leading therapy and less in the reflective therapy; a similar pattern was discovered for clients who entered therapy with tendencies to be more deferent. Clients who entered therapy with more need for autonomy tended to feel less defensive in leading therapy.

The view that individual therapists create different effects on their clients *independent of the type of therapy given* was partially supported by these studies. Therapists differed significantly in the defensive and positive feelings they elicited from their clients, regardless of treatment method. This was also true for the amount of guarded verbal behavior they produced in their clients in the first four interviews.

It was in Core Group II that it first became apparent that interaction was an important fact to consider; this group of studies was the first to examine the interaction of the therapist as an individual and the type of therapy he was employing, and the results were affirmative. Clients felt significantly more defensive or more positive in one type of therapy than did other clients for the same therapist when employing the second type of therapy. For some therapists, this increase in client defensiveness or positive feelings was in the leading therapy, and for others in the reflective.

In 1957 four more studies, known as *Core Group III*, were completed, and were identical in conception with Core Group II, except that different hypotheses were considered. Karmiol (1957) was able to demonstrate a relationship between the degree of therapists' preference for a leading or reflective type of therapy and (1) the clients' positive or defensive responses to therapy, or (2) the therapists' positive or negative response to the client. A statistically significant negative correlation was found between the reflective scale of the Therapists' Conception of Good Therapeutic Handling and the negative scale of the Therapists' Personal Reaction Questionnaire.[2] This seems to indicate that therapists who prefer a client-centered therapy did not tend to express negative feelings toward their clients in the early stages of therapy. This evidence gives some support to the idea that there is a relationship between a therapist's preference for therapy method and his response to his clients.

[2]These are two unpublished scales developed by the Second Core Psychotherapy Research Group at Pennsylvania State University under my direction. The scales were later incorporated, in part, into my *Client's Affect Scale* and *Therapist's Affect Scale*, described later in this chapter.

Kahn (1957) found that, insofar as therapist perception of client dynamics and behavior is concerned, the therapist who is more negatively disposed toward one client than another perceives the dynamics and behavior of the former less accurately in reflective therapy, and there is a similar trend in the leading therapy. The passive–active qualities of a therapist were related to the accuracy of his perceptions of the client in a leading-type therapy. Preference for a type of therapy was related to therapists' ability to judge and/or empathize with the client. Leading and reflective therapies differentially influence the accuracy of therapists' perceptions of their client's dynamics.

A study by Baker (1957) was directed at the problem of varying the therapeutic technique. The major purpose of the study was the investigation of the differential effects of a leading and of a reflective psychotherapeutic approach on clients' indiscriminate perceptions and resistance to analyzing problems. The statistical analyses supported the hypothesis that a leading psychotherapy is more effective than a reflective therapy in reducing personal overgeneralizations. Persons who discontinue therapy reveal more resistance to analyzing problems than those who continue it.

Some other studies using the Snyder Therapy Classification system should be reviewed briefly here. In 1964 Russell and Snyder reported a dramatic study demonstrating that counselors showed a good bit of anxiety in response to the amount of hostility their clients displayed toward them in simulated therapy interviews. A counseling paradigm employed two actors role-playing as clients, and 20 counselors. Independent variables were hostile or friendly client behavior and amount of counselor experience. There were four dependent measures of counselor anxiety: palmar sweating, eyeblink rate, client–actor estimates of counselor anxiety, and independent judgments of verbal anxiety of counselors' protocols. Results revealed that hostile client behavior led to significantly greater anxiety than did friendly behavior. Amount of graduate training and counseling experience had little effect on the degree of counselor anxiety in either hostile or friendly interviews. Modifications of some of the measures, lengthening the interviews, increasing group sizes, or finding more discriminate groups might have changed this last finding. Palmar sweating was of questionable utility as a measure of anxiety.

In a subsequent study, Heller, Myers, and Kline (1963) employed client actors in simulated therapy interviews, and demonstrated that dominant client behavior will evoke dependent therapist behavior, whereas dependent client behavior will evoke dominant therapist behavior. They also showed that hostile client behavior will evoke hostile therapist behavior, and friendly client behavior will evoke friendly therapist behavior.

Frank and Sweetland (1962), using Snyder's system and a method almost identical with it, studied the verbal interaction in client-centered psychotherapy during four interviews for each of forty clients. Their results showed that therapists' statements definitely have a selective influence on the character of clients' responses. Clarification of feeling and Forcing Insight (the latter somewhat comparable to Snyder's Interpretation) both produced significant increases in the number of Understanding and Insight responses. Direct Questioning and Interpretation were antithetical in their effects. Interpretation resulted in increased Understanding and Insight and a decrease in Statement of Problems, but Direct Questions produced the reverse effect. The consistency of Snyder's "sequel relationships" was demonstrated, and there was support for the behaviorist's argument that client behavior is amenable to modification as a result of the therapist's responses.[3]

Gordon (1957) studied the effect of a "Leading" and a "Following" psychotherapeutic technique in dealing with hypnotically induced repression and hostility. "Miniature neuroses" were induced under hypnosis, and the discriminative difference between the results of leading and following (directive and nondirective) therapists were studied. He found the leading therapy more effective than the following for lifting repression. It was also found that therapist's experience that might lead to formulation of incorrect hypotheses about a client has a deleterious effect on the lifting of repression, and is also associated with stronger expressions of transference hostility by the client. Techniques were classified as leading or following on the basis of Snyder's Classification System of responses.

Harway and Iker (1964) used Snyder's classification system (and others) to devise a way of programming psychotherapy interviews into a computer, so as to evaluate temporal relationships between individual words in different phases of therapy, thus leading to possible measures that might better reveal the nature of psychotherapy change. Apparently, little has been done to follow up this rather imaginative approach, however.

Cannon (1964) was one of the few researchers to use those of Snyder's *Affect* Scales appearing in Snyder's 1961/63 revision. Cannon attempted to determine, as Snyder had, the similarity of personality of counselors and clients expressing positive attitudes toward each other, but the results were somewhat inconclusive. (See Snyder's results below.)

---

[3]The sequel relationships referred to the matter of what types of clients' statements (e.g., statements of the problem, understanding and insight, etc.) tended to follow most frequently each of the different types of therapists' statements (e.g., clarification of feeling, interpretation, etc.).

The final study to be reported in this survey is that of 1961, in which Snyder and I added to the original coding system a more detailed system of measuring the interpersonal relationship, by developing a Therapist's Affect Scale and a Client Affect Scale, administered to the therapist and the client after every interview.[4] Twenty therapy cases, of an average length of 25.5 interviews, were recorded on tapes. After each interview, all 20 clients filled out a 200-item scale reporting their attitudes toward the therapy and the therapist. The therapist also filled out a different 196-item scale regarding his attitudes toward the client, his estimate of the client's feeling toward him, of the client's progress in therapy, and the client's postinterview need structure. After every fifth interview, the client filled out the Edwards PPS test, and once, at the beginning of therapy, he took the MMPI. The therapist took the Edwards twice, and at the end of therapy made six rankings on the client: rapport, hostility, dependency, guardedness, success of the case, and amount he thought he was liked by the therapist. From one to three years after therapy, the therapist also rated the clients on (1) type of value systems they held; (2) affect; (3) affect from the therapist; (4) controllingness; (5) self-disclosure (toward the therapist); (6) estimates of maladjustment present at the beginning of therapy; and (7) Leary's "circle" of personality traits. The clients were also dichotomized into "better" and "poorer" clients on the basis of a multiple criterion of seven from the above measures. (The therapist had not seen test scores or rankings on the clients while their therapy was in progress.)

The data were analyzed by a series of thirteen factor analyses, and point-biserial correlations of each item with the factors. In the factor analyses, from one to four factors were obtained for representative interviews on both the Therapist's Affect Scale and the Client's Affect Scale items. Intercorrelations of these factors on different interviews revealed that we were dealing with three factors on each scale, one positive and two negative. There was a considerable amount of evidence that on both affect scales two partially correlated negative factors appeared: on the Client's Affect Scale, we found a factor of active resistance or hostility,

---

[4]Each of these scales is 200 items long. They appear and are described in our 1961 book *The Psychotherapy Relationship* (New York: Macmillan & Co.). The flavor of the scales can be learned from the following sample items:

From the Therapist Affect Scale (or Personal Reaction Questionnaire):
  (1) Today I felt that we had a pretty relaxed, understanding kind of relationship.
  (11) Today I found that I knew what the client was trying to express even before he finished his statement.
From the Client Affect Scale
  (27) My counselor and I are somewhat like companions, searching together for new meanings in my experiences.
  (54) Today I would have to admit that my counselor hurt me.

and one of passive resistance or withdrawal. On the Therapist's Affect Scale, the two negative factors were one of impatience with the client and one of anger or irritation with him. These four, plus a positive factor on each scale, that is, primarily therapist empathy and client trust, are the ones that held up statistically.

There were definite personality differences between the clients in the better group and those in the poorer. Better clients tended to fall in the MMPI hypomanic and obsessive group, while poorer ones were in the depressive or schizoid groups. The changes which occurred in therapy seemed to be in the direction of a more healthy adjustment, which related to specific need structures of the individual client. Four of the clients *least* like the therapist in personality at the beginning of therapy (because of their strong dependency needs) were ranked as the most successful clients, and as exhibiting the best rapport with the therapist.

There is strong evidence that the clients in the Factor-Group I (uninhibited, energetic, suggestible people) were the ones who showed the strongest affection for the therapist, and he for them. They were also more frequently the better clients. On the other hand, the clients in the Factor-Group IV (depressive but suggestible) were the ones whose affect toward the therapist was more negative, as was his toward them. The therapist showed a marked preference for cooperative, suggestible, alert, nonhostile, compulsively hard-working neurotics of superior intelligence. He was much less satisfied with the therapeutic relationship with the more hostile, unmotivated, resistant, schizoid, or sociopathic persons. The better clients proved to exhibit more signs of compulsivity and dependency, and this caused them to be dissimilar to the therapist in need structure. On the other hand, the poorer clients showed consistent signs of being more independent, and therefore more like the therapist in personality. We see in these facts some evidence for the concept of a desirable reciprocity of personality between client and therapist, individuals tending to "pull" from others responses opposite from their own. At least it appeared, in our study, that therapist and client had a better relationship when their need structures tended to complement each other, rather than to be similar.

We also found that the clients' positive affect toward the therapist tended to increase throughout therapy, while the negative affect tended to rise to a high point at the middle of therapy, and then to decline to a lower level than at the beginning. The composite of these two trends is one of overall affect rising in the second half of therapy. However, when the affect trends for better and poorer clients are differentiated, we find that transference for the better clients became more negative around the middle of therapy, but later in therapy rose to a higher level than at any previous time. In the poorer cases, however, the transference tended to fluctuate at a considerably lower level than for the better clients, tending to drop off after the middle of therapy, but at the end rising to a level comparable to the better clients' lowest level.

Concerning countertransference for the clients as a whole, there was almost no variation in positive affect, but negative affect showed a noticeable tendency to increase. Considering the better clients alone, the therapist's positive affect was in the direction of a slight rise. Toward the poorer clients, there was a fairly pronounced fluctuation, but with a pronounced increase in negative affect at the end of therapy.

There was a fair amount of evidence that our clients tended to cluster into two groups, those whose attitudes toward the therapist were primarily positive, and those who felt essentially more negative. One special measure of countertransference we obtained was the correlation of the clients' scores on the Client Affect Scale with the therapist's scores on the same test, filled out after each interview the way the therapist believed the client had probably filled out the test. For twelve of the clients, the therapist's scores correlated significantly with the client's; these twelve cases were equally divided between better and poorer clients. A check on whether the therapist could approximate the better clients' replies on the Client Affect Scale more accurately than the poorer clients' replies revealed that he could do so.

Probably the most significant finding of the entire study was a correlation between the scores on the Client Affect Scale and the Therapist Affect Scale of $.70 \pm .12$. This constitutes a numerical index of the character of the therapy relationship. We found it almost incontrovertably conclusive that therapist affect and client affect tended to covary highly with each other, possibly supporting the psychoanalytic "Law of Talion," that for every aspect of therapeutic transference there is a comparable and parallel phenomenon of change in countertransference. This phenomenon is also revealed in Figure 1, showing the mean trends of therapist's and client's affect for better and for poorer clients.

SUMMARY

In 1943, I developed a system for the classification of the verbal interactions of clients and therapists in psychotherapy interviews, which has been widely used both for training in psychotherapy and for much research on that process. This system classified both the interactional components of therapist and client responses and the affective quality of the client productions. I also showed the frequencies of these different categories of responses occurring in fairly typical client-centered (Rogerian) psychotherapy at that time. The system was slightly

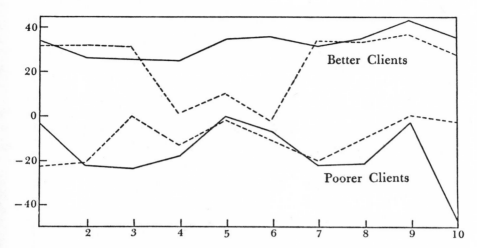

FIGURE 1. Mean trends in therapist's and client's affect for better and poorer clients. Solid lines are for therapist; broken lines are for clients. A constant correction of −45 has been subtracted from all clients' scores so as to equate the therapist's and clients' means.

revised in 1963 to add a method of classifying the direction and the object of the affect being reported by the client.

Among the various researches which have employed the Snyder system, the most important are probably those attempting to describe the character of certain therapeutic systems—particularly the client-centered method of Rogers. Another major group of studies has evaluated certain psychological phenomena evidenced by the clients in therapy, such as resistance, repression, defensiveness, passivity, anxiety, hostility, and verbal productivity. Also studied has been the relationship of the therapists' and the clients' affective responses to each other, including client-generated hostility toward the therapist. The effects of certain therapist personality characteristics on their methods of therapy have been examined. Another important variable which has been studied is the sequel relationship between certain types of therapeutic interventions and the subsequent client responses. Finally, there have been a number of studies which have compared or contrasted two different systems of psychotherapy—particularly, the client-centered system and a more directive one based on Dollard and Miller's learning theory therapy.

Any of the above areas of study would certainly be open to further exploration in the future. Particularly appropriate might be studies further analyzing the personalities of therapists and clients, and their effects on the therapeutic process. More specific studies of the sequel relationship between therapist intervention and client response would certainly be in order.

It is also possible that this system, or one modified from it, might be applied to other types of interpersonal interactions. The fields of industrial supervision, classroom teaching, and retail selling suggest themselves. The analysis of the methods of conducting courtroom interviews or interrogation might be studied in a manner of this sort. Group and family interactions and their dynamics might be susceptible to a study using similar methods. In other words, almost any interpersonal interaction involving two or more persons would probably lend itself to this sort of analysis.

REFERENCES

Ashby, J. D., Ford, D. H., Guerney, B. G. Jr., & Guerney, L. F. (1957). The effects on clients of therapists administering a reflective and a leading type of psychotherapy. *Psychological Monographs, 71,* 453.

Aronson, M. (1957). A study of the relationship between certain counselor and client characteristics in client-centered therapy. In Snyder, W. U. (Ed.), *Group report of a program of research in psychotherapy* (pp. 39–54). State College, PA.: Pennsylvania State University.

Baker, E. (1953). *The differential effects of two psychotherapeutic approaches on client perceptions.* Unpublished doctoral dissertation, Pennsylvania State University.

Blau, B. A. (1953). A comparison of more improved with less improved clients treated by client-centered methods. In Snyder, W. U. (Ed.) *Group report of a program of research in psychotherapy* (pp. 120–126). State College, Pa.: Pennsylvania State University.

Cannon, H. J. (1964). Personality variables and counselor–client affect. *Journal of Counseling Psychology, 11,* 35–41.

Edwards, A. L. (1959). *Edwards Personal Preference Schedule.* New York: Psychological Corporation.

Frank, G. H., & Sweetland, A. (1962). A study of the process of psychotherapy: The verbal interaction. *Journal of Consulting Psychology, 26,* 135–138.

Gillespie, J. F. Jr. (1953). Verbal signs of resistance in client-centered therapy. In Snyder, W. U. (Ed.) *Group report of a program of research in psychotherapy* (pp. 105–119). State College, PA.: Pennsylvania State University.

Gordon, J. E. (1957). Leading and following psychotherapeutic techniques with hypnotically induced repression and hostility. *Journal of Abnormal and Social Psychology, 54,* 405–410.

Harway, N. I., & Iker, H. P. (1964). Computer analysis of content in psychotherapy. *Psychological Reports, 14,* 720–722.

Hathaway, S. R. & McKinley, J. C. (1951). *Minnesota Multiphasic Personality Inventory.* New York: Psychological Corporation.

Heller, K., Myers, R. A., & Kline, L. V. (1963). Interview behavior as a function of standardized client roles. *Journal of Consulting Psychology, 27,* 117–122.

Kahn, M. W. (1953). The role of perceptual consistence and generalization change in Rorschach and psychotherapy behavior. In Snyder, W. U. (Ed.) *Group report of a program of research in psychotherapy* (pp. 75–87). State College, PA.: Pennsylvania State University.

Kahn, R. K. (1957). *Therapist discomfort in two psychotherapies.* Unpublished doctoral dissertation, Pennsylvania State University.

Karmiol, E. (1957). *The effect of the therapist's acceptance of therapeutic role on client-therapist relationship in a reflective and a leading type of psychotherapy.* Unpublished doctoral dissertation, Pennsylvania State University.

Page, H. A. (1953). An assessment and predictive value of certain language measures in psychotherapeutic counseling. In Snyder, W. U. (Ed.), *Group report of a program of research in psychotherapy* (pp. 88–93). State College, PA.: Pennsylvania State University.

Rakusin, J. M. (1953). The role of Rorschach variability in the prediction of client behavior during psychotherapy. In Snyder, W. U. (Ed.), *Group report of a program of research in psychotherapy* (pp. 60–74). State College, PA.: Pennsylvania State University.

Rausch, H. L. & Bordin, E. S. (1957). Warmth in personality development and in psychotherapy. *Psychiatry, 20,* 351–363.

Roshal, J. G. (1953). The type-token ratio as a measure of change in behavior variability during psychotherapy. In Snyder, W. U. (Ed.) *Group report of a program of research in psychotherapy* (pp. 94–104). State College PA.: Pennsylvania State University.

Russell, P. D. & Snyder, W. U. (1964). Counselor anxiety in relation to amount of clinical experience and quality of affect demonstrated by clients. *Journal of Consulting Psychology, 27,* 358–363.

Seeman, J. (1949). A study of the process of nondirective therapy. *Journal of Consulting Psychology, 13,* 157–168.

Snyder, W. U. (1945). An investigation of the nature of nondirective psychotherapy. *Journal of General Psychology, 33,* 193–223.

Snyder, W. U. & Snyder, B. J. (1961). *The psychotherapy relationship.* New York: Macmillan & Co.

Snyder, W. U. (1963). *Dependency in psychotherapy.* New York: Macmillan & Co.

Tucker, J. E. (1953). Measuring client progress in client-centered therapy. In Snyder, W. U. (Ed.) *Group report of a program of research in psychotherapy* (pp. 55–59). State College, PA.: Pennsylvania State University.

4

Verbal Response Modes as Intersubjective Categories

William B. Stiles

INTRODUCTION

The three-channel hypothesis (Russell & Stiles, 1979) distinguishes three classes of verbal process-coding categories and proposes that each class taps a different channel of interpersonal communication in psychotherapy. *Content* categories, such as *body parts* or *separation anxiety*, concern denotative or connotative meaning of discourse units. The content channel carries information about the speaker's current concerns, attitudes, and personality dynamics. *Extralinguistic* categories, such as *laughter* or *hesitation*, concern speaking behaviors that accompany or modify language, but are themselves neither semantic nor syntactic. The extralinguistic channel carries information about the speaker's current (and usually transitory) emotional state—a momentary state of anger, for example, in contrast to an enduring attitude of hostility toward someone. *Intersubjective* categories, such as *question* or *blame*, concern brief relationships of the speaker to the intended recipient; that is, unlike content or extralinguistic categories, intersubjective categories imply the existence of another person (e.g., one questions *another person*; one blames *another person*). The intersubjective channel carries information about interpersonal relationships and social roles, and, in psychotherapeutic communication, about the therapist's technique.

The three-channel hypothesis does not require that any type of information be carried *exclusively* in one channel (nor are these three an exhaustive listing of possible channels). For example, information about

WILLIAM B. STILES • Department of Psychology, Miami University, Oxford, OH 45056.

transitory emotional states can be drawn from content categories (cf. Gottschalk & Gleser, 1969), and information about personality characteristics can be drawn from intersubjective categories (McDaniel, 1979). Nevertheless, the associations of types of categories with types of information are strong enough to recommend that investigators choose a coding system corresponding to the type of information they are interested in (Russell & Stiles, 1979).

The verbal response mode (VRM) taxonomy (Stiles, 1978b, 1978–79, 1979) is a purely intersubjective system. Each of its eight basic categories, Disclosure, Advisement, Edification, Confirmation, Question, Interpretation, Acknowledgment, and Reflection, implies a particular "microrelationship" of speaker to other. For example, a Disclosure reveals thoughts or feelings to the other; an Advisement guides the other's behavior. This taxonomy has evolved from a list of modes (Goodman & Dooley, 1976) identified from naturalistic observation of help-intended interaction by Gerald Goodman (Goodman, 1972). It is in a tradition that traces to Carl Rogers and his students, notably Snyder (1945 and this volume). The discipline of conducting nondirective psychotherapy apparently calls attention to the intersubjective details of verbal process. This tradition has been influenced also by the work of Bales (1950, 1970) on small-group interactions, an influence brought into psychotherapy research especially by Strupp (1955, 1957a,b).

This chapter will examine the VRM system in relation to the three-channel hypothesis. Specifically, it will consider the hypothesis that VRMs, which are intersubjective categories, reflect primarily social roles, relationships, and therapeutic technique. The chapter includes (1) a description of the VRM system, (2) an application of the system to two excerpts of psychotherapy from contrasting schools (client-centered and gestalt), and (3) a review of VRM research on psychotherapy and other relationships.

TAXONOMY OF VERBAL RESPONSE MODES

A single communicative act can be construed as conveying information about one point on a temporal continuum of experience from one center of experience to another. In order to refer to two distinct points of experience, two communicative acts are needed.

The grammatical realization of the communicative act is the utterance, which is the scoring unit for the VRM taxonomy. Each independent clause, nonrestrictive dependent clause, compound predicate, or term of acknowledgment or address is counted as a separate utterance

(Stiles, 1978a). This grammatical definition has been developed to avoid units whose sense demands two different codes.

Principles of Classification

This taxonomy's major distinguishing feature is that its categories are defined by conceptual principles of classification. The three principles are called *source of experience, frame of reference,* and *focus.* Each principle can have the value "speaker" or "other." Each of the eight modes represents a unique combination of "speaker" and "other" values of the principles; thus, the taxonomy can be summarized as 2 × 2 × 2 matrix, as shown in Table 1, or three-dimensionally as a cube. (Imagine the top half of Table 1 in front of the bottom half.)

Source of experience concerns whose experience (ideas, feelings, information) is the central topic of the utterance. Disclosures, Advisements, Edifications, and Confirmations concern the speaker's experience, whereas Questions, Interpretations, Acknowledgments, and Reflections concern the other's experience.

Frame of reference concerns whose viewpoint is used in making the utterance. A frame of reference is the constellation of associated experiences (information, ideas, memories, etc.) that gives the central experience the meaning it has in a particular utterance. The relation of an experience to its frame of reference is like that of figure to ground. An utterance can use either speaker's or other's frame of reference. (Strictly speaking, if speakers are to understand their own utterances, they cannot use a frame of reference that is *exclusively* the other's. The taxonomic issue is thus whether a speaker uses only his or her own private frame of reference or instead uses a frame of reference that is *shared* with the other.) Disclosures, Advisements, Questions, and Interpretations use the speaker's frame of reference, whereas Edifications, Confirmations, Acknowledgments, and Reflections use a frame of reference that is shared with the other.

Focus concerns whether the speaker, in making the utterance, implicitly presumes to know what the other's experience or frame of reference is or should be. An utterance is focused on the speaker if no such presumption is required; an utterance is focused on the other if such a presumption is necessary in order for it to have the meaning that it does have. Disclosures, Edifications, Questions, and Acknowledgments do not require such a presumption, and are focused on the speaker. Advisements, Confirmations, Interpretations, and Reflections do require such a presumption, and are focused on the other.

The body of Table 1 gives descriptions of the eight mode intents and

TABLE 1
Taxonomy of Verbal Response Modes

Source of experience	Frame of reference	Focus	
		Speaker	Other
Speaker	Speaker	*Disclosure (D)* Reveals thoughts, feelings, perceptions, intentions. Form: first person singular ("I") or first person plural ("we") where the other is not a referent.	*Advisement (A)* Attempts to guide other's behavior; commands, suggestions, permission, prohibition. Form: imperative or second person ("you") and verb of permission, prohibition, or obligation.
Speaker	Other	*Edification (E)* States objective information (need not be true or emotionally neutral). Form: declarative and third person.	*Confirmation (C)* Compares speaker's experience with other's; agreement, disagreement, shared experience or intention. Form: first person plural ("we") where the other is a referent; compound subjects that include speaker and other ("you and I").
Other	Speaker	*Question (Q)* Requests information or guidance. Form: interrogative, with inverted subject-verb order or interrogative words such as who, what, when, where, why, or how.	*Interpretation (I)* Explains or labels the other; judgments or evaluations of the other's experience or behavior. Form: second person ("you") with verb that implies an attribute or ability of the other.
Other	Other	*Acknowledgment (K)* Conveys reception of or receptiveness to communications from other; simple acceptance, salutations. Form: nonlexical utterances ("mm-hm"), contentless lexical utterances ("yes," "no," "well") terms of address ("hello").	*Reflection (R)* Puts other's experience into words; repetitions, restatements, clarifications. Form: second person ("you") with verb that implies internal experience or volitional action of the other.

of sets of grammatical features that are associated with each intent. The intent descriptions are only approximations, of course, since the definitions are given by the intersections of the taxonomic principles. The form descriptions reflect a rough consensus of myself, my collaborators, and a large number of coders as to which grammatical features characteristically express each of the eight mode intents.

Development of the Taxonomy

The progenitor of the present taxonomy (Goodman & Dooley, 1976) included descriptions of 5 of the present 8 modes. Goodman's sixth category, *silence* (an extralinguistic category), was replaced by Acknowledgment, and two categories were added, Edification and Confirmation. The two added modes are rarely used by psychotherapists (Stiles, 1979), which may explain why Goodman, whose concern was with help-intended communication, did not consider them as distinct categories. However, as shown in Table 1, their existence is "predicted" by the intersection of the principles of classification.

Goodman has developed a series of tape-recorded lectures and directed exercises designed to teach response modes to professional and paraprofessional helpers (Goodman, 1978). His students have developed modifications of his response mode system and have applied them in research on the training of helpers and on the detailed process of psychotherapy (see Elliott, Stiles, Shiffman, Barker, Burstein, & Goodman, 1982).

The present taxonomy's principles began as ways to make fine discriminations among Goodman's intuitively distinctive categories of utterances. However, with the principles articulated, this process has been turned around, so that in the present version the principles formally define the modes—in effect, the taxonomy is pulling itself up by its own conceptual bootstraps. Thus, strictly speaking, the names of the modes are only mnemonics for the principle-defined interpersonal "microrelationships." On the other hand, the categories defined in this way correspond closely to natural families of utterances that have been used as categories by many previous taxonomists. In particular, surprisingly little adjustment is necessary to reconcile the principle-based definitions of the five modes retained from the Goodman system with their original descriptions (Goodman & Dooley, 1976). For example, utterances that presume knowledge of the other's experience (focus on other) and express it (other's experience) from the speaker's viewpoint (speaker's frame of reference), such as "You are being defensive," are classed as Interpretations. However, such utterances would also be called "interpretations" by most process scoring systems that use only descriptive definitions, including Goodman's.

Advantages of the Taxonomy

The advantages of a principle-based system over a system of categories defined by descriptions or sets of examples include guarantees of mutual exclusivity, exhaustiveness, and a systematic basis for grouping related categories, all of which are standard desiderata (cf. Butler, Rice, & Wagstaff, 1962; Holsti, 1969; Lazarsfeld & Barton, 1951; Russell & Stiles, 1979).

VRM categories are mutually exclusive because the principles require forced choices. Coders can ask: Whose experience is the topic? Whose frame of reference is used? and On whom is it focused? about each utterance's intent. The answers, restricted to "speaker" or "other," place the utterance in a unique category, as shown in Table 1.

VRM categories are exhaustive insofar as "speaker" and "other" exhausts the membership of the interacting dyad. No new modes can be discovered, because all possible combinations of "speaker" and "other" values are accounted for; all possible results of the three forced choices yield one of the modes in Table 1. (However, the taxonomy does not exhaustively classify microrelationships among three or more people. For example, it does not classify the impact on person C of what person A says to person B.)

The principles are also a basis for articulating similarities and differences among modes and for grouping modes that are alike. For example, Reflection and Interpretation are similar modes, but they differ in whose frame of reference is uses to view the other's experience.

Another advantage of the VRM taxonomy is that it is a general purpose system, not tied to any one kind of interaction (such as psychotherapy) or to any one position about how interactions *should* be conducted (i.e., its categories are not value laden). Most other intersubjective systems used to study psychotherapy have been constructed from empirically—or theoretically—derived ideas about psychotherapy. Consequently, categories may reflect specifically psychotherapeutic purposes (e.g., *minimal encourages* in Ivey's 1971 system; *forcing client to choose and develop topic* in Snyder's 1945, system; *exploratory operations; focal probes* in Strupp's 1957a system), or the distribution of categories may reflect peculiarities of psychotherapeutic interaction (e.g., the absence of an Edification category—one of the commonest modes in everyday conversation—in Goodman & Dooley's, 1976, framework of help-intended communication). The VRM system does not share these distortions (or, from another viewpoint, these specializations) because the principles of classification assume only that two people (two centers of experience) are interacting, without reference to the setting or purpose of the interaction. As a result, the VRM system is applicable to any discourse in which a communicator and an intended recipient can be identified, even when one or both are diffuse collectivities, such as the readership to whom the utterances in this book are addressed. Consequently, the system can be used for direct, quantitative comparisons of psychotherapy with other kinds of verbal interactions.

The taxonomic principles show why VRM measures reflect intersubjective phenomena: the values of each principle are *speaker* and *other*, that is, the "subjects" whom the microrelationship is between. The three principles, and the taxonomy's enumeration of the 8 ways they can connect two centers of experience, may offer the beginnings of a terminology to describe human relatedness.

This prototheory's central concept, "experience," is a venerable one in humanistic psychology (Gendlin, 1962, 1964; Mahrer, 1978; Rogers, 1958, 1959). The taxonomy's formulation suggests that points in experience are packaged as linguistic units, and that these units can be classified and counted. The modes used in exchanging experience measure a central aspect of the interactants' relationship with each other.

The three principles also have theoretical implications about the organization of experience within individuals. For example, the frame of reference principle implies that the *meaning* of an experience is not intrinsic to the experience itself. The meaning consists of the context of other, associated experiences in which the central experience is placed. The "same" experience might be recast in any number of frames of reference, within either speaker or other.

Relations to Speech Act Theory

The study of speech acts by linguists, philosophers, and ethnographers (Austin, 1975; Bach & Harnish, 1979; Brown & Levinson, 1978; Cole & Morgan, 1975; Dore, 1979; Searle, 1969) has developed parallel to, but largely independent of, the study of intersubjective categories by psychologists. Central to speech act theory is the concept of the *illocutionary*, articulated by Austin (1975).

An illocutionary act is the speech act performed *in* making an utterance. For example, in uttering, "Who was that masked man?" one asks a question; in uttering, "Please answer the telephone," one makes a request; in uttering, "The tide is going out," one makes an assertion. Questioning, requesting, and asserting are illocutionary acts. Austin distinguished illocutionary acts from *locutionary* acts, which consist of simply uttering words, and from *perlocutionary* acts, which consist of producing some effect on the actions or attitudes of others. In making an utterance, one typically performs all three types of acts—locutionary, illocutionary, and perlocutionary—simultaneously. For example, in saying "Please answer the telephone," one may simultaneously utter those words (locutionary act), make a request (an illocutionary act), and induce someone to comply (a perlocutionary act). I have elsewhere argued that all illocutionary acts have an intersubjective component (Stiles, 1981); that is, an utterance's illocutionary force presupposes an other on whom that force acts. Conversely, all intersubjective categories—including but by no means limited to verbal response modes—can be construed as classes of illocutionary acts. That is, these two lines of research—the linguistic-philosophical study of speech acts and psychotherapy process research—seem to me to share a common domain.

For psychotherapy process research, the fruits of interdisciplinary cross-fertilization may include application of the speech act concept of *felicity* to intersubjective categories. As Austin recognized, different families of illocutionary acts must meet different social and epistemological conditions in order to be felicitous, or "happy." Utterances that fail to meet appropriate felicity conditions may be said to be "flawed" or to "misfire," or to be infelicitous in some other way. Perhaps the most familiar felicity condition is *truth*, that is, a false assertion is infelicitous. However, truth is irrelevant to the "happiness" of questions or directives, whose felicity conditions might be better described as "answerability" and "feasibility," respectively. Truth, as a felicity condition, seems best reserved for Edifications, as classified by the VRM taxonomy. Even a Disclosure's felicity seems better described as *sincerity* than as truth, since there is no way to demonstrate an objective correspondence between a Disclosure and a state of the world.

The present system's taxonomic principles may help specify epistemological felicity conditions that each of the eight mode intents is required to meet in order to be felicitious (e.g., an Edification must be true; a Disclosure must be sincere; an Advisement must be feasible; a Reflection must be empathic). In each case, felicity depends on the congruence of the experience with the frame of reference, given the presumptions specified by the focus. For example, a felicitous Reflection is one in which the other's experience, as expressed by the speaker, is congruent with the other's internal frame of reference (of which the speaker must presume some knowledge).

Taxonomic Categories

Review of each of the eight basic categories may elucidate the taxonomic principles (cf. Table 1). It may be helpful to recall that the category names formally refer to the principle-defined categories, so that they may have slightly different meanings than in some other systems.

Disclosures concern the speaker's experience, use the speaker's private frame of reference, and presume no specific knowledge of the other (focus on speaker). One would need access to the speaker's private experience to determine whether a Disclosure was true. Note that the criterion is the privateness of the information, and not its intimacy, its emotional charge, or its psychological depth, in contrast to self-disclosure categories in some systems defined by description or example. Thus, revealing intimate facts or describing emotionally significant events is *not* Disclosure in this taxonomy, if the facts or events are (or were) objectively observable in principle. However, telling mundane perceptions or intentions is Disclosure, because perceptions and intentions are, in principle, private events. Examples include:

- I love you.
- I hear something ticking.
- I'm going to fix some coffee.
- I've never felt comfortable with her.
- I think he's the best man for the job.

Advisements also concern the speaker's experience and use the speaker's frame of reference, but they presume to impose these (i.e., to focus) on the other. In effect, the speaker attempts to provide an experience for the other by guiding the other's behavior.

- You shouldn't work so hard.
- Take me to the airport.
- Tell me more about it.
- You may come out when you're ready to behave yourself.
- Imagine your father is sitting in that chair.

Edifications, like Disclosures, concern the speaker's experience, and they presume no knowledge of the other (focus on speaker). However, they use a frame of reference that is *shared* with the other. To use a shared frame of reference without presuming knowledge of the other is to use a common or neutral frame of reference, meaning one shared with any other. Objective reality is such a frame of reference. Thus Edifications are statements of fact—information that is, in principle, public, or accessible to an external observer in the right place at the right time with the right skills. However, a third party's private experiences are considered objective from the viewpoint of the speaker–other dyad (access to the *speaker's* private frame of reference would not be decisive). Consequently, statements like "He feels unhappy" are scored Edification in this taxonomy. Utterances need not be true or emotionally neutral to be scored Edification.

- The book is on the table.
- Something is ticking.
- He went to fix some coffee.
- She has never felt comfortable with me.
- My ankle is sprained.

Confirmations, like Edifications, concern the speaker's experience and use the other's frame of reference, but they *do* presume knowledge of the other (focus on other). That is, the speaker presumes to share the other's private frame of reference and to compare his or her own experience with the other's. The term "Confirmation" was chosen to connote existential confirmation—sharing a frame of reference. It does *not* mean affirmation; for example, disagreements are also served as Confirmation.

- We agree that the plan is sound.
- You and I disagree about everything.
- We believe in a strong America.
- We've about exhausted that topic.
- We always have a terrible time when we visit them.

Questions concern the other's experience but use the speaker's frame of reference and presume no specific knowledge of the other (focus on speaker). In effect, the speaker seeks information from the other to add to his or her own frame of reference. No presumption of knowledge is necessary; if the speaker knew, there would be no need to ask.

- Who was that masked man?
- Are you the owner of the blue station wagon?
- What does it make you think of?
- What is the capital of Ohio?
- Has the game started yet?

Interpretations, like Questions, concern the other's experience and use the speaker's frame of reference, but they presume knowledge of what the other's experience is. The speaker imposes his or her own viewpoint on the other's experience. Psychoanalytic theory, or some other theory of personality or psychotherapy, may serve as a therapist's frame of reference for making an Interpretation. The term Interpretation in this taxonomy has a more restricted meaning than in colloquial usage, since it refers only to statements about the other's private experience or volitional behavior. Thus, judgments about a third party, a work of art or literature, or any other external state of affairs would not be scored Interpretation in this taxonomy even though they might be called "one person's interpretation" colloquially.

- You're probably right.
- You lay tile like a professional.
- You have obsessive-compulsive tendencies.
- You are a nincompoop.
- You are exaggerating its importance.

Acknowledgments concern the other's experience and use the other's frame of reference but presume knowledge of neither. This paradox makes Acknowledgment something of a null category. Acknowledgments have no explicit content; all of their meaning comes from their immediate context. In effect, the speaker indicates reception of or receptiveness to the other's experience without necessarily presuming to know what that experience is. Acknowledgments are thus often used to facilitate—to encourage a more complete exposition by the other.

- Mm-hm.
- Yeah.
- Oh.
- Hello.
- Nancy!
- Well . . .

Reflections, like Acknowledgments, concern the other's experience and use the other's frame of reference. However, unlike Acknowledgments, Reflections presume knowledge of (focus on) the other. The speaker explicitly communicates his or her understanding of the other by putting the other's experience into words. In contrast to an Interpretation, the criterion of accuracy of a Reflection is the *other's* view of the matter. For example, "You are angry" is a Reflection if the speaker is communicating an understanding that the other is privately and consciously experiencing anger. However, it is an Interpretation if it communicates an inference that the speaker might continue to hold despite denials by the other. Repetitions, restatements, and summaries of the other's communication are generally Reflections, but statements that go well beyond what the other has stated are still Reflections, so long as the speaker's intent is to express the other's experience or volitional behavior *as it is viewed by the other.* As with other modes, it is the speaker's intent, and not the accuracy or truth (felicity) of the utterance, that determines whether it is Reflection.

- You wish you had a lollipop.
- You went to the store.
- You feel ashamed and yet determined to show that your choice was reasonable.
- You're planning to vote against him.
- You say you did that already.

Mixed Modes

The descriptions of the grammatical forms of the modes given in Table 1—and in more detail in the VRM coding manual (Stiles, 1978a)—are only indirectly based on the principles of classification. The forms can be scored independently of the mode intents, and in fact quite commonly the form of one mode is used to express the intent of a different mode. For example, "I believe you are projecting aspects of your father onto me" uses a Disclosure form to convey an Interpretation intent. This is abbreviated D(I)—the intent symbol is enclosed in parentheses (see Table 1 for mode symbols)—which is read, "Disclosure in service of Interpretation." With 8 forms and 8 intents, the taxonomy permits 64 possible form–intent combinations—8 *pure modes*, in which form and intent coincide, and 56 *mixed modes*, in which form and intent differ.

Some other examples of mixed modes are:

- You felt anxious?   R(Q)
- It's probably too hard for you.   E(I)
- Would you roll up your sleeves?   Q(A)
- Hmm?   K(Q)
- I walked all the way.   D(E)
- I see.   D(K)
- He upset me.   E(D)
- (Have you eaten yet?) No.   K(E)
- (Are you hungry?) No.   K(D)

It must be emphasized that utterances are coded in context, and that knowledge of the immediately preceding utterances is often necessary to accurately infer an utterance's intent.

Mixed modes carry the intersubjective force of their form as well as their intent. Theoretically, form and intent reflect two levels of the interpersonal relationship, a *formal* level that is explicit and superficial, and an *intentional* level that is implicit and deeper. For example, "I wish you would open the window" D(A) formally reveals a wish, whereas intentionally it directs the other to do something. Using the Disclosure form seems to soften the presumptuous, directive intent of the utterances, in contrast to the command, "Open the window" A(A). The separation of form from intent may reflect a partial independence of the early ontogenetic development of linguistic and social-communicative capacities (cf. Dore, 1979).

Scoring, Contextual, and Summarizing Units

Following the distinctions made by previous writers and reviewers (Dollard & Auld, 1959; Kiesler, 1973; Marsden, 1971), the *scoring unit* for the VRM system is the utterance, defined grammatically (above). The *contextual unit,*—the information which coders are instructed to consider in coding—could in principle include the entire history of the speaker–other relationship. That is, identifying the intent (though not the form) of an utterance might require special knowledge of interactions that have taken place previously. In practice, however, the preceding few utterances are sufficient context to decide most utterances' VRM intent unambiguously.

It is worth pointing out here that, as Bach and Harnish (1979; see also Grice, 1957) have noted, communicative intent (or illocutionary force) is a *reflexive intent*—intended to be recognized *as* intended to be recognized. *Hints,* which are only intended to be recognized as intended (not as intended to be recognized), *manipulations,* which are only intended to be recognized (but not as intended), and *deceptions,* which are private experiences not intended to be recognized, carry reduced illocutionary force and are not scorable as VRM intent, even though a perceptive coder may sometimes discern them. Reflexive intents are thus "on record" in Brown and Levinson's (1978) sense, so that in scoring intent VRM coders are not required to read the speaker's mind any more than the utterance's intended recipient is.

The VRM *summarizing unit,* "the stretch of interaction about which some statement is made or the unit in terms of which quantification is performed" (Kiesler, 1973, p. 39), has usually been the *encounter* or some distinct segment of an encounter. Most VRM studies have summarized over each individual's utterances in a conversation (or part of a conversation), although it would be possible to summarize over dyadic units as well (e.g., see Stiles, Putnam, Wolf, & James, 1979a).

Reliability of VRM Coding

Coding reliability of the VRM system varies with the coder, with the material coded, and with the procedures used to assess coding reliability. Perhaps the conceptually simplest measure is the percentage of utterances in a transcript on which two independent coders agree. Typical levels of this kind of pairwise agreement have been about 85% for form and about 75% for intent, for undergraduate volunteer coders working from transcripts (i.e., without audio- or videotapes), who have had at least 20–30 hours of practice, feedback, and discussion on the type of transcript (e.g., psychotherapy, medical interviews, student–professor conversations) on which they are tested. To give some idea of the range of variation from study to study, agreement was only 80.9% for form and 65.8% for intent on transcripts of parents and children interacting in a modified revealed differences procedure (Stiles & White, 1981; some results of this research are described below). This relatively low agreement reflects the high incidence of fragmented sentences and ambiguous utterances in these interactions. On the other hand, average agreement was 91.2% for form and 80.3% for intent in a study of conversations involving college students and professors in the laboratory (Cansler, 1979; Cansler & Stiles, 1981). As is the case for any coding system, reliability can be improved by careful attention to transcription and punctuation (reducing errors in unitizing), and by systematic monitoring and feedback for coders during coding.

These levels of agreement, while adequate, are lower than desirable. Furthermore, they underestimate the "information value" of the codes for the following reason: even when coders disagree on the form or intent of an utterance, they usually agree that it is one of two modes. For example, coders might disagree as to whether an utterance's intent was Reflection or Interpretation, but none would call it Disclosure, Question, or any of the other modes. To make use of this latent information, in most VRM studies three people have independently coded each transcript, and their work has been combined on a two-out-of-three basis. That is, a code is included in a final composite set if any two coders agree; otherwise the utterance is coded "disagreement." By this method, two-out-of-three agreement has typically been over 95% for both form and intent; that is, fewer than 5% of utterances have typically been coded "disagreement." Even the unusually unreliable codes in the parent–child study (Stiles & White, 1981) yielded two-out-of-three agreement of 96.9% for form and 92.2% for intent. The Cansler (1979; Cansler & Stiles, 1981) student–professor study had two-out-of-three agreement of 99.2% for form and 97.6% for intent.

Of course, any summary measure of agreement across all codes obscures differences in the reliability of particular codes. Experience with VRM coding has shown that common modes in a particular set of transcripts tend to be coded more reliably than rare modes. This apparently reflects differential coder vigilance rather than category definitions, since different modes attain high and low reliability in different studies.

For assessing utterance-by-utterance intercoder agreement for particular categories, the index of choice is Cohen's kappa (Cohen, 1960), a measure that is corrected for chance agreement and is interpretable as an intraclass correlation coefficient (Fleiss, 1975). For assessing intercoder agreement on summary measures, such as the frequency or percentage of a person's utterances in a category, a product-moment reliability coefficient (comparing two coders' results across a set of transcripts) can be calculated.

Table 2 gives examples of these two reliability measures, taken from a study by Premo (1978), which coded half-hour conversations of mar-

TABLE 2
Mean Intercoder Agreement (Kappas) and Reliability (Pearson Product–Moment Correlations) for Mode Forms and Intents in Half-hour Conversations of Married Couples and Strangers[a]

Mode	Cohen's kappa		Reliability of conversation totals	
	Form	Intent	Form	Intent
Disclosure	.93	.63	.94	.78
Advisement	.63	.46	.88	.88
Edification	.88	.75	.98	.91
Confirmation	.58	.30	.96	.51
Question	.90	.89	.93	.93
Interpretation	.56	.36	.77	.74
Acknowledgment	.96	.77	.99	.91
Reflection	.74	.54	.88	.63

Note. From *Verbal Respone Mode Use in Married Couples versus Stranger Dyads: Acquaintance and Familiarity* by B. E. Premo, 1978. Chapel Hill: University of North Carolina (Doctoral Dissertation). Reprinted by permission.
[a]Means are based on comparing three complete sets of codes of 48 speakers' utterances.

ried couples and of dyads whose members were initially strangers. The first two columns give values of kappa, and the second two columns give reliability coefficients based on the frequency of utterances in each mode across 48 speakers (two participants in each of 24 transcribed conversations). Note that both measures are *pairwise* comparisons (actually, the average of three pairwise comparisons). The level of agreement for the two-out-of-three composites that Premo (1978) used in analyzing results was, as usual, substantially higher.

In most VRM studies so far, coders have worked from verbatim transcripts. However, direct audiotape coding may be adequately reliable, at least when attention is focused on a restricted number of codes. McDaniel (1980; McDaniel, Stiles, & McGaughey, 1981) focused on six categories of client VRM used in psychotherapy, D(D), E(D), D(E), E(E), K—defined as any utterance with Acknowledgment form or intent—, and Other. Coders working directly from audiotapes tallied these six categories for each 5-min segment, identified by tones placed on the tape. To assess intercoder reliability, five therapy sessions (including 54 5-min segments) were coded independently by all four coders. In addition, verbatim transcripts of three of these sessions (including 33 5-min segments) were coded independently by two other coders. Table 3

TABLE 3
Intercoder Reliability of Client Verbal Response
Mode Percentages in 5-min Segments
of Psychotherapy

Mode[a]	Audiotape versus audiotape[b]	Audiotape versus transcript[c]	Transcript versus transcript[d]
D(D)	.81	.84	.86
E(D)	.54	.63	.85
D(E)	.66	.62	.83
E(E)	.84	.87	.88
K	.88	.81	.97
Other	.79	.57	.88

Note. From *Clients Verbal Response Mode Use and Its Relationship to Measures of Psychopathology and Change in Brief Psychotherapy* by S. H. McDaniel, 1979. Chapel Hill: University of North Carolina (Doctoral Dissertation). Reprinted by permission.
[a]Mode abbreviations: D = Disclosure, E = Edification; form is written first, intent second in parentheses. K = Acknowledgment form or intent.
[b]Median of the six correlations among four audiotape coders, based on 54 segments (five sessions).
[c]Median of the eight correlations between four audiotape coders and two transcript coders, based on 33 segments (three sessions).
[d]Correlation between two transcript coders, based on 33 segments (three sessions).

shows median reliability coefficients (Pearson *r*s) between pairs of coders for the percentage of client utterances in each VRM category in 5-min segments for (a) audiotape coding, (b) audiotapes versus transcript, and (c) transcript coding. As the table indicates, transcript coding was slightly more reliable than direct audiotape coding; however, audiotape reliability was adequate.

Quantitative Indices of Interactions

The intersecting classifications of utterances by the three principles and by form and intent given the VRM taxonomy considerable versatility in quantitatively representing discourse. Possible indices include the percentage (or frequency) of each of the 64 form–intent combinations (a "VRM profile"), and the percentage (or frequency) of each of the eight forms (regardless of intent) and the eight intents (regardless of form).

It is also possible to calculate the proportion of a person's utterances that concern the speaker's (or other's) experience, regardless of their frame of reference or focus, and similarly for the other principles. These proportions, or "role dimensions," have been given names (Stiles, 1978b). The proportion of utterances concerning the other's experience (i.e., Question, Interpretation, Acknowledgment, or Reflection) is called *attentiveness* (versus informativeness); the proportion of utterances using the other's frame of reference (i.e., Edification, Confirmation, Acknowledgment, or Reflection) is called *acquiescence* or nondirectiveness (versus control or directiveness); and the proportion of utterances focused on the other (i.e., Advisement, Confirmation, Interpretation, or Reflection) is called *presumptuousness* (versus unassumingness or deference). Research investigating these indices has supported their construct validity (Cansler, 1979; Cansler & Stiles, 1981; Stiles, 1979; Stiles, Putnam, James, & Wolf, 1979; Stiles, Waszak, & Barton, 1979). Still other VRM indices based on theoretical arrangements of modes have been used successfully (Premo, 1978; Premo & Stiles, 1983).

VRM data can be used to explore the influence of interactants on each other. To illustrate, in brief segments of interactions, strangers' attentiveness (use of other as source of experience) was negatively correlated (i.e., if one member was attentive, the other tended to be informative; Cansler, 1979; Cansler & Stiles, 1981; Premo, 1978), whereas when longer conversations were considered as a whole, no such relationship was found (Premo, 1978). This suggests that strangers take turns (cf. Duncan, 1972, 1974; Duncan, Brunner, & Fiske, 1979) in being attentive or informative, but that over longer stretches of dialogue, they take roughly equal numbers and lengths of turns.

Interactants' modes can also be grouped empirically by factor analysis into "verbal exchanges," that is, sets of modes that tend to be used together across encounters. Factor scores for such exchanges show how much a *dyad* engaged in a particular type of exchange. (For an example, see Stiles, Putnam, Wolf, & James, 1979a; results of this study are reviewed below.)

VRMs have not yet been used in a Markov chain analysis of the sequential dependencies within conversation (cf. Brent & Sykes, 1979; Gottman, 1979; Raush, 1972); however, the VRM system has some advantages for such an investigation. A major methodological hurdle in applying Markov techniques is the very large number of utterances needed to obtain stable estimates of transition probabilities from each category to each other category (e.g., the probability that a therapist Acknowledgment will follow a client Question). This number increases geometrically with the number of categories used and the chain length considered, so that most investigators have had to condense their coding systems to two to four categories per interactant (e.g., Brent & Sykes, 1979; Gottman, 1979). The VRM system's basis in dichotomous principles of classification makes it well adapted to such condensation.

For example, all utterances could be considered only with respect to their source of experience—whether their intent was attentive or informative. The resulting four categories (speaker's or other's experience × two dyad members) could be subjected to Markov-type analysis using a reasonably sized sample of interaction. Parallel analyses could then be performed using other principles of classification to give additional perspectives.

The VRM system is supported by computer programs, documented in the coding manual (Stiles, 1978a), that give intercoder agreement statistics, prepare detailed feedback for coders (for use in training and in monitoring reliability to prevent "coder drift"), and calculate profiles and the other VRM indices described above. Such software is essential for efficient handling of the large volume of data and numerous alternative indices generated by VRM coding.

ANALYSIS OF PSYCHOTHERAPEUTIC INTERACTION

This section includes an application of the VRM system to excerpts of transcripts of two contrasting types of verbal psychotherapy. The results of coding these excerpts illustrate some of the findings of previous VRM studies of psychotherapy (McDaniel, 1980; McDaniel, Stiles, & McGaughey, 1981; Stiles, 1979; Stiles, McDaniel, & McGaughey, 1979; Stiles & Sultan, 1979).

To show how the VRM system is applied, I have coded some published sample dialogue from *Client-Centered Therapy* by Carl R. Rogers (1951, p. 152) and *Gestalt Therapy Verbatim* by Fredrik S. (Fritz) Perls (1969, pp. 108–109). The excerpts are fairly clear examples of the respective therapeutic techniques (cf. Stiles, 1979), although, of course, they are far too short to be truly representative. The excerpts are also fairly typical illustrations of the issues encountered in VRM coding of psychotherapeutic dialogue. Although a majority of utterances can be coded unambiguously, a substantial minority require exercise of judgment about coding or unitizing. In my commentary, I have tried to draw attention to the problems and to explain how I arrived at my judgment.

My judgments reflect a body of "lore" that includes "litmus tests" for deciding between alternative codes and standard resolutions for common problems of unitizing and coding fragmentary utterances and ungrammatical constructions. Much of this lore is embodied in the current version of the VRM manual (Stiles, 1978a). In developing standard resolutions and litmus tests, the overriding consideration has been consistency with the taxonomic principles. Thus, insofar as possible, "rules" articulated in the manual are shorthand summaries of reasoning from the principles, rather than arbitrary or intuitive decisions.

Client-Centered Therapy

In the first excerpt (from Rogers, 1951, p. 152), the young woman client ("S"), in her second interview, senses some sort of discrepancy between her present values and values introjected in an earlier period of life. In this and the following excerpt, it may be helpful to read through the dialogue first, skipping my commentary, to gain an overview of the interaction.

S 102: *It seems–*   E(D)
   This is a false start, but it is unitized because it has a complete verb. The subject is third person, so the form is Edification. The intent is not completely clear, but from the way the thought is eventually finished, "it" apparently refers to the speaker's feelings or values, that is, experiences viewed from within her private frame of reference. Hence the intent is coded Disclosure. An alternative code would be E(*), where "*" means that the intent is unscorable due to insufficient information. VRM coders are routinely instructed to avoid the "*" code if a reasonable inference can be made.
I don't know–   D(D)
   This process comment is a complete, grammatical utterance and must be coded. The form is first person, and the source of experience, frame of reference, and focus are the speaker's. Despite their apparently minimal *content*, such process comments may have a substantial impact on the speaker–other relationship.
It probably goes all the way back into my childhood.   E(D)
   "It" apparently refers to the client's private feelings, so the intent is Disclosure. Note that the "probably" is *not* relevant to making this determination. In general, levels of probability or confidence do not bear on VRM scoring.
I've—for some reason I've—   NOT CODED
   These false starts are not unitized because they do not contain a *complete* verb, even though they do contain the auxiliary "have."
my mother told me that I was the pet of my father.   E(E)
   The subject is "mother," which is third person. The verb is "told." The *that*-clause is the object of "told" and not unitized separately. What her mother told her is an objective matter, which could, in principle, have been determined by an objective observer in the right place at the right time; hence the intent is Edification.
Although I never realized it—   D(D)
   Realizing takes place in the speaker's private frame of reference.
I mean,   D(E)
   This is a filler. Like the ubiquitous "you know," it seems to be a form with no intent. After much discussion of such utterances with collaborators and coders, I have come around to taking the *intent* of such fillers from the parent clause—in this case the following utterance (an Edification). Scored in this way, a filler has the force of a repetition—intensifying the effect of the parent clause.
they never treated me as a pet at all.   E(E)
   The subject, "they," is third person, so the form is Edification. The intent appears to be Edification because (as the succeeding sentences make clear), the speaker is trying to describe the objective state of affairs in her early family life—not merely that she didn't *feel* like a pet.
And other people always seemed to think I was sort of a privileged one in the family.   E(E)
   The utterance's subject is third person—"people"—so the form is Edification. The intent is difficult to code because it is not clear whether "seemed" refers to the

speaker's private perceptions (in which case the intent would be Disclosure) or to the speaker's somewhat limited confidence that her statement is objectively true (as I have judged). Note that the reference to third parties' subjective experience does *not* make the intent Disclosure. That is, access to the speaker's private frame of reference would not help decide the truth of a statement about what "other people" thought.

But I never had any reason to think so.   D(E)

This intent is also difficult. "Reason" apparently refers to objective evidence, so that the sentence's truth depends on objective circumstances (Edification intent), that is, that the speaker was not given special privileges. However, if the sentence is interpreted as reporting only "I never thought so," it should be coded D(D).

And as far as I can see looking back on it now, it's just that the family let the other kids get away with more than they usually did me.   E(E)

The subject is "it," and the speaker describes what the family did, so the utterance is a pure Edification. Two possible traps in coding this utterance are (1) the opening dependent clause, which does not make a separate assertion but merely indicates the speaker's level of confidence in the main clause, and (2) the obvious emotional importance of the situation. Neither is a basis for coding Disclosure intent. Whether "the family let the other kids get away with more" is an objective matter that, in principle, could have been determined by an external observer.

And it seems for some reason to have held me to a more rigid standard than they did the other children.   E(E)

Again, I judged that "seems" conveys the speaker's less than perfect confidence rather than her revealing subjective experience. That is, the implied criterion of truth is what they actually did rather than what she thought.

C 103: *You're not so sure you were a pet in any sense,*   R(R)

The subject is second person ("you"). The sentence concerns the other's experience, views it from the other's perspective, and presumes knowledge of the other, so it is coded Reflection.

but more that the family situation seemed to hold you to pretty high standards.   E(R)

The subject is "situation," which is third person, so the form is Edification. The intent is clearly to convey the counselor's empathy (i.e., the counselor presumes to express the client's experience as viewed by the client).

S 103: *M-hm.*   K(C)

The form is obviously Acknowledgment. However, the intent does more than convey receipt of the counselor's Reflection. It conveys the sense that the speaker's experience was *correctly* depicted by the counselor. That is, the speaker's "M-hm" *concerns her own experience* and presumes that the counselor understands it in approximately the same way as she does—that is, that they share a frame of reference. It is an *agreement* on the meaning as Reflected by the counselor. Thus it is scored Confirmation intent.

That's just what occurred to me;   E(C)

This utterance similarly presumes knowledge of what the counselor is thinking. In effect it says, "We are thinking alike"; thus, the intent is Confirmation.

and that the other people could sorta make mistakes   E(E)

In scoring this Edification intent I have assumed that "could sorta make mistakes" meant that others did not elicit censure for their misbehavior—an objective matter. Note that it is irrelevant, for VRM scoring purposes, that this memory may be distorted, as the subject herself begins to realize in the next speech. The point is that (in my judgment) the subject *intended* to use an external frame of reference.

or do things as children that were naughty or "that was just a boyish prank" or "that was just what
you might expect"   E(E)
>   This is scored separately from the preceding utterance as a compound predicate,
>   even though the main verbs, "make" and "do," share the same auxiliary, "could."
>   The subject is "people" for both utterances. Quoted material is not unitized sepa-
>   rately; in this case they are equivalents of the adjective "naughty." In general,
>   quoted material is not part of the speaker–other relationship.

but Alice wasn't supposed to do those things.   E(E)
>   "Alice" is third person, even though it refers to the speaker. "Supposed to" appar-
>   ently describes the attitudes of third parties (i.e., neither speaker nor other), that is, it
>   is placed in a frame of reference external to speaker and other—hence the intent is
>   Edification.

C 104: *M-hm.*   K(K)
>   This is a clear example of a pure Acknowledgment; it indicates receipt of the other's
>   communication.

With somebody else it would just be—oh, be a little naughtiness;   E(R)
>   The subject is third person, "it"; the intent is to restate the other's communication.
>   Note that the "oh" in this position is treated as a dysfluency (i.e., as extra-linguistic),
>   rather than as an Acknowledgment form, so it is not coded. I have bent a unitizing
>   rule here by not separating this into two utterances, since the main verb, "be" is
>   repeated.

but as far as you were concerned, it shouldn't be done.   E(R)
>   Again, the utterance's subject is "it," and the intent is to restate the other's
>   communication.

S 104: *That's really the idea I've had.*   E(C)
>   Again, the speaker puts her own experience in a shared frame of reference, in effect
>   saying, "we think alike."

I think the whole business of my standards, or my values, is one I need to think about rather carefully,
>   D(D)
since I've been doubting for a long time whether I even have any sincere ones.   D(D)
>   These first-person utterances obviously reveal private experiences. In general, causal
>   clauses introduced by "since" or "because" are utilized separately because they
>   make an additional assertion.

C 105: *M-hm.*   K(K)
Not sure whether you really have any deep values which you are sure of.   R(R)
>   This is technically a fragment, without either a subject or a verb. However, the intent
>   is clearly Reflection. In determining the form of such utterances, coders are in-
>   structed to code the *understood* subject and verb, if these can be determined unam-
>   biguously from context. In this utterance, "you are" is clearly understood. In some
>   other cases, parallel construction can be used to determine what form is understood.
>   In cases where two or more different forms are equally plausible, but the intent is
>   clear, coders are instructed to score pure modes.

S 105: *M-hm.*   K(C)
M-hm.   K(C)
>   Again, these Acknowledgment forms indicate agreement with the counselor's Re-
>   flection (Confirmation intent) rather than merely receipt.

C 106: *You've been doubting that for some time*   R(R)
An obvious pure Reflection (other's experience, other's frame of reference, focus on other).

S 106: *Well,*   K(K)
The word "well" is contentless; it gains all of its meaning from context, a characteristic of Acknowledgment forms. This utterance concerns the other's communication (the preceding Reflection) and does not express agreement or disagreement. Unlike many Acknowledgments, "well" usually holds the floor for the speaker, rather than returning the floor to the other, as "m-hm" and "yeah" do.
I've experienced that before.   D(D)
Speaker's experience, speaker's frame of reference, focus on speaker.
Though one thing, when I make decisions I don't have—   D(D)
The "I don't have" is unitized as a false start with a complete verb. I treated the opening phrase as "Though *for* one thing," which is not unitized, rather than as "Though *there is* one thing," which would have been a separate utterance. In general, it seems prudent to avoid reconstructing as much as possible.
I don't think—   D(D)
Another false start whose intent is obvious.
It seems that some people have—have quite steady values that they can weigh things against when they make a decision.   E(D)
I scored this as the speaker intentionally revealing her private beliefs. That is, I judged that whether or not people really have such values is irrelevant to the truth (sincerity) of the utterance.
Well,   K(K)
I don't,   D(D)
and I haven't had,   D(D)
and I guess I'm an opportunist (laughing),   D(D)
These utterances reveal private experiences. Note that the extralinguistic laughing has no effect on VRM codes.
I do what seems to be the best thing to do at the moment,   D(D)
and let it go at that.   D(D)
The two parts of the compound predicate are unitized separately.

C 107: *You have no measuring rods that you can use.*   R(R)

S 107: *Yes.*   K(C)
M-hm.   K(C)
That's the way I feel. (Pause)   E(C)
All Confirmation intent—responses to the counselor's accurate Reflection.
Is our time about up,   Q(Q)
Mr. L.?   K(Q)
The use of a proper name or title to address someone is scored as Acknowledgment form. In this utterance, the "Mr. L." is scored as a filler, taking its intent from the parent clause. It thus has the effect of intensifying the Question.

C 108: *Well,*   K(K)
I think there are several minutes more.   D(E)
Despite the use of "I think," the speaker's intent is to Edify. That is, the implied criterion of truth is clock time rather than the speaker's private belief. The word "think" is used to communicate a level of confidence rather than to reveal internal experience.

Gestalt Therapy

The following interchange between Fritz Perls (F) and "May" (M) took place in a "Dreamwork Seminar," in front of a small audience of other seminar participants (Perls, 1969, pp. 108–109).

M: *I feel afraid*   D(D)

and I'm shaking   D(E)

Fear is a subjective experience (Disclosure intent); shaking is an objectively observable sign (Edification intent).

and it's hard for me to breathe   E(D)

Difficulty in breathing is subjective.

and when I started talking, I began to tense up.   D(E)

"Tensing up" could be either objective or subjective, either muscle tension or nervousness. I judged that May meant the former, that is, I assumed that her report was, in principle, falsifiable by objective measurements (Edification intent).

F: *Close your eyes*   A(A)

and tense up.   A(A)

These are obvious Advisements; Fritz is imposing an experience on May by directing her behavior.

Take responsibility for tensing up.   A(A)

See how you tense up;   A(A)

These are Advisements even though the prescribed action is internal and unobservable by anyone except the other.

Which muscles tighten?   Q(Q)

M: *It's in the top part of my body and in my chest and arms and hands.*   E(E)

And it restricts my voice.   E(E)

Again, these could be taken as subjective—in which case the codes should be E(D)—but I judged May's intent to be reporting the state of her musculature. I was guided in part by the question, which was "Which muscles tighten?" rather than "Which muscles feel tight?"

F: *Can you tighten still more?*   Q(A)

Fritz here directs May to increase her tension. He is not seeking an answer about the ability (i.e., the intent is Advisement, not Question).

Yah.   K(I)

I take this to be a judgment that May has performed correctly, not merely an Acknowledgment that Fritz has observed the performance—which would be K(K).

Okeh,   I(K)

Conversely, I take this to be (in intent) an Acknowledgment that May has performed the task and *not* a judgment that the performance was okay—which would be I(I).

Now interrupt this, a little bit at least   A(A)

Now you see what you're doing to yourself?   R(Q)

The intent is evidently Question (presumably the transcriber used the question mark to signal a rising inflection), but there is no inverted subject-verb order or interrogative word, so the form is Reflection.

We are often doing many things to ourselves instead of doing these to the world.   C(I)

The subject "we" apparently includes both Fritz and May—hence it is Confirmation form. The intent, however, seems to be an explanation of May's volitional behavior in Fritz's frame of reference (Interpretation intent).

Now let's make an experiment.   A(A)

"Let's" has an understood second-person subject ("You let us"), which is an Advisement form. The intent is problematic because it is not completely clear just what Fritz is directing May to do. If the utterance is taken to reveal only Fritz's *intention* to "make an experiment," it could be coded A(D).

Could you stand up, please,	Q(A)
May.	K(A)

In the first utterance, the subject-verb order is inverted, so the form is Question though there is no question mark. The intent is obviously a directive; Fritz is requesting action, not an answer. The second utterance is a term of address, which is Acknowledgment form. In this use, it is a filler that takes its intent from the parent clause; it has the effect of intensifying the Advisement.

Now could you tense—tighten me as you tightened yourself up.	Q(A)

Again, this instruction uses an inverted subject-verb order, which is Question form.

Now just crush me	A(A)
. . . crush me . . . (May crushes Fritz, then sighs).	A(A)

The nonverbal behavior (crushing) and the extralinguistic behavior (sighing) are not coded.

Now sit down.	A(A)
How do you feel now?	Q(Q)
M: (breathes heavily) *I can't stand it.*	D(D)
F: *Yah?*	K(Q)
What happened?	Q(Q)
M: *There were lights flashing in my eyes.*	E(D)

This is evidently a report of subjective experience (i.e., Disclosure intent)—not of external, physical lights.

and I got so tense I just snapped.	D(D)

Clearly this does not refer to physiological muscle tension.

F: *Stay with your hands.*	A(A)
M: *They're trembling.*	E(E)

I assume May is reporting a physical movement here.

F: *Let them tremble.*	A(A)
What else do you feel?	Q(Q)
M: *I feel numb.*	D(D)

Numbness is a private sensation.

F: *Say this again.*	A(A)
M: *I don't feel anything.*	D(D)
I'm numb.	D(D)
F: *Now close your eyes*	A(A)
and get into the numbness.	A(A)
How do you feel numb?	Q(Q)
M: (whispers) *I feel grey, greyish cold.*	D(D)
I still feel closed in.	D(D)
It's just all grey.	E(D)
F: *You look as if you're in a hypnotic trance.*	I(I)

Fritz places May's behavior in his own frame of reference.

Results of Coding Psychotherapeutic Interaction

Table 4 gives the VRM profiles for the excerpts coded above. Although the samples were necessarily brief and arbitrarily selected, the results illustrate findings of previous VRM studies of psychotherapeutic dialogue (Stiles, 1979; Stiles & Sultan, 1979). Briefly, (1) in both excerpts,

TABLE 4
Verbal Response Mode Profiles for Excerpts of Client-Centered
and Gestalt Therapy

Therapist mode	Client-centered		Gestalt	
	Percentage	Frequency	Percentage	Frequency
R(R)	36.4	4	0	0
E(R)	27.3	3	0	0
K(K)	27.3	3	0	0
A(A)	0	0	48.3	14
Q(Q)	0	0	17.2	5
Q(A)	0	0	10.3	3
Other[a]	9.1	1	24.1	7
Total[b]	100.1	11	99.9	29
Client mode				
D(D)	33.3	12	50.0	8
E(E)	22.2	8	18.8	3
E(D)	8.3	3	18.8	3
D(E)	5.5	2	12.6	2
K(C)	13.9	5	0	0
E(C)	8.3	3	0	0
Other[a]	8.3	3	0	0
Total[b]	99.8	36	100.2	16

Note. Mode abbreviations are Disclosure (D), Advisement (A), Edification (E), Confirmation (C), Question (Q), Interpretation (I), Acknowledgment (K), and Reflection (R). Form is written first, intent second in parentheses.
[a]Includes modes used only once by a speaker.
[b]Percentage totals differ from 100 because of rounding errors.

the client's VRM profile was grossly different from the therapist's, (2) the two therapists' profiles were grossly different from each other, and (3) the two clients' profiles were very similar to each other.

The virtual lack of overlap in mode use between therapists and clients contrasts with the similarity of *content* within each excerpt. For example, in the client-centered excerpt, both therapist and client referred to being a family "pet"; in the gestalt excerpt, both referred to being "tense." Presumably, applying a *content* coding system to these excerpts would reveal these therapist–client similarities. To use other words, the VRM profiles sharply distinguish the *roles* of the participants, independently of the topic of their conversation; this is, of course, consistent with the three-channel hypothesis (Russell & Stiles, 1979).

The therapists' profiles in these excerpts were completely different from each other and almost completely in conformity with the prescriptions and proscriptions of their respective schools of psychotherapy. The theory of client-centered therapy explicitly admonishes therapists to assume "the internal frame of reference of the client" (Rogers, 1951, p. 29), which permits them to use only Reflection, Acknowledgment, Confirmation, and Edification (see Table 1), the *nondirective* or *acquiescent* modes (cf. Stiles, 1978b). In gestalt therapy, "the therapist stays absolutely in the now" (Perls, 1969, p. 53), where "the now" may be understood as the therapist's own existential frame of reference. Gestalt therapists are thus enjoined to use the other four modes—Advisement, Disclosure, Interpretation, and Question, which are the *directive* or *controlling* modes.

The extent to which the therapists conformed to these theoretical prescriptions in the excerpts coded above is shown in Table 5. Both in form and intent, most of the client-centered therapist's utterances were nondirective (other's frame of reference), and the gestalt therapist's utterances were directive (speaker's frame of reference). This systematic difference is not merely an artifact of preferences for particular favorite responses; even if utterances in the "favored" mode—R(R) for the client-centered therapist, A(A) for the gestalt therapist—is ignored, a large majority of the remaining utterances still conform to the prescriptions. This pattern also held true in a study of a substantially larger sample of teaching examples of client-centered and gestalt therapy (Stiles, 1979).

Psychoanalytic theory prescribes still a different "slice" of the 2 × 2 × 2 taxonomic "cube" (Table 1), modes concerning the patient's experience, that is, Question, Interpretation, Acknowledgment, and Reflection. This prescription follows from the insistence that the therapist attend entirely to the patient's thoughts and verbal productions while refusing to use "treatment by suggestion" (Advisement) or to divulge

TABLE 5
Therapists' Use of Directive (Speaker's Frame of Reference) and Nondirective (Other's Frame of Reference) Modes in Coded Excerpts of Client-Centered and Gestalt Psychotherapy

Therapist utterances	Client-centered		Gestalt	
	Percentage	Frequency	Percentage	Frequency
Form				
Directive modes	9.1	1	82.8	24
Nondirective modes	90.9	10	17.2	5
Intent				
Directive modes	0	0	96.6	28
Nondirective modes	100.0	11	3.4	1

Note. Directive modes (speaker's frame of reference) are Disclosure, Advisement, Question, and Interpretation. Nondirective modes (other's frame of reference) are Edification, Confirmation, Acknowledgment, and Reflection.

his own experience (Disclosure, Edification). "The doctor should be opaque to his patients and, like a mirror, should show them nothing but what is shown to him" (Freud, 1958, p. 118). VRM coding of teaching examples of psychoanalytic therapy confirmed that a preponderance of therapist utterances conformed to this prescription (Stiles, 1979).

The taxonomic principles thus form a bridge between psychotherapeutic theory and technique. That is, the theory describes the therapist's task in terms that are understandable as "frame of reference" and "source of experience," and these principles in the taxonomy specify particular classes of utterances. In this formulation, neither the theories nor the mode prescriptions specify the *content* of the interaction. Instead, they specify a particular *relationship* of the therapist to the client, in which any content might be discussed.

Despite the systematic therapist differences and the different topics of conversation, the clients' VRM profiles, shown in Table 4, are remarkably similar to each other. Most client utterances were in the four *exposition modes:* D(D), E(E), E(D), and D(E). That is, both clients talked primarily about their own private experience (Disclosure intent) and secondarily about objective matters (Edification intent), using first- or third-person declarative sentences. Clients' consistent reliance on the exposition modes, particularly D(D), despite dramatic differences in their therapists' mode use, appears characteristic of verbal psychotherapy (Stiles & Sultan, 1979). In the client-centered excerpt, the client used K(C) and E(C) to express agreement with therapist Reflections. This secondary pattern—the use of brief Confirmation-intent utterances to express agreement (or disagreement) with therapists' presumptuous utterances (Reflections, Interpretations, Advisements)—is also common in client behavior across schools of therapy (Stiles & Sultan, 1979), although it did not appear in the brief gestalt excerpt above.

VRM RESEARCH FINDINGS

VRM Research on Psychotherapeutic Process

The systematic differences in VRM use found among therapists of different schools (Stiles, 1979), and illustrated in the above excerpts, converge with similar findings by other investigators using other intersubjective systems (Brunink & Schroeder, 1979; Cartwright, 1966; Hill, Thames, & Rardin, 1979; Snyder, 1945; Strupp, 1955, 1957). The consistency of these results suggests that if there is a common core to psychotherapeutic process, it is unlikely to be found in the therapists' verbal techniques. However, the similarity of client VRM profiles across schools suggests that there might be a common "active ingredient" in the client's verbal behavior.

The most obvious candidate is client Disclosure—D(D). In using D(D) a client explores his or her own internal frame of reference using the first person ("I") to take personal responsibility for subjective experiences (i.e., to "own" or "accept" them). D(D) may thus be a central, defining feature of "good process." Of course, no single intersubjective category could alone be an adequate characterization of good psychotherapeutic process, as the other chapters in this volume demonstrate. Any complete characterization must include not only content and extralinguistic aspects, but other nonverbal, sequential, and situational processes, as well as the attitudes and numerous other personal characteristics of the participants (cf. Kiesler, 1980). Nevertheless, the prominence of D(D) in the client profile and the theoretical relevance of subjective "I" statements to the *self* suggest that client Disclosures may play a very important role.

As a first test of the hypothesis that client Disclosure is an active ingredient in psychotherapy, client VRM use in interview segments was compared with more global ratings of good process on the Experiencing (EXP) scale (Stiles, McDaniel, & McGaughey, 1979). The EXP scale (Klein, Mathieu, Gendlin, & Kiesler, 1969) is a fully anchored 7-point Likert-type rating scale developed to measure the primary client process variable in the client-centered theory of personality change (Gendlin, 1962, 1964; Rogers, 1958; see reviews by Gendlin, Beebe, Cassens, Klein, & Oberlander, 1969; Kiesler, 1971; Klein *et al.*, 1969). The strongest VRM correlate of EXP was the percentage of D(D) ($r = .58$), suggesting that raters relied heavily on client Disclosure in their judgments of good process (Stiles, McDaniel, & McGaughey, 1979).

If client D(D) is a major active ingredient in psychotherapy, then clients' use of D(D) in psychotherapy should be positively correlated with therapeutic benefit. However, a first test of this hypothesis failed to show this effect (McDaniel, 1980; McDaniel, Stiles, & McGaughey, 1981). Three sessions each from the brief (average, 17 sessions) psychotherapy of 31 clients—anxious, depressed, introverted male college students—were coded using the VRM system, and the resulting VRM profiles (percentage of utterances in each mode) were compared with measures of psychopathology and psychological distress taken at intake, at termination, and at follow-up, and with ratings of change in therapy. The interviews and outcome measures were collected as part of the Vanderbilt Psychotherapy Project (Strupp & Hadley, 1979). Results of the VRM-outcome comparison showed no clear or consistent relationship between client D(D)—or any other client mode—and measures of improvement. However, client D(D) was positively correlated (*rs* were about .5) with measures of psychological disturbance, including the MMPI depression scale and therapist ratings of overall severity of disturbance and of psychic distress, taken at intake and at termination. That is, clients who were more severely disturbed or distressed tended to use a higher proportion of D(D) in their psychotherapy sessions.

This relation of an intersubjective category with an enduring individual difference variable was unexpected from the perspective of the three-channel hypothesis (Russell & Stiles, 1979). However, finding an association of excessive self-disclosure with psychopathology is not unprecedented (Anchor, Vojtisek, & Patterson, 1973; Mayo, 1968; Persons & Marks, 1970; Stanley & Bownes, 1966), nor is it inconsistent with the hypothesis that clients' use of D(D) is therapeutic. The relationship of client Disclosures to psychopathology might be construed as analogous to the relationship of fever or white blood cell count to infection in some physical illnesses. Fever and white cell count are reliable indices of infection; however, their function is not to signal or promote disease but to fight it. Raised temperature and leucocytes are components of the immune system's protective response to invading microorganisms. Analogously, Disclosure may be a protective response to psychological distress; by exposing and exploring private experience with another person, clients can come to terms with internal and external stresses.

Since D(D) was not related to outcome, it is worth noting that the average VRM profile in the McDaniel (1980) study most closely resembled the profile for level 2 on the EXP scale (see Stiles, McDaniel, & McGaughey, 1979, for VRM profiles of each EXP level), including only 27.8% D(D) and 14.9% E(D). By contrast, the average VRM profile in the earlier study of assorted psychotherapy sessions, including five teaching examples and five tapes of graduate student therapists working in community settings (Stiles & Sultan, 1979), most closely resembled the profile for level 5 on the EXP scale, with 37.9% D(D) and 22.3% E(D). According to Gendlin (1969; Gendlin et al., 1968), an EXP level of 4 to 6 is essential for progress to occur in psychotherapy. Thus the Vanderbilt clients' level of Disclosure may have been insufficient to produce large therapeutic benefits. Strupp and Hadley (1979) report that these clients' gains averaged significantly more than untreated controls on some measures; however, the differences were modest, and they may have been overshadowed by individual differences in degree of disturbance, that is, in the measures that did correlate with D(D). In order to show a correlation of D(D) with change in therapy, the change attributable to therapy must be substantial, at least for some clients. An adequate test of the hypothesis that D(D) promotes therapeutic gain will require either that large, clear gains be demonstrated or that high levels of D(D) were attained.

VRM Research on Other Discourse

Although the VRM taxonomy evolved from research on psychotherapy, it can be applied equally well to any discourse in which a sender and an intended recipient can be identified. It has been used to study conversations of college students with each other and with professors (Cansler, 1979; Cansler & Stiles, 1981; Stiles, Waszak, & Barton, 1979), parents and children (Stiles & White, 1981), married couples (Premo, 1978; Premo & Stiles, 1983), and medical interviews (Stiles, Putnam, James, & Wolf, 1979; Stiles, Putnam, Wolf, & James, 1979a,b). Applications to political campaign speeches and courtroom interrogation of rape victims are in progress. VRM indices have also been compared with rating measures of dialogue (Stiles, 1980a).

A general finding in this research has been a powerful effect of role and task on VRM use. This effect is, of course, consistent with the three-channel hypothesis and the implication that VRM indices measure communication in the intersubjective channel (Russell & Stiles, 1979).

VRM profiles drawn from two studies, one of parent–child interaction (Stiles & White, 1981), and one of patient–physician interaction (Stiles, Putnam, Wolf, & James, 1979a, 1979b), illustrate the effects of role and task. Both studies involved individuals with complementary roles performing different interpersonal tasks, so that both influences could be assessed. In addition, both the doctor–patient relationship and the parent–child relationship have been proposed as prototypes of the psychotherapist–client relationship, so it is instructive to make direct comparisons.

Table 6 shows the VRM profiles of 62 parents and their 4th-, 5th-, or 6th-grade children interacting in a modified revealed-differences procedure. The procedure had two phases: in the first phase, each parent–child dyad was told to "reach agreement" on some mutually problematic situation identified by the interviewer in consultation with both parties. Typical "situations" were disagreements about bedtimes, TV watching, and chores. In the second phase, dyad members were told to "Tell how you feel" about the problematic situation. Thus, whereas the first phase instructions focused on problem-solving, the second phase instructions focused on affect expression. Each parent–child dyad completed the two-phase procedure for two different problematic situations. The profiles in Table 6 are thus means of two situations for each of the 62 dyads. (Approximately equal numbers of father–son, father–daughter, mother–son, and mother–daughter dyads were included.) Further details of setting, sample, and procedure are given elsewhere (Martin & Hetherington, 1971; Stiles & White, 1981).

The VRM profiles in Table 6 show that parents directed both phases

TABLE 6

Mean Verbal Response Mode Profiles for Parents and Children in
Phase 1 (Reach Agreement) and Phase 2 (Tell How You Feel) of a
Modified Revealed Difference Task

Parent mode[a]	Phase 1	Phase 2	Test of difference between phases t values
Q(Q)	23.2	24.7	.85
D(D)	7.2	15.5	6.83***
I(I)	6.1	4.7	−1.96
A(A)	5.3	3.1	−3.01**
E(E)	4.7	2.0	−3.60***
K(K)	3.3	3.8	.79
R(Q)	1.8	3.2	2.50*
E(D)	1.7	4.5	4.34***
Other[b]	42.0	32.9	
Total	100.0	100.0	
Number of utterances	28.8	19.6	
Child mode[a]			
D(D)	24.1	38.0	5.09***
K(D)	16.3	19.4	1.49
K(C)	7.5	5.6	−1.73
E(E)	6.4	3.3	−2.42*
D(E)	4.9	3.0	−1.89
K(K)	4.4	5.0	.77
I(C)	3.5	.4	−4.00***
E(D)	3.3	5.8	2.12*
Other[b]	25.1	17.6	
Total	100.0	100.0	
Number of utterances	14.0	9.2	

Note. From "Parent-Child Interaction in the Laboratory: Effects of Role, Task, and Child Behavior Pathology on Verbal Response Mode Use" by W. B. Stiles and M. L. White, 1981, Journal of Abnormal Child Psychology, 47. Copyright 1981 by Plenum Press. Reprinted by permission..
[a]Mode abbreviations: Disclosure (D), Question (Q), Edification (E), Acknowledgment (K), Advisement (A), Interpretation (I), Confirmation (C), Reflection (R). Form is written first, intent second; for example, E(D) means Edification form with Disclosure intent.
  Means for each phase based on two interactions by each of 62 parent–child dyads.
[b]Includes modes used less than 3% in both phases and utterances coded unscorable or disagreement.
*p < .05 by two-tailed t test for correlated samples, df = 61. **p < .01 by two-tailed t test for correlated samples, df = 61. ***p < .001 by two-tailed t test for correlated samples, df = 61.

of the interaction with Questions and Advisements, and made judgments about their children (Interpretations); they also expressed their own thoughts and feelings (Disclosures). The children mostly told of their own reactions, using K(D)—"yes" and "no" answers to questions—and D(D). They also gave some objective information (Edification intent) and indications of agreement or disagreement (Confirmation intent).

The differences between phases can be summarized as an increase in the proportion of Disclosure intents in the second phase by both parents and children, with a consequent decrease in the proportions of other modes. This, of course, is exactly what the instructions to "tell how you feel" called for.

Table 7 shows the VRM profiles of physicians and adult outpatients in 52 initial interviews in a general medical clinic of a university hospital. Patients were seen for a wide variety of problems, such as musculoskeletal pain, upper respiratory tract infection, genitourinary tract infection, headaches, and abdominal pain, typical of a primary care practice. Details of setting, sample, and procedure are described elsewhere (Stiles, Putnam, Wolf, & James, 1979a,b). Interviews were transcribed, VRM coded, and divided into three segments: (1) the medical history, in which the patient describes reasons for coming, and the

TABLE 7
Verbal Response Mode Profiles (Mean Percentage of Utterances in Each Mode) for Patients and Physicians of 52 Initial Interviews

Physician mode[a]	Medical history	Physical examination	Conclusion
Q(Q)	42.8	22.1	13.1
K(K)	16.7	5.0	5.2
I(K)	11.0	13.2	8.1
R(R)	8.7	4.4	1.8
A(A)	1.7	23.0	9.4
D(D)	2.4	7.9	11.6
E(E)	2.6	3.2	15.9
Patient mode[a]			
E(E)	18.5	14.5	10.9
D(E)	17.7	10.2	9.9
D(D)	16.6	11.5	17.1
E(D)	15.4	15.8	8.3
K(E)	9.7	11.2	4.7
K(D)	6.8	15.8	7.1
I(K)	*	2.3	11.3
K(K)	*	2.2	9.4
Q(Q)	1.1	4.6	7.1

Note. From "Verbal Response Mode Profiles of Patients and Physicians in Medical Screening Interviews" by W. B. Stiles, S. M. Putnam, M. H. Wolf, and S. A. James, 1979b, *Journal of Medical Education, 54.* Copyright 1979 by the American Medical Colleges. Reprinted by permission.
[a]Mode abbreviations are Disclosure (D), Question (Q), Edification (E), Acknowledgment (K), Advisement (A), Interpretation (I), Confirmation (C), and Reflection (R). Table includes modes used 5% or more in at least one segment.
*Less than 1%.

physician gathers background data, (2) the physical examination, and (3) the conclusion segment, in which the physician gives explanations and instructions.

The profiles of the three segments correspond to clinical experience and to descriptions given in texts on medical interviewing (e.g., Enelow & Swisher, 1972; Morgan & Engel, 1969). In the medical history, most physician utterances were Questions—Q(Q)—or Acknowledgments— K(K) ("mm-hm," "yeah") or I(K) ("right," "okay," with no judgment or evaluation intended). Patient utterances were almost all Edification or Disclosure in intent, that is, giving objective or subjective information. However, a substantial minority were Acknowledgment in *form:* K(E) and K(D)—"yes" or "no" answers that communicate objective or subjective information, respectively.

- (Did you have a rash?) Yes.   K(E)
- (Did it itch?) Yes.   K(D)

These modes show a transfer of information from patient to physician during the history.

In the physical examination, physicians continued to ask Questions, but used more Advisements ("Open your mouth") and Disclosures ("I'm going to check your throat") to direct patients through examination procedures. Patients continued to give information, but with relatively more K(E) and K(D)—more "yes" and "no" answers.

In the conclusion, physicians continued to gather information from patients, shown by physician Questions and Acknowledgments and patient Edifications and Disclosures, but in addition there was a substantial flow of information from physicians to patients, including explanations of illness and treatment, shown by physician Edifications and Disclosures and patient Acknowledgments and Questions. Comparison of these profiles with verbal interaction data from other studies (Davis, 1971; Freemon, Negrete, Davis, & Korsch, 1971; Bain, 1976) suggests, insofar as comparisons across coding systems are possible, that medical interviews tend to be conducted similarly, despite differences in setting and patient population (Stiles, Putnam, Wolf, & James, 1979b).

Factor analysis of mode frequencies was used to test the hypothesis that each segment might consist of a mixture of several types of "verbal exchange" between patient and physician. Patient and physician modes involved in one type of exchange would tend to be correlated with each other across interviews, and so they should appear together on a factor (see Stiles, Putnam, Wolf, & James, 1979a).

The factor analyses showed that each interview segment had a clear and simple structure, consisting of two or three distinct verbal exchange factors, each of which had an identifiable medical function. For example, the medical history consisted primarily of two types of verbal exchange. In the *exposition exchanges*, with high loadings for patient E(E), D(E), E(D), and D(D), and for physician K(K), patients told their story in their own words (Edification and Disclosure forms), while physicians facilitated with "mm-hms." In the *closed question exchanges*, with high loadings for physician Q(Q) and R(R), and for patient K(E) and K(D), physicians asked Questions and Reflected the sense of answers, while patients answered "yes" or "no."

Factor scores for all seven verbal exchange factors (two from the history, two from the physical examination, and three from the conclusion) were computed for each interview; these scores represented the extent to which a patient–physician pair engaged in each type of exchange. Two of the exchanges were significantly correlated with patient satisfaction measured by a postinterview questionnaire (Wolf, Putnam, James, & Stiles, 1978). Exposition exchanges in the history segment were associated with affective satisfaction (feelings of warmth and acceptance; trust in the doctor). *Feedback exchanges* in the conclusion segment, which consisted mainly in physician E(E), that is, pure Edifications, and patient K(K)—Acknowledgments—and Q(Q)—Questions—were associated with cognitive satisfaction (understanding of illness and treatment).

The strong association of satisfaction with Edifications found in this study supports the emphasis by Waitzkin and others (Waitzkin & Stoeckle, 1972, 1976; Waitzkin & Waterman, 1974) on the importance of information exchange in medical care, and it is consistent with surveys showing patients' desire for more information from their doctors (Kincey, Bradshaw, & Ley, 1975; Reader, Pratt, & Mudd, 1956; Ware & Snyder, 1975), and with the association of recalled explanations with satisfaction in patients' reports (Korsch, Gozzi, & Francis, 1968). This emphasis on objective information contrasts with the emphasis on subjective information (exploring attitudes and feelings) in psychotherapy.

Comparison of Role Relationships

The doctor–patient and parent–child profiles are consistent with the psychotherapist–client profiles in showing gross role differences, even though within each dyad members were talking about the same things (i.e., their utterances had similar content). The profiles are also consistent in showing that VRM use changes systematically with task requirements. On the other hand, within a particular role and task, different individuals tend to use similar mixtures of modes, despite variations in content. This pattern of results supports the three-channel hypothesis.

Of course, it is no surprise that people act differently when they are engaged in different tasks, or that people engaged in similar tasks act similarly. The point is that the VRM taxonomy provides a common metric on which different verbal roles and tasks can be quantitatively compared, and with which individual variations in the performance on a particular task can be measured.

One common feature of the parent–child, doctor–patient, and psychotherapist–client relationships is the asymmetry with respect to status. The status discrepancy is reflected in the relatively greater use of *presumptuous* (focus on other) modes by the superior role (compare Tables 4, 6, and 7), which has been found to be an extremely reliable pattern of VRM use (Cansler, 1979; Cansler & Stiles, 1981; Stiles, Putnam, James, & Wolf, 1979; Stiles, Waszak, & Barton, 1979). Theoretically, higher status implies a social assumption of greater knowledge, wisdom, or authority, so that a higher status person can appropriately presume knowledge of what a lower status person's experience is or should be, as required for Reflections, Interpretations, Confirmations, and Advisements. For a lower status person, such presumption would be socially inappropriate.

Comparison of Tables 4, 6, and 7 also shows a heavy use of the informative exposition modes—D(D), E(D), D(E), and E(E)—by clients, children, and patients, whereas therapists, parents, and physicians used relatively more of the attentive modes—Question, Acknowledgment, Interpretation, and Reflection. This pattern reflects a common requirement of the tasks studied, that the superior role gather information from the inferior role.

Comparison of the psychotherapy client profiles with the profiles for children and medical patients emphasizes the predominance of pure Disclosures in clients' discourse. By contrast, children and patients used more Edification intents and more Acknowledgment forms ("yes" and "no" responses). Interestingly, the child "tell how you feel" profile (phase 2) is quite similar to the client profile; "telling how you feel" about a problematic situation is, of course, a reasonable description of the psychotherapy client role.

The generalization that different individuals use similar mixtures of VRMs when acting in the same social role contrasts with the finding that psychotherapists of different theoretical persuasions use systematically different VRM profiles. Evidently, different schools of therapy prescribe different kinds of relationships as beneficial, so that there are many different psychotherapist roles. The role of psychotherapist is guided by theory—rather than by immediate social factors such as relative status and intimacy—far more than most other roles in society.

A researchable possibility is that different psychotherapies produce systematically different kinds of therapeutic benefits (Stiles, 1980b). Psychological health may be best construed as a multiplicity of patterns of growth and adjustment rather than as conformity to a uniform "normality," so that successful clients may diverge from each other in directions that are partly determined by the role their therapist takes. On the other hand, it is a central and curious feature that all of the therapist roles seem to elicit roughly the same client role as a complement. Thus, another tenable hypothesis is that each school of therapy has developed a different means to promote client self-exploration through Disclosure.

SUMMARY

The VRM taxonomy is a purely intersubjective coding system. Research on psychotherapy and other interpersonal interactions has shown that VRM indices are very sensitive to the roles of interactants and the tasks that they are engaged in, as proposed by the three-channel hypothesis. Psychotherapists are especially systematic in their use of VRMs; their VRM profiles differ depending on the theory they espouse, and their VRM use is logically related to their particular theoretical position. Client VRM use is remarkably consistent, despite therapist differences; this narrowly defined client verbal role may be the "common core" to the otherwise diverse collections of interpersonal encounters known as psychotherapy. Indirect evidence suggests that the critical "therapeutic" element within the common client VRM profile may be use of Disclosure. This mode is the predominant one in client speech, and its relative proportion within an interview segment is highly correlated with raters' judgments of good process (on the Experiencing scale). However, it remains to be shown whether greater client Disclosure leads to better outcomes.

The VRM system's advantage over other intersubjective systems is its derivation of conceptual principles. These principles show some promise as terms or dimensions in a general theory of the contribution of language to interpersonal relationships.

REFERENCES

Anchor, K. N., Vojtisek, J. E., & Patterson, R. L. (1973). Trait anxiety, initial structuring, and self-disclosure in groups of schizophrenic patients. *Psychotherapy: Theory, Research, and Practice, 10,* 255–258.
Austin, J. L. (1975). *How to do things with words* (2nd ed.). Oxford: Clarendon Press.
Bach, K., & Harnish, R. M. (1979). *Linguistic communication and speech acts.* Cambridge: M.I.T. Press.

Bain, D. J. G. (1976). Doctor-patient communication in general practice consultations. *Medical Education, 10,* 125–131.

Bales, R. F. (1950). *Interaction process analysis: A method for the study of small groups.* Reading, MA: Addison-Wesley.

Bales, R. F. (1970). *Personality and interpersonal behavior.* New York: Holt, Rinehart, & Winston.

Brent, E. E., & Sykes, R. E. (1979). A mathematical model of symbolic interaction between police and suspects. *Behavioral Science, 24,* 388–402.

Brown, P., & Levinson, S. (1978). Universals in language usage: Politeness phenomena. In E. N. Goody (Ed.), *Questions and politeness: Strategies in social interaction.* Cambridge, England: Cambridge University Press.

Brunink, S. A., & Schroeder, H. E. (1979). Verbal therapeutic behavior of expert psycho-analytically oriented, gestalt, and behavior therapists. *Journal of Consulting and Clinical Psychology, 47,* 567–574.

Butler, J. M., Rice, L. N., & Wagstaff, A. K. (1962). On the naturalistic definition of variables: An analogue of clinical analysis. In H. H. Strupp & L. Luborsky (Eds.), *Research in psychotherapy* (Vol. 2). Washington, D.C.: American Psychological Association.

Cansler, D. C. (1979). Effects of status on verbal behavior (Doctoral dissertation, University of North Carolina at Chapel Hill, 1979). *Dissertation Abstracts International, 40,* 2355B. (University Microfilms No. 7925895).

Cansler, D. C., & Stiles, W. B. (1981). Relative status and interpersonal presumptuous-ness. *Journal of Experimental Social Psychology, 17,* 459–471.

Cartwright, R. D. (1966). A comparison of the response to psychoanalytic and client-centered psychotherapy. In L. A. Gottschalk & A. H. Auerbach (Eds.), *Methods of research in psychotherapy.* New York: Appleton-Century-Crofts.

Cohen, J. (1960). A coefficient of agreement for nominal scales. *Educational and Psychological Measurement, 20,* 37–46.

Cole, P., & Morgan, J. L. (Eds.). (1975). *Syntax and semantics, Vol. 3: Speech acts.* New York: Academic Press.

Davis, M. S. (1971). Variations in patients' compliance with doctors' orders: Medical practice and doctor-patient interaction. *Psychiatry in Medicine, 2,* 31–54.

Dollard, J., & Auld, F., Jr. (1959). *Scoring human motives: A manual.* New Haven: Yale University Press.

Dore, J. (1979). Conversational acts and the acquisition of language. In E. Ochs & B. B. Schieffelin (Eds.), *Developmental pragmatics.* New York: Academic Press.

Duncan, S., Jr. (1972). Some signals and rules for taking turns in conversations. *Journal of Personality and Social Psychology, 23,* 283–292.

Duncan, S., Jr. (1974). On the structure of speaker-auditor interaction during speaking turns. *Language in Society, 2,* 161–180.

Duncan, S., Jr., Brunner, L. J., & Fiske, D. W. (1979). Strategy signals in face-to-face interaction. *Journal of Personality and Social Psychology, 37,* 301–313.

Elliott, R., Stiles, W. B., Shiffman, S., Barker, C. B., Burstein, B., & Goodman, G. (1982). The empirical analysis of help-intended communications: Conceptual framework and recent research. In T. A. Wills (Ed.), *Basic processes in helping relationships* (pp. 333–356). New York: Academic Press.

Enelow, A. J., & Swisher, S. N. (1972). *Interviewing and patient care.* New York: Oxford University Press.

Fleiss, J. L. (1975). Measuring agreement between two judges on the presence or absence of a trait. *Biometrics, 31,* 651–659.

Freemon, B., Negrete, V. F., Davis, M., & Korsch, B. M. (1971). Gaps in doctor-patient communication: Doctor-patient interaction analysis. *Pediatric Research, 5,* 298–311.

Freud, S. (1958). Recommendations to physicians practicing psycho-analysis. In J. Strachey (Ed. and Trans.), *The standard edition of the complete psychological works of Sigmund Freud* (Vol. 12). London: Hogarth Press.

Gendlin, E. T. (1962). *Experiencing and the creation of meaning.* New York: Free Press of Glencoe.

Gendlin, E. T. (1964). A theory of personality change. In P. Worchel & D. Byrne (Eds.), *Personality change.* New York: Wiley.

Gendlin, E. T. (1969). Focusing. *Psychotherapy: Theory, Research, and Practice, 6,* 3–15.

Gendlin, E. T., Beebe, J., III, Cassens, J., Klein, M., & Oberlander, M. (1968). Focusing ability in psychotherapy, personality, and creativity. In J. M. Shlein (Ed.), *Research in psychotherapy* (Vol. 3). Washington, DC: American Psychological Association.

Goodman, G. (1972). *Companionship therapy: Studies in structured intimacy.* San Francisco: Jossey-Bass.

Goodman, G. (1978). *SASHATapes: Self-led automated series on helping alternatives.* Los Angeles, CA: UCLA Extension.

Goodman, G., & Dooley, D. (1976). A framework for help-intended communication. *Psychotherapy: Theory, Research, and Practice, 13,* 106–117.

Gottman, J. M. (1979). *Marital interaction: Experimental investigations.* New York: Academic Press.

Gottschalk, L. A., & Gleser, G. D. (1969). *The measurement of psychological states through the content analysis of verbal behavior.* Berkeley: University of California Press.

Grice, H. P. (1957). Meaning. *Philosophical Review, 66,* 377–388.

Hill, C. E., Thames, T. B., & Rardin, D. K. (1979). Comparison of Rogers, Perls, and Ellis on the Hill Counselor Verbal Response Category System. *Journal of Counseling Psychology, 26,* 198–203.

Holsti, O. R. (1969). *Content analysis for the social sciences and the humanities.* Reading, MA: Addison-Wesley.

Ivey, A. E. (1971). *Microcounseling: Innovations in interviewing training.* Springfield, IL: Charles C Thomas.

Kiesler, D. J. (1971). Patient experiencing and successful outcome in individual psychotherapy of schizophrenics and psychoneurotics. *Journal of Consulting and Clinical Psychology, 37,* 370–385.

Kiesler, D. J. (1973). *The process of psychotherapy: Empirical foundations and systems of analysis.* Chicago: Aldine.

Kincey, J., Bradshaw, P., & Ley, P. (1975). Patients' satisfaction and reported acceptance of advice in general practice. *Journal of the Royal College of General Practice, 25,* 558–566.

Klein, M. J., Mathieu, P. L., Gendlin, E. T., & Kiesler, D. J. (1969). *The experiencing scale: A research and training manual* (Volume 1). Madison, Wisc.: Wisconsin Psychiatric Institute.

Korsch, B. M., Gozzi, E., & Francis, V. (1968). Gaps in doctor-patient communication. I. Doctor-patient interaction and patient satisfaction. *Pediatrics, 42,* 855–871.

Lazarsfeld, P. F., & Barton, A. H. (1951). Qualitative measurement in the social sciences: Classification, typologies, and indices. In D. Lerner & H. D. Lasswell (Eds.), *The policy sciences: Recent developments in scope and method.* Stanford, CA: Stanford University Press.

Mahrer, A. R. (1978). *Experiencing: A humanistic theory of psychology and psychiatry.* New York: Brunner/Mazel.

Marsden, G. (1971). Content-analysis studies of psychotherapy: 1954 through 1968. In A. E. Bergin & S. L. Garfield (Eds.), *Handbook of psychotherapy and behavior change: An empirical analysis.* New York: Wiley.

Martin, B., & Hetherington, E. M. (1971). *Family interaction and aggression, withdrawal, and nondeviancy in children.* Terminal Progress Report on Grant No. MH 12474, National Institute of Mental Health.

Mayo, P. R. (1968). Self-disclosure and neurosis. *British Journal of Social and Clinical Psychology, 7,* 140–148.

McDaniel, S. H. (1980). Clients' verbal response mode use and its relationship to measures of psychopathology and change in brief psychotherapy (Doctoral dissertation, University of North Carolina at Chapel Hill, 1979). *Dissertation Abstracts International, 41,* 359B. (University Microfilms No. 8013966)

McDaniel, S. H., Stiles, W. B., & McGaughey, K. J. (1981). Correlations of male college students' verbal response mode use in psychotherapy with measures of psychological disturbance and psychotherapy outcome. *Journal of Consulting and Clinical Psychology, 49,* 571–582.

Morgan, W. L., & Engel, G. L. (1969). *The clinical approach to the patient.* Philadelphia: W. B. Saunders.

Perls, F. S. (1969). *Gestalt therapy verbatim.* Layfayette, CA: Real People Press, 1969.

Persons, R. W., & Marks, P. A. (1970). Self-disclosure with recidivists: Optimum interviewer-interviewee matching. *Journal of Abnormal Psychology, 76,* 387–391.

Premo, B. E. (1978). Verbal response mode use in married couples versus stranger dyads: Acquaintance and familiarity (Doctoral dissertation, University of North Carolina at Chapel Hill, 1978). *Dissertation Abstracts International, 40,* 498B. (University Microfilms No. 7914395)

Premo, B. E., & Stiles, W. B. (1983). Familiarity in verbal interactions of married couples versus strangers. *Journal of Social and Clinical Psychology, 1,* 209–230.

Raush, H. L. (1972). Process and change—A Markov model for interaction. *Family Process, 11,* 275–298.

Reader, G. G., Pratt, L., & Mudd, M. C. (1957). What patients expect from their doctors. *Modern Hospital, 89*(1), 88–94.

Rogers, C. R. (1951). *Client-centered therapy.* Boston: Houghton-Mifflin.

Rogers, C. R. (1958). A process conception of psychotherapy. *American Psychologist, 13,* 142–149.

Rogers, C. R. (1959). A theory of therapy, personality, and interpersonal relationships, as developed in the client-centered framework. In S. Koch (Ed.), *Psychology: A study of a science* (Vol. 3). New York: McGraw-Hill.

Russell, R. L., & Stiles, W. B. (1979). Categories for classifying language in psychotherapy. *Psychological Bulletin, 86,* 404–419.

Searle, J. R. (1969). *Speech acts: An essay in the philosophy of language.* Cambridge: Cambridge University Press.

Snyder, W. U. (1945). An investigation of the nature of nondirective psychotherapy. *Journal of General Psychology, 33,* 193–223.

Stanley, G., & Bownes, A. F. (1966). Self-disclosure and neuroticism. *Psychological Reports, 18,* 350.

Stiles, W. B. (1978a). *Manual for a taxonomy of verbal response modes.* Chapel Hill: Institute for Research in Social Science, University of North Carolina at Chapel Hill.

Stiles, W. B. (1978b). Verbal response modes and dimensions of interpersonal roles: A method of discourse analysis. *Journal of Personality and Social Psychology, 36,* 693–703.

Stiles, W. B. (1978–79). Discourse analysis and the doctor-patient relationship. *International Journal of Psychiatry in Medicine, 9,* 263–274.

Stiles, W. B. (1979). Verbal response modes and psychotherapeutic technique. *Psychiatry, 42,* 49–62.

Stiles, W. B. (1980a). Comparison of dimensions derived from rating versus coding of dialogue. *Journal of Personality and Social Psychology, 38,* 359–374.

Stiles, W. B. (1980b, September). *Psychotherapeutic process: Is there a common core?* Symposium presentation, American Psychological Association Convention, Montreal, Quebec, Canada.

Stiles, W. B. (1981). Classification of intersubjective illocutionary acts. *Language in Society, 10,* 227–249.

Stiles, W. B., & Sultan, F. E. (1979). Verbal response mode use by clients in psychotherapy. *Journal of Consulting and Clinical Psychology, 47,* 611–613.

Stiles, W. B., & White, M. L. (1981). Parent-child interaction in the laboratory: Effects of role, task, and child behavior pathology on verbal response mode use. *Journal of Abnormal Child Psychology, 9,* 229–241.

Stiles, W. B., McDaniel, S. H., & McGaughey, K. (1979). Verbal response mode correlates of experiencing. *Journal of Consulting and Clinical Psychology, 47,* 795–797.

Stiles, W. B., Putnam, S. M., James, S. A., & Wolf, M. H. (1979). Dimensions of patient and physician roles in medical screening interviews. *Social Science & Medicine, 13A,* 335–341.

Stiles, W. B., Putnam, S. M., Wolf, M. H., & James, S. A. (1979a). Interaction exchange structure and patient satisfaction with medical interviews. *Medical Care, 17,* 667–681.

Stiles, W. B., Putnam, S. M., Wolf, M. H., & James, S. A. (1979b). Verbal Response Mode profiles of patients and physicians in medical screening interviews. *Journal of Medical Education, 54,* 81–89.

Stiles, W. B., Waszak, C. S., & Barton, L. R. (1979). Professorial presumptuousness in verbal interactions with university students. *Journal of Experimental Social Psychology, 15,* 158–169.

Strupp, H. H. (1955). An objective comparison of Rogerian and psychoanalytic techniques. *Journal of Consulting Psychology, 19,* 1–7.

Strupp, H. H. (1957a). A multidimensional analysis of therapist activity in analytic and client-centered therapy. *Journal of Consulting Psychology, 21,* 301–308.

Strupp, H. H. (1957b). A multidimensional system for analysing psychotherapeutic techniques. *Psychiatry, 20,* 293–306.

Strupp, H. H., & Hadley, S. W. (1979). Specific versus nonspecific factors in psychotherapy: A controlled study of outcome. *Archives of General Psychiatry, 36,* 1125–1136.

Waitzkin, H., & Stoeckle, J. D. (1972). The communication of information about illness: Clinical, sociological, and methodological considerations. *Advances in Psychosomatic Medicine, 8,* 180–215.

Waitzkin, H., & Stoeckle, J. D. (1976). Information control and the micropolitics of health care: Summary of an ongoing research project. *Social Science and Medicine, 10,* 263–276.

Waitzkin, H., & Waterman, B. (1974). *The exploitation of illness in capitalist society.* Indianapolis: Bobbs-Merrill.

Ware, J. E., & Snyder, M. K. (1975). Dimensions of patient attitudes regarding doctors and medical care services. *Medical Care, 13,* 669–682.

Wolf, M. H., Putnam, S. M., James, S. A., & Stiles, W. B. (1979). The medical interview satisfaction scale: Development of a scale to measure patient perceptions of physician behavior. *Journal of Behavioral Medicine, 1,* 391–401.

III
Extralinguistic Category Strategies

5

A Speech Interaction System

Joseph D. Matarazzo, Donald J. Kiesler, and Arthur N. Wiens

DEVELOPMENT OF THE SYSTEM

In collaboration initially with G. Saslow, R. Matarazzo, and J. Phillips and more recently with A. Wiens and others, we have been concerned since 1955 with the analysis of interview material, focusing on the formal or interactional components of communication. We assume that "the very essence of diagnostic interview and psychotherapy material—interview content—is carried by durations of communicative action (utterances) and silence. Nevertheless, only in the very recent past have investigators seemed to concern themselves with the form (and other normative characteristics) of the distributions of these two basic and highly stable interview variables" (Matarazzo, Wiens, Matarazzo, & Saslow, 1968, p. 353).

Both the rationale and methodology derived initially from Chapple's Interaction Chronograph method (Chapple, 1939; Chapple & Donald 1946) and his interaction theory of personality.

> The basis of Chapple's interaction method is an analysis of the time variable during the interview. After considerable work in the field, Chapple arrived at his conclusion that time was an important variable for describing human

Portions of this chapter were excerpted from J. D. Matarazzo and A. N. Wiens, *Behavior Modification*, 1977, *1*, 453–480, and D. J. Kiesler, *The process of psychotherapy: Empirical foundations and systems of analysis.* Chicago: Aldine, 1973, pp. 128–146.

JOSEPH D. MATARAZZO and ARTHUR N. WIENS • Department of Medical Psychology, Oregon Health Sciences University, Portland, OR 97201.   DONALD J. KIESLER • Department of Psychology, Virginia Commonwealth University, Richmond, VA 23284.

relations. He and his early collaborator, Arensberg, found that their field work as anthropologists was unduly hampered by the lack of precision and communicability of the various "subjective" variables which anthropologists (and other behavior scientists) were then using to describe human relations, in the family, tribe, interview-situation, etc. (Matarazzo, Saslow, & Matarazzo, 1956, pp. 349–350)

From an examination of our previous studies in evaluation of personality, we concluded that one measurable factor that seemed highly significant was time. The question then arose: What traits of personality express themselves in time? (Chapple & Donald, 1946, p. 199)

We all know, as a matter of observation, that people have different rates (timing) of interaction. Some of our friends or acquaintances seem to talk and act very speedily as compared to ourselves; others are slow and deliberate. These characteristics of individuals are something we intuitively recognize, and we often are at variance with the rates at which others act. (Chapple & Arensberg, 1940, p. 31)

If the reader sharpens his powers of observation, he will see that in many cases people whom he does not like or cannot get along with say exactly the same things that the people he does like say. So actors frequently take a short play, play it first as a tragedy and then, using the same words, play it as a comedy. Here the language is seen as unimportant, and the timing is the factor which makes the difference in its effect on the audience. (Chapple & Arensberg, 1940, p. 33)

[Chapple, thus,] has taken the (behavioristic) position that personality can be assessed without recourse to intrapsychic and other currently popular psychodynamic formulations, and further that this assessment involves merely the process of observing the *time relations* in the interaction patterns of people. Accordingly, Chapple has indicated that this method, because of its objectivity, can lead to a *science* of personality. (Matarazzo *et al.*, 1956, p. 350)

Utilizing Chapple's rationale, we set out to apply his measurement methodology to the study of clinical interviews, in both naturalistic and experimental settings.

Many investigators have used the interview as their instrument of assessment (change in behavior). The advantages of the clinical interview are its obvious flexibility and uniqueness, so that every patient has an opportunity to manifest his own, presumably learned, interpersonal behavior patterns. Its major disadvantage as a research instrument is its notorious unreliability. . . . It has long seemed to us that some standardization of the interviewer's behavior in the clinical interview, combined with suitably precise recording of predefined variables, could enable one to surmount its major handicap of unreliability while preserving its dynamic nature (spontaneity, richness, multidimensionality, transference potentialities, etc.). Chapple laid the groundword for just such an approach. (Saslow & Matarazzo, 1959, p. 125)

Thus, the two major goals of our research program were defined: first, to develop a standardized interview format, an experimental analogue of the clinical interview, for studying dyadic interaction; and second, to modify and use Chapple's interaction chronograph procedure for measuring the basic temporal factors of participants' behavior in the interview.

DESCRIPTION OF THE SCORING SYSTEM

The earliest research, summarized in Saslow and Matarazzo (1959), concerned itself with a series of five studies designed to test one of the critical questions on which any long-term research program on the interview, such as we proposed, would depend: Is the interview speech behavior of an interviewee sufficiently *reliable* or *stable* for him or her so that such speech behavior could form the basis for further study? In answering this question, we initially employed Chapple's Interaction Chronograph and the ten speech variables that it generated (Matarazzo *et al.*, 1956). However, a subsequent factor analysis (Matarazzo, Saslow, & Hare, 1958) revealed that many of these ten variables were redundant, and that two variables (speech and silence durations), and possibly a third (a speaker's interruption of his partner or similar "maladjustment" in synchrony), more than adequately recorded what previously had required ten separate measures. We then developed our own successor to the Chapple chronograph, the Interaction Recorder (Johnston, Jansen, Weitman, Hess, Matarazzo, & Saslow, 1961; Wiens, Matarazzo, & Saslow, 1965). Later, the system was expanded into a Group Interaction Recorder, which records a whole group of interacting participants (up to 24 persons) involved in group psychotherapy or sensitivity training sessions (Morris, Johnston, Bailey, & Wiens, 1968). However, when only several channels of this latter 24—channel recording device are used, it, too, is a two-person Interaction Recorder.

The basic unit in the recording system is the length of each interviewer's and interviewee's speech and silence units as they occur in ordinary conversation and are recorded on the Interaction Recorder (Wiens *et al.*, 1965). The Interaction Recorder is an electronic device that time-records on paper or magnetic tape an account of the time when either person in an interview is speaking or silent. These recordings are binary coded and acceptable to a modern computer. An interview is recorded "live" through a one-way mirror by an observer who depresses (on the Interaction Recorder) either the interviewer or the interviewee key, depending upon who is talking. Both keys are depressed if both participants are talking at the same time. Each key is released at the completion of an utterance, providing for a sequential analysis of the interview, which is automatically provided by the computer printout.

Three speech variables are derived from the interview data: (1) *mean speech duration*, the total time in seconds the interviewee (or interviewer) speaks divided by his or her total number of speech units; (2) *mean speech late cy*, the total latency time (the period of silence separating two different peech units) divided by the number of units of interviewee (or inter iewer) latency; and (3) *percentage interruption*, the total number of times the interviewee (or interviewer) speaks divided into the number of these same speech units that were interruptions of his or her partner. Hence, the system has as its basic units the duration of each interview participant's unit of speech, his or her reaction time before each unit of speech, and the number of these units that are interruptions of his or her conversational partner.

DATA COLLECTION CONTEXT

By far the majority of our studies using the Interaction Recorder focused on interview behaviors occurring in a live, clinical, but nominally standardized interview. Examples of the real-life interviews we have utilized are (1) initial psychiatric interviews with inpatients and outpatients; (2) employment interviews with applicants applying for civil-service positions, and so forth; and (3) interviews with administrators. However, in one major investigation, built upon years of preliminary research, we studied seven full psychotherapy cases involving naturally occurring, live psychotherapy interviews (Matarazzo *et al.*, 1968). In all studies but the latter, we have shown that interview research such as ours can be carried out by employing a basic research design dividing the real life interview into three parts, each typically lasting fifteen minutes: a baseline period, an experimental period, and a return to the baseline period. The interviewer is instructed to interview in his normal manner in Periods 1 and 3, and to introduce a planned change in his own speech behavior in Period 2. Thus, for example, in a 5-10-5 study, the interviewer conducted his nondirective interviewing in Periods 1 and 3—utilizing open-ended utterances of approximately 5-seconds duration—but doubled these utterances to approximately 10 seconds in the experimental period. The effect was a similar *increase* in the interviewee's average speech durations in Period 2. Other tactics similarly investigated were head nods, the use of "mm-hmm" and similar verbal reinforcers, increases in the interviewer's own reaction time, and so forth. (See a review of these studies in Matarazzo *et al.*, 1968, and Figure 1 in this chapter.)

DATA FORM

The typical form of interview material judged by the observer who presses the key of the Interaction Recorder has been the in-progress, live interview observed through a one-way mirror. However, a later study indicated that the same speech measures can be taken directly from tape recordings of interviews yielding scores equally reliable and equivalent to those obtained by an observer of the live interview. Three observers were used for this study (Wiens, Molde, Holman, & Matarazzo, 1966), an experienced observer who recorded live from behind a one-way mirror, and two beginning students who later recorded from tape recordings of the same interviews.

> When our overall findings are reviewed, . . . it is apparent that comparable data were obtained among the different observer-recorders (whether they recorded live or from tape). . . . This comparability was evident in the high correlations (0.94 to 0.99 for the two interviewee speech measures and also for one of the two interviewer speech measures) and similar mean values for the different observers when they recorded the interviewee's duration of utterance and latency, and the interviewer's duration of utterance. Even when the more difficult variable, interviewer latency, was dealt with—with numerical values of less than one second and undoubtedly involving individual differences in observer reaction time—gross comparability for all practical purposes was evident in mean values that ranged from 0.55 to 0.75 seconds, and in correlations between observers that were significant in two out of three cases. Nevertheless, reliability is less for this variable and it may be necessary to utilize some recording aids that will enhance comparability of data recorded for this variable and thereby decrease to a considerable degree the variance among observers, live or tape. We conclude from our findings that it is feasible to collect data initially by tape-recording interviews and subsequently recording them on the Interaction Recorder or similar devices for analysis of speech and silence duration characteristics. (pp. 258–259)

For individuals wishing a more modern and relatively inexpensive computer system for recording speech variables such as those studied by us, Hargrove and Martin (1982) describe a simple system utilizing an Apple II microcomputer system that they adapted to facilitate this type of research.

For individual investigators not wishing to utilize an electronic recording system, Matarazzo, Holman and Wiens (1967) have shown that

> a word count from a typescript of an interview is all that an investigator needs to derive [our] variables . . . since the correlation between average duration of utterance for each speaker as recorded by stopwatch or other chronographic device and the average number of words spoken per utterance by this same person in that interview is of the order of 0.92. Thus, any investigator can now tape record a therapy interview, transcribe it, count the number of words spoken in each utterance by each speaker, compute the

mean number of words per utterance for both speakers, and thereby have data for his own cases comparable to [ours]. (Matarazzo *et al.*, 1968, p. 391)

CHOICE OF UNITS

We define our basic speech unit as the "utterance," which is "merely what an experienced or naive observer would record if he or she used the conventions appropriate to ordinary conversational behavior in our society" (Matarazzo *et al.*, 1968, p. 353).

> [The utterance is] separated at either end by two silence periods—one silence following the other participant's last comment (that is, the speaker's latency), the second silence following the speaker's own comment and preceding the listener's next comment (that is, the listener's latency). Pauses for breathing, for choosing words, for reflection, etc., are included in the speech unit when the context clearly suggests that the speaker has not yet completed that utterance. . . . However, pauses (again determined by context) which precede the introduction of new ideas or thoughts by the same individual, without an intervening comment by the other interview participant, signal the onset of a new speech unit. (Wiens, Molde, *et al.*, 1966, p. 253)

We have not explicitly discussed the different units involved in process measurement. From the preceding paragraph and the published references we use as examples of their scoring unit (Rogers' and Wolberg's transcribed verbatim speech units for therapist and patient), it is clear that our scoring unit is the utterance, for both patient and therapist. In scoring a particular utterance in a session, the observer has as context the preceding interview interaction to that point. Furthermore, in making decisions about interruptions, silences, and other variables in the system, the observer must keep in mind some part of the immediately succeeding interaction. The most relevant context (which would define the "contextual unit" for the system) is the interaction immediately preceding and immediately following the utterance, all of which occurs in a matter of seconds. Finally, the most frequently employed "summarizing unit" is the total session. An individual's score on a particular variable is calculated for the entire session, and represents an average of his or her scores for the numerous individual utterances occurring within that session. The evidence we have published on observer reliability in recording out scoring unit adds substance to our claim that the scoring unit is reliably and objectively described (Phillips, Matarazzo, Matarazzo, & Saslow, 1957; Wiens, Molde, *et al.*, 1966).

PARTICIPANT–CONTEXT RESTRICTIONS

Some of the Interview Speech Interaction measures by definition (for example, latency) require assessment of the verbal interaction of both participants. However, in a monologue situation, some of the measures (for example, duration of utterance or latency between successive utterances) could easily be obtained. Goldman-Eisler (1968), among other investigators, has done just this type of analysis of such single-person speech behavior (for example, during a lecture, reciting a standardized passage, etc.).

TYPE OF SAMPLING INDICATED

We typically have applied our system to entire interview sessions (either a 45- or 50-minute standardized experimental interview or live therapy sessions). However, we have concerned ourselves with the issue of the kind of sampling necessary, random or stratified. Our results show that the speech measures derived from a 15-minute segment of a 45-minute interview correlate between 0.70 and 0.90, with comparable measures based on the whole 45-minute interview (for example, Matarazzo, Wiens, Saslow, Allen, & Weitman, 1964, p. 112). Interview samples shorter than 15 minutes are not recommended; 10-minute samples were found to be less reliable (Matarazzo, 1962, pp. 497–499).

SAMPLE LOCATION WITHIN THE INTERVIEW

We have not specifically addressed the problem of from where (in the hour) samples of interaction can be extracted that will yield speech scores representative of therapist and patient behavior during the entire interview hour. However, the research referred to in the last section would suggest that, when samples must be utilized, a 15-minute segment can be taken from any part of the interview.

SAMPLE LOCATION OVER THERAPY INTERVIEWS

In one study of live psychotherapy (Matarazzo *et al.*, 1968), we studied seven psychoneurotic patients whose total therapy interviews ranged from 11 to 50, with an average of 23 sessions. Since speech

measures were obtained by an observer who witnessed each live therapy session for each case, the issue of where and in what manner (randomly or systematically) to sample over the continuum from initiation to
termination did not rise. Whether the different sampling procedures
yield different results for the speech variable scores in different phases
of psychotherapy remains an unanswered question. However, we have
published a number of graphs for a whole therapy (up to 50 sessions);
these clearly reveal marked changes from session to session in the
speech behavior of both the patient and the therapist (Matarazzo et al.,
1968). Interesting correlates of these session-to-session changes were
described in the same study.

CLINICAL SOPHISTICATION OF JUDGES

It seems quite likely that clinical sophistication is totally unrelated to
one's skill as an observer and recorder for the Interview Speech Interaction procedure, since only the temporal factors of the interaction are
considered. Several studies have, in fact, revealed that even the most
inexperienced observers can generate data comparable to a highly skilled
clinician-observer (Wiens, Molde, Holman, Matarazzo, 1966; Matarazzo,
Holman & Wiens, 1967).

TRAINING REQUIRED OF JUDGES

We reported an early study where two observers made simultaneous but independent live recordings of the same standardized interviews. "One of the observers had had approximately two years of
experience (involving many hundreds of interviews) observing the standardized interview in an employment setting. The second observer was
relatively inexperienced, having recorded only some ten practice interviews, and these in a psychiatric rather than a department store setting"
(Saslow & Matarazzo, 1959, p. 132; see also Phillips et al., 1957). The
results were striking evidence that one obtains reliable and equivalent
interview speech scores from an inexperienced observer. The intrarater
reliabilities for nine speech scores for the inexperienced observer ranged
from 0.71 to 1.00, with eight of the nine variables having coefficients
above 0.94. The means and standard deviations of each measure for the
two observers were almost identical, and the scores for the two observers ranged in intercorrelation from 0.94 to 1.00. Later studies showed
that observers having no more than several hours practice with this

procedure can apply the system as well as others who have had extensive experience (Wiens, Molde, et al., 1966; Matarazzo, Holman, & Wiens, 1967).

TRAINING MANUAL

We (Matarazzo & Wiens, 1972) have put much of the published research of our group in book form. In addition to a definition of each of the three speech variables, the book contains a verbatim transcript of an interview that clearly delineates each speech unit and also identifies interruptions as scored in this system.

INTERRATER AND INTRARATER RELIABILITIES REPORTED

We have given considerable attention to the reliability of various aspects of our scoring and interview procedure. In the study described in this section, very high *interobserver* consistency was obtained for two observers independently recording the same interviews. From this study we concluded that "the observation and recording of interaction patterns during the partially standardized interview is a highly reliable undertaking . . . the observer's task is largely a mechanical one once he has read, understood, and practiced the published rules as to what constitutes an action and an inaction (Matarazzo, Saslow, & Matarazzo, 1956, pp. 362–364). Observer response-sets or biases "appear to have little effect upon the interview interaction record finally obtained" (Saslow & Matarazzo, 1959, p. 135). Later research confirmed and extended these results (Wiens et al., 1966; Matarazzo, Holman, & Wiens, 1967).

We have also examined various aspects of reliability vis-à-vis our standardized interview procedure. The results show that a single interviewer "is able both to learn and to follow the rules of the standardized interview to a reasonably high degree" (Saslow & Matarazzo, 1959, p. 137). A related but separate question is: How reliably can two interviewers carry out the standardized interview with a given sample of subjects? Results from another study indicated that two interviewers can perform comparably in the standardized format. We concluded that "the ability to learn and follow the rules is not limited to one interviewer. . . . Interviewers can, with a little practice, become research instruments of considerable reliability" (Saslow & Matarazzo, 1959, pp. 138–139).

A final aspect of reliability has to do with the interviewee's interaction patterns as they occur in the standardized interview. The results of various studies suggest that

> interviewee interaction patterns have the following characteristics. First, there are wide individual differences in interaction patterns among subjects. Second, the interviewee interaction characteristics for any given subject are highly stable across two different interviewers when the latter standardize their interviewing behavior along the minimal predefined dimensions of our standardized method; and at the same time, these interviewee characteristics are modifiable by planned changes in the intrainterview behavior of either interviewer. Third, the marked stability and modifiability of an individual's interaction patterns, found for our first sample of subjects, were cross-validated in a second sample. And fourth, the stability and modifiability were equally striking when only a single interview was used and the test–retest interval was extended to several days, five weeks, and eight months, in contrast to the first two studies, which employed a test–retest interval of a few minutes. (Matarazzo, Saslow, & Hare, 1958, p. 419)

Thus, the interaction variables reflect stable and invariant personality characteristics under the real-life but minimally standardized interview conditions in which subjects were studied:

> We have studied and established as having extremely high reliability the following aspects of interview interaction behavior: the reliability of the interviewer who serves as the independent variable by conducting the standardized interview; the reliability of the interviewee interaction patterns, the dependent variables; the reliability of the observer who observes the interviewer–interviewee interaction and records his observations by pressing separate keys for each participant; and finally, the reliability of the scorer who scores the final interaction chronograph record. (p. 419)

DIMENSIONALITY CONSIDERATIONS

We (Matarazzo, Saslow, & Hare, 1958) conducted a factor analysis of twelve of the interview interaction measures recorded by the earlier-employed Chapple Interaction Chronograph. This factor analysis of the data of 60 subjects, as well as a replication study, revealed the presence of four independent factors: two major (speech and silence) and two weaker (initiative and interruption-maladjustment).

> The results indicate that as viewed from an interaction chronograph framework, doctor–patient interactions (and possibly most other two-person interactions) consist of two very stable factors for any given individual: (a) how long on the average he or she waits or remains silent before communicating (response latency), and (b) the number and average duration of each of these communicative interactions. A third [weak] factor [is] the frequency with which one initiates or starts again with another communication unit of his [or her] own when his [or her] partner has not answered. . . . A fourth [also

weak] factor [is] the efficiency with which a member of the communicating pair synchronizes and adjusts (or maladjusts) to his [or her] partner. (pp. 427–28)

As a result of this study, we have stopped analysing all [fourteen of the] Chapple variables and their numerous derivative variables, and have focused our attention, instead, on the two strongest factors, speech and silence [latency] duration [for patient and therapist]. Together these . . . account for about 88 percent of the variance of the 14 interview interaction measures recorded by the Interaction Chronograph. (Matarazzo, Wiens, & Saslow, 1965, p. 190)

VALIDITY STUDIES

The various validity studies of interaction process in the quasi-experimental interview, as well as the later study of psychotherapy interviews and the earliest saliency studies, are summarized in several places (Matarazzo, 1965; Matarazzo, Wiens, & Saslow, 1965; Matarazzo, Wiens, Matarazzo, and Saslow, 1968; Saslow & Matarazzo, 1959; Matarazzo and Wiens, 1972; Jackson, Wiens, Manaugh, & Matarazzo, 1972; Matarazzo, Wiens, & Manaugh, 1975; and Wiens, Manaugh, & Matarazzo, 1976). Our earlier reliability studies revealed that: (1) there are *wide individual differences* across persons in speech, silence, and interruption behavior; and (2) despite these individual differences, the speech behavior of any given individual is *highly stable,* for him or her from one interview situation to another, providing the interviewer maintains a fairly consistent interviewing style. Subsequent studies in this program of research indicated that these objective, noncontent dimensions of interviewee speech also show a number of modest personality and other validity correlates, and are subject to control by the interviewer. Thus, in one study involving real-life employment interviews, we (Matarazzo *et al.,* 1968), found that by doubling or halving the duration of each of his own single speech units in each of three 15-minute periods of an otherwise free 45-minute interview, the interviewer was able to influence the mean speech duration of twenty job applicant interviewees in the three comparable periods of the interview (see Figure 1). The positive results of this study were cross-validated in two additional studies, in which the interviewer unobtrusively controlled his single speech unit durations to approximately roughly 10-5-10-second and 5-15-5-second durations in the three parts of his planned interview. These findings have since been independently confirmed in analogous studies by Simpkins (1967) and Lauver, Kelley, and Froehle (1971).

That such interview-control effects are not limited to face-to-face employment interviews was revealed in another study (Matarazzo, Wiens, Saslow, Dunham, & Voas, 1964), in which we discovered that the speech behavior of an orbiting astronaut could be "controlled" by changes in the speech behavior of the ground communicator. In an ingenious extension of this study, Ray and Webb (1966) showed that how much or how little President Kennedy talked in response to a reporter's questions in his 1961–1963 series of press conferences was clearly related to the length, or shortness, of the question posed by the reporter. Effects such as these are clearly out of the realm of conscious awareness.

Research carried out on our silence measure also demonstrated that planned changes in the interviewer's own latency (reaction time before he answers his conversational partner) also quite dramatically produced the predicted increases and decreases in the corresponding latency behavior of the interviewee (Matarazzo & Wiens, 1967). The third speech variable, frequency of an interviewer's *interruption* of the interviewee, also revealed that the corresponding interruption rate of the interviewee could be brought under the control of the interviewer with surprising regularity (Wiens, Saslow, & Matarazzo, 1966).

Concurrent with these studies, the research program was extended to a study of a situation, psychotherapy, in which the two conversational partners met not merely for one encounter (a single employment interview), but for a series of encounters. We studied three psychotherapists who were paired with two patients, two patients, and three patients respectively (that is, seven patient–therapist individual psychotherapies). The results of this research (Matarazzo, Wiens, Matarazzo, and Saslow, 1968) revealed a heretofore unsuspected "synchrony" or "tracking" over sessions in the speech behavior of one speaker in relation to the speech behavior of his conversational partner. That is, the study of one person's durations of pauses before answering his or her conversational partner showed sizable differences in average pause length from one day to the next and also a remarkable correlation between one person's session ups and downs in pause lengths and similar increases and decreases in the same variable in his or her conversational partner on these same days. Frequency of interrupting behavior likewise showed this "tracking" or "synchrony" across numerous face-to-face encounters (see section on empathy below).

It appeared to us that, in order to increase our knowledge in this area (for basic personality theory and study) even further, the results of this first decade of research on speech and silence measures should next be applied in natural settings, so as to better test their potential as indexes of underlying attitudinal, mood, and motivational states. The tenability of such an application was suggested by an earlier study, revealing that an experimentally induced "expectancy" in an interviewee that he would talk to either a "cold" or "warm" interviewer markedly influenced the interviewee's latency before answering the interviewer in an otherwise free employment interview (Allen, Wiens, Weitman, & Saslow, 1965). Likewise, a study by Craig (1966) revealed that the increased accuracy of an interviewer's statements about an interviewee's underlying personality and attitudinal attributes very clearly affected (increased) the length of the subsequent verbal responses by the interviewee.

These two studies, and a third one (Wiens, Matarazzo, Saslow, Thompson, & Matarazzo, 1965) demonstrating that "supervisory" versus "nonsupervisory" status was reflected in the speech characteristics of these two classes of interviewee-respondents, suggested that speech and silence indexes deserved to be examined for their potential (theoretical and practical) to reveal a respondent's underlying moods, attitudes, or motivational characteristics in real life situations. If these speech measures were found to be viable indexes of such motivational characteristics, that finding would be an important contribution to psychological science, especially personality theory.

Contribution to basic personality theory is thus the primary purpose of a direction we began to take in 1967. This basic goal served as the framework for five studies completed subsequently. In the first (Manaugh, Wiens, & Matarazzo, 1970), we learned, despite our initial methodological attempts to control for such an effect, that four groups of young college students, interviewed one at a time, showed *differential* and statistically significant changes in their speech and silence behavior when discussing a topic (their individual *educational* background) that was *salient* in their current collegiate life situation, relative to discussion of two less salient topic areas (their family background and their occupational background).

In a follow-up study (Matarazzo, Wiens, Jackson, & Manaugh, 1970a) designed to remove or otherwise control for this differential content saliency in four similar groups of undergraduate subjects, we utilized interviews involving discussion of two presumably (*a priori*) *equally* salient interview content categories, each subject's *college major* and his *present living setting* (home, dormitory, apartment, etc.). Contrary to expectation, the overriding result of this study, consistent with that of its predecessor, was the finding, again in both the two control and two experimental groups, that *college major* was a content topic of apparent higher intrinsic saliency (as revealed by differences in their speech behavior) for these eighty subjects than was *living setting*.

Concurrent with the execution of these first two studies, we conducted and published another study (Matarazzo, Wiens, Jackson, &

Manaugh, 1970b), a variant of the first study. Sixty job applicants for the position of patrolman in Portland, Oregon were each given a 45-minute interview unobtrusively divided into three 15-minute segments. During each segment, a different content area (education, occupation, and family history) was discussed. The results, when compared with twenty job applicants in a control group, showed that their noncontent dimensions of speech behavior again *were* differentially affected by the content being discussed by the interviewer. The *job applicants* spoke with a statistically significantly shorter reaction time and with a longer mean utterance during content conditions involving a discussion of their *occupational* histories. These results, cross-validated on a second group of thirty applicants, were interpreted to suggest that the content category *occupation* was tapping a higher level of saliency in these job applicants in this content area than was either the content category of education or family. This finding was consistent with our twice-confirmed finding in the first two studies, in which education (or its derivative, college major) was found to be a content area with differential sensitivity or saliency in interviewees who were current college students.

These studies led to the postulation that discussion of the topic area *education* with college-student interviewees and the topic area *occupation* with job-applicant interviewees tapped, in each group, an already present, differentially viable (salient) motivational state appropriate to each subject's own life space, as this motivational or personality-emotional state was being revealed in each subject's interview, noncontent speech behavior.

As a more direct check of this hypothesis, we developed an approach which would allow us to abandon further searches for evidence of saliency in the speech of target *groups* of subjects (collegiate versus job applicant groups) but, instead, would allow us to search for interview content areas which are salient for each individual. We (Jackson, Manaugh, Wiens, & Matarazzo, 1971), developed a questionnaire-type scale, the Topic Importance Scale, or TIS, which consists of 45 items. Each individual is to rate on a 7-point scale, for four separate subdimensions, the importance to him or her of each of these 45 topic areas, for example, his or her interest in drugs, the Vietnam War, marriage, goal in life, feelings about self, and so forth. The first results with this scale revealed that (1) the TIS saliency ratings show the usual and necessary levels of reliability, and (2) the TIS saliency ratings show early evidence of being *valid* indexes of "saliency" as revealed by their potential to differentiate: (a) married from unmarried subjects; (b) draft-exempt from draft-eligible subjects; and (c) subjects majoring in different undergraduate disciplines. These TIS saliency results were obtained by comparing subgroups of subjects differing in the ways indicated by these initial validity studies.

   As a more direct study of the validity of the TIS to reflect or mirror the content area(s) or highest saliency in the *individual* case, we (Jackson, Wiens, Manaugh, & Matarazzo, 1972) completed two studies directly relating an individual's areas of high (or low) saliency, as a motivational state, to the speech behavior of this same subject in an interview situation not related to the independently obtained saliency ratings. The two studies tested this relationship between duration of utterance, reaction time, and interruption and the saliency of the content being discussed by an interviewee, first in terms of group differences, and subsequently for each individual subject studied uniquely. In the first study, 40 male college students were interviewed in a 30-minute interview about one topic of known high saliency (goals in life) and one of known low saliency (interior decorating) for 15 minutes per topic. In the second study, 50 male college students were interviewed about two topics that were specifically selected to be of high or low saliency for each interviewee, based on his own TIS saliency ratings months earlier. The results of both studies indicate that interviewees talk with a longer average duration of utterance (but content-specific either high or low latency) when talking about a high saliency topic relative to a low saliency topic. Interestingly, the topic discussed *first*, irrespective of its own saliency value, was characterized by a relatively lower duration of utterance.

   It was clear to us that our earlier psychotherapy research, despite the interesting synchrony obtained, had failed to yield clues for a full understanding of the empirically observed ups and downs from one session to another in a patient's speech behavior. Unfortunately, the development of a content saliency measure yielded mixed validity findings and thus did not easily permit us and others to more effectively relate the content of an interview with the formal speech and silence measures we had so extensively studied. These same speech and silence variables were, however, being studied in another context as well, that concerned with interviewer empathy and outcome in psychotherapy (see Matarazzo & Wiens, 1977, for review). One basis for our interest in this area is the increasing belief today that the interpersonal dynamics and therapeutic processes involved in *psychotherapy* and in *behavior modification* are not as totally dissimilar as they appeared a decade or two ago. Although empirical evidence to support such possible commonality of processes, dynamics, and related features is sparse, typical of today's rethinking of the issues, as well as the problems still remaining in this area, are the following observations by Morganstern (1976):

> It is often assumed that behaviorists are cold, mechanistic, uncaring laboratory technicians, with little regard for the "therapeutic relationship." On numerous occasions, students and clients have indicated surprise that the behaviorists they have seen or heard (or have been treated by) have been concerned, warm, and "human." (pp. 59–60)

It could be argued that there is a huge literature to attest to the fact that such variables as empathy, warmth, and genuineness do relate to interview content (by increasing, for example, self-exploration and self-disclosure, Truax & Carkhuff, 1967), and in turn, to treatment outcome. The reliability of such measures, however, and the validity of the outcome variables in these studies are questionable. . . . This is not to suggest that such variables as empathy, warmth, genuineness, openness, honesty, etc. are *unimportant* in behavioral interviewing. On the contrary, it is strongly felt by the author that under some circumstances certain relationship variables will facilitate assessment and enhance treatment outcome. The point, however, is that very little is known about the effects of particular therapist characteristics on assessment information, continuance in therapy, compliance, and outcome measures in behavior therapy.

Our view of research on the speech and silence behavior of the therapist and patient in both behavior therapy and psychotherapy, as well as interview research, is that such a beginning base of empirical data as Morganstern and others have been seeking has appeared in the literature. It also is of interest to note that the speech behavior of the two participants in therapy may provide advocates of behavior modification and of psychotherapy a common behavioral link, inasmuch as talking involves both content and form, that is, *what* one says (psychodynamics) and *how* one transmits this content (behavioral dynamics).

Sanford (1942, p. 813), in his extensive review of the literature on speech and personality, quotes Ben Jonson, who wrote that "language most showeth a man; speak that I may see thee." In the three decades since Sanford's review, thousands of studies were published by investigators who have studied the verbal content, linguistic noncontent, and gestural aspects of each speaker in the face-to-face interaction of initial interviews, psychotherapy interviews, and other two-person conversations. Excellent reviews of this literature are available in Matarazzo (1965a), Goldstein, Heller, and Sechrest (1966), Truax and Carkhuff (1967), Goldman-Eisler (1968), Duncan (1969), Jaffe and Feldstein (1970), Bergin and Garfield (1971), Matarazzo and Wiens (1972), Mehrabian (1972), Siegman and Pope (1972), Bergin and Strupp (1972), Kiesler (1973), Strupp (1973), Weitz (1974) among other sources.

The studies reported in the first two decades of this research resulted in a disappointing yield, considering the massive effort involved. Investigators became disillusioned, and many abandoned these research tributaries to pursue other, potentially more rewarding, problems. However, accumulating evidence suggests that this state of affairs has been changing during the past decade as, bit by bit, a few seemingly robust variables have been emerging. One of these variables has been designated by the term *empathy*. Inasmuch as it is no doubt found in all human conversational experiences (e.g., parent–child, peer–peer, spouse–spouse, and so on), it is surprising that research on its nature and characteristics received impetus only after a theoretical notion and framework for understanding empathy was published in a paper entitled "The Necessary and Sufficient Conditions of Therapeutic Personality Change" by Rogers (1957). In this paper, Rogers proposed that three personal characteristics of the therapist, when communicated to, or otherwise sensed by, the patient, represent the necessary and sufficient conditions for client personality change to occur. Rogers wrote that these three core conditions are that the therapist be a *genuine* person within the therapeutic hour; that he experience an *unconditional regard* for his client; and that he himself experience and concurrently communicate a sensitively *empathic understanding* of his client's personal world. During the subsequent decade many investigators, notably Rogers and his younger collaborators (Rogers, Gendlin, Kiesler, & Truax, 1967), developed appropriate rating scales and also, collectively at first and then individually, subjected these three variables or core ingredients for successful psychotherapy to intensive investigative scrutiny. The results of their own research efforts and those of other investigators have been reviewed by Truax and Carkhuff (1967), Bierman (1969), Truax and Mitchell (1971), Kiesler (1973), and others. Additionally, objective rating scales, with numerous verbatim examples, for use by judges in assessing how much or how little any given interviewer or psychotherapist evidences each of these three facilitative core conditions in his verbalizations, have been published by Truax and Carkhuff (1967), and the contents of these three scales have been collated for easy reference by Kiesler (1973, pp. 428–431). Although questions have been raised by Chinsky and Rappaport (1970) and Rappaport and Chinsky (1972) about the meaning of one of these core process variables, Truax's construct of accurate empathy, researchers continue to find this process variable useful—as judged by the continuing flow of research on it. A comprehensive review of the reliability of judges' use of these three scales also was published by Truax and Mitchell (1971, pp. 320–321), and numerous validity studies on them are reviewed by Truax and his collaborator in this same publication, as well as in the various reviews by him and others cited above.

No attempt will be made to duplicate these reliability and validity literature reviews here. Rather the intent is to review the accumulating literature on one of these variables, *empathy,* as this literature relates to our own program of investigative interest and the more general issue of focus in this review. Many writers cited in the reviews above have attempted to define this process or phenomenon of empathy. Here, we will cite only one of these sources, Truax and Mitchell (1971, pp. 317–319), who describe it as follows:

Accurate empathic understanding involves the ability to *perceive* and *communicate* accurately and with sensitivity both the feelings and experiences of another person and their meaning and significance. . . . This allows us to contribute to the expansion and clarification of the other person's own awareness of his experiences and feelings. This is the essence of the fine balance between identification with the other person and objectivity that is the hallmark of an accurately empathic person. Being empathic, we assume the role of the other person, and in that role initiate ourselves the process of self-exploration as if we were the other person himself. In dealing with the disturbed person, it is as if we were providing *a model for him to follow* [emphasis added], as if we were saying by our example "even fearful or terrifying experiences or feelings are not so terrible that they cannot be touched and looked at."

Intensive focusing on the other person, of course, is central to the perceptive aspect of deep empathic understanding, since it allows us to note subtle nonverbal communications—the minute facial, postural, and gestural clues that often contradict or multiply the meaning of another person's verbal communications.

As we have all learned in life, people are not always what they seem. All of us have been conditioned from childhood to present social facades so that we often say in a polite manner when we are insulted or hurt and are asked about it, "Oh no, that doesn't matter." Even with a minimal empathic grasp, the other person should be able to see that it does indeed bother us a great deal. Thus, to be empathic we must separate the meaningful communications from another person from those arising from a defensive screen or social facade.

Most basically, of course, we rely upon the moment-by-moment changes in the other person as a sign of what is most meaningful. . . . Thus hurried and empty laughter can communicate as deeply and as clearly as moistened eyes; the overly strong denial tells us as much as the halting and strained confrontation. Often a blush, a stammer, a flood of words, a change in breathing, a tensing of posture, or a lack of socially appropriate feeling, may be much more important than what the other person at that moment is saying in words.

In one sense we help clarify another person's understanding of himself by serving as a mirror to his emotional and phenomenological self. Just as he learns about his physical self by seeing his image in a mirror, he learns about his emotional and phenomenological self by hearing these aspects of him reflected by us.

When empathy is defined in terms of operational scales measuring the therapist's responses to the client, it becomes clear that what is being measured is an *interpersonal* skill [emphasis added] rather than simply an attitude or a personality attribute.

As noted above, empathy is a characteristic of humans which manifests itself in a communicational interpersonal encounter, be the encounter with one's parent, peer, spouse, teacher, neighbor, or other person. All humans possess a capacity for some empathic understanding of their conversational partner. The Truax Empathy Scale (Truax &

Carkhuff, 1967, pp. 46–58) permits a judge to assign an objective rating on empathic understanding of what is and has been transpiring, from very low to very high (1 to 9, respectively), to individual units of communication emitted by one person to another.

Although our own research on the interview during the past two decades has focused primarily on such noncontent variables of the two-person communication as each person's single units of duration of utterance, reaction time latency, and interruption behavior, we nevertheless early discerned, although we were not able to identify it as such at the time, that a process (e.g., synchrony) akin to empathy was becoming evident in the results of our research. Thus, in our earliest studies (as reported briefly above), we discovered that a change in the interviewer's speech and silence behavior was followed by comparable changes in the speech behavior of his interviewees. This early serendipitous finding led to a whole series of new studies (summarized years later by Matarazzo & Wiens, 1972, p. 91; p. 103; and in the present Figures 1 and 2) designed to investigate this phenomenon in more detail. The first of these was a study in which an interviewer, interviewing 20 *bona fide* job applicants, was asked to conduct his typical 45-minute nondirective, clinically oriented employment interview with each applicant, but to introduce one investigative constraint—namely, to restrict all his open-ended nondirective inquiries to 5 seconds each time he spoke during the first 15 minutes of the interview, to double these to 10 seconds in the next 15 minutes, and, finally, to return to the 5-second utterance baseline level in the last 15 minutes. The results of this 5-10-5 study, cross-validated in a subsequent study of 20 similar subjects (Ss) this time utilizing a 10-5-10 design (Matarazzo, Weitman, Saslow & Wiens, 1963), were quite striking. As the experimenter (E) increased or decreased his own speech duration (from 5.3 to 9.9 to 6.1 seconds) there was a comparable increase or decrease in the speech duration of the interviewee (from 24.3 to 46.9 to 26.6 seconds, $p < .001$). In an attempt to explain this dramatic finding of a 93% increase in Ss' duration of utterance when the interviewer doubled his own duration of utterance, and a cross-validation of this finding with 20 additional Ss in a 10-5-10-second study, we wrote:

> One hint of a mechanism other than duration as such for the interviewer's influence on duration of speech of the interviewee comes from the research of Lennard and Bernstein (1960, pp. 180–182). From the study of four therapists in eight psychotherapy experiences which lasted for a period of eight months, these investigators present evidence that patients report greater satisfaction with individual therapy sessions in which the therapist was more verbally active (i.e., spoke in longer average utterances) than for those in which he was less active verbally. The possibility suggested by this is that the 40 Ss of our (5-10-5 and 10-5-10) study talked more during the 10-sec periods because they experienced "more satisfaction" as a result of E's greater verbal

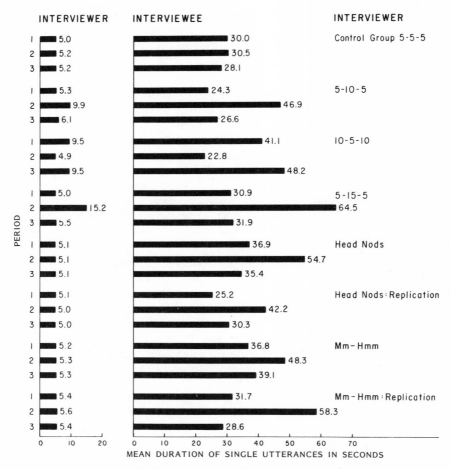

FIGURE 1. Interviewer influence on duration of interviewee speech.

participation during these periods. If this is the case, we may have found that greater participation by E (longer durations of single utterances) is a variable which correlated with a change in S's mood, which change in turn is followed by a longer verbalization on the part of S. If this mechanism accounts for all the duration effects we have cited above from our own and other studies, the modification of the mood of the interviewees by very short increments in duration of utterance (of the order of 5 sec) is surprising. (Matarazzo *et al.*, 1963, pp. 456–457)

During the next several years we extended our inquiry into the influence of increases in the interviewer's degree of activity on the duration of speech of his interviewee by: (1) an extension of these first two

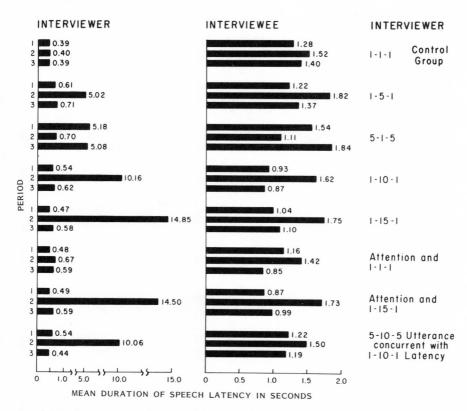

FIGURE 2. Interviewer influence on duration of interviewee reaction time latencies.

studies to a 5-15-5-second duration of utterance paradigm; (2) having our interviewer maintain his utterance durations unchanging throughout the three periods of the interview, but instructing him to *head nod* each time the interviewee began to speak in period 2; and (3) a repetition of this last design, except that the interviewer was instructed to substitute repeated Mm-Hmms for nodding in period 2. The results with each of these three increases in interviewer activity were as striking as those obtained in our first 5-10-5 study.

In subsequent research with similar job applicants, we instructed our interviewer to maintain a constant 5-5-5 duration of utterance during the 45-minute interview, but this time to vary his reaction time latency (RTL) before responding to the applicant's last utterance. A control group and four experimental groups were interviewed, utilizing the following interviewer RTLs across the three periods of the interview: 1-1-1, 1-5-1, 5-1-5, 1-10-1, and 1-15-1 seconds, respectively. The results revealed that, just as the case for the duration of utterance variable, there was a one-to-one synchrony between the latency behavior of the interviewees relative to that of the interviewer (see Figure 2).

These results appeared to be striking evidence that one human could influence the speech behavior of his or her conversational partner with no apparent conscious awareness of this on the part of the latter, nor, might we add, on the part of a host of experienced observers viewing these interviews from the other side of a one-way mirror. We reasoned that this latter lack of recognition of these subtle but striking changes may occur because we each have been conditioned to pay more conscious attention to the *content* of a conversation than to the formal properties of speech (DOU, RTL) which convey this content.

In 1967 we offered the following explanation of the results of the just described studies on interviewer and interviewee latency, and the earlier duration of utterance studies:

> To date our search for an explanation of the mechanism underlying the interviewer's ability to influence the interviewee's speech (utterance) duration has led us to postulate that any of a number of classes of behavior constituting greater activity by the interviewer (e.g., head nodding, saying Mm-Hmm, increasing his own speech durations) is interpreted by the interviewee as indicating that the interviewer is more interested in, or more *empathic* [emphasis added] toward, the interviewee, or that he otherwise values the interviewee more. That is, these interviewer tactics may be functioning as social reinforcing stimuli, each of them being "pleasing" to the interviewee in that they suggest to him that the interviewer is interested in him, or is satisfied with him. This perception of the interviewer's more positive attitude leads to a postulated state of "greater satisfaction" on the part of the interviewee in the dynamic two-person exchange and this hypothetical state in turn leads to greater activity (longer durations of single utterances) on the part of the interviewee.

> The results (of the RTL modifiability research) are still consistent with this hypothesis in that . . . short latencies on the part of the interviewer (and his concomitant greater talking) quite possibly are "pleasing" to the interviewee, whereas longer ones may be "anxiety-arousing" or otherwise "displeasing" to him, resulting in comparable short and long reaction times, respectively, on his part. (Matarazzo & Wiens, 1967, p. 65)

Although the design and methodology of our research on interview interaction had led us to describe the direction of the above influence process as emanating from the interviewer (whose behavior we were experimentally controlling) to the interviewee, we nevertheless were aware that the phenonemon of empathic influence was *reciprocal* and universal in all humans and not the province only of interviewers. Just this, in fact, was shown by Lauver, Kelley and Froehle (1971), who reversed the E and S roles used by us in a replication of our 1967 RTL study, making their "client" the E and their counselor the S, and who found results similar to ours. We stated our belief that empathy, albeit differing in levels, was universal when we wrote, in an annual review chapter, that psychotherapy

> is a natural framework within which to apply some of the vast store of knowledge in social psychology which appears to have immediate relevance to psychotherapy theory, practice, and research. For example, the social psychology of 'influence' or 'decision-making' as seen in two-person (and group) behavior; or the social psychology of 'communication processes'; the psychology of 'affiliation'; or 'cognitive dissonance'; etc. Those psychologists who heretofore have seemed to make a fetish of such concepts as 'the process' of psychotherapy, or who exalted 'the transference' relationship to a position of almost religious pre-eminence will learn, to their surprise I believe, that such mystical phenomena are probably little more that what occurs in most, if not all, social interactions; and that the same general laws and principles which are relevant to the study of other behavior also apply to the study of psychotherapy." (Matarazzo, 1965, pp. 217–218)

Nevertheless, the clinically oriented psychotherapy sessions, with each participant behaving freely and without instruction from us, were the principal sources of research data available to our research team, and thus we searched for evidence of these reciprocal relationships there. In fact, we found considerable evidence of such reciprocal as well as synchronous relationships (doctor to patient and patient to doctor, with neither one identifiable as cause or effect) in the first seven therapist–patient pairs of psychotherapy cases we studied (Matarazzo et al., 1968).

It was evident as we studied these seven psychotherapist–patient dyads that one or another of our seven therapist–patient pairs showed marked reciprocal "tracking" or "synchrony" in their interruption and silence behavior over sessions, whereas another pair among the seven, involving the same therapist paired with another patient, did not show such synchrony or reciprocal influence. These and the finding (Matarazzo et al., 1968, Tables 3, 4, 5, and 6) of other intrapair correlations on still other speech–speech behaviors for some of these seven pairs on still other variables, but no such finding for one or another of the seven pairs on the same variable, led us to express the hope that

> the results from our seven therapy cases with the duration of latency and percentage of interruption variables, presented earlier in this paper, along with the duration of utterance variable just discussed, will lead other investigators interested in "process" in psychotherapy (or parent–child, peer–peer, or other significant human interactions) to include measures of these three (speech) variables along with each investigator's own variables (ambiguity, type token ratio, empathy, focusing ability, positive regard, depth of interpretation, etc.).

> In our opinions, the types of data presented in this paper for the latency, interruption, and duration of utterance variables, collected concurrent with

comparably potentially rich variables now also being studied in isolation by other investigators, quite conceivably and in combination, could suggest heretofore unsuspected outcome measures which are derivatives of these various process measures and also have a higher probability of proving their validity and usefulness than any measures heretofore used or proposed. We believe the various evidences (albeit mostly empirical and not theoretically based, at this point) of "synchrony," "tracking," "modeling," and other forms of "reciprocal influence" demonstrated above for our seven therapy cases may hold just such promise for the student of "outcome" as well as the investigator interested in the "process" involved in many other human-to-human communication and interaction networks. (Matarazzo et al., 1968, pp. 392–393)

Only four years later, we found, and already were able to review, several studies demonstrating a relationship between one or another of our three mechanically recorded speech measures and one or another of the psychotherapy measures (specifically "experiencing" and "empathy") introduced by the Rogers, Gendlin, Kiesler, and Truax team (1967) and derived by judges listening to the actual content in the tape-recorded segments of psychotherapy interactions. Based on these preliminary findings with these two process variables, we wrote:

Inasmuch as duration of utterance as a measure can be derived quickly and efficiently from a tape recording merely by counting the words in an utterance, and latency and interruption derived almost as easily, these [just-reviewed studies relating process and formal speech characteristics] indicate that studies simultaneously using process measures from *each* of these content and noncontent systems are now possible. (Matarazzo & Wiens, 1972, p. 127)

These remarks were clearly a product of the *Zeitgeist*, for studies of the type being called for in the above quote and utilizing speech and silence measures concurrent with other process measures (such as empathy), and outcome measures already were underway. Other such studies would soon be reported. In the hope of furthering this area of investigative effort, we reviewed those studies involving both the process variable of *empathy* and speech and silence measures similar to our own and here summarize the correlations reported between empathy and speech in Table 1.

The Strupp and Wallach (1965) study shown at the top of Table 1 utilized 59 physician–psychotherapist Ss who were asked to *dictate* their own next verbal response to the patient's last comment while viewing two psychotherapy films developed by the investigators. The film was stopped at the same preselected points for each S, and this permitted Strupp and Wallach to record, among many other variables, such noncontent variables as whether S did or did not make a comment at each point (frequency of no talk), when he or she did speak each S's reaction

TABLE 1
Speech and Silence Correlates of Speaker's Rated Level of Empathy

	Interviewer							Interviewee				
	Mean duration of utterance[1]	Total talk time[a]	Proportion of total talk time	Frequency of no talk (total silence)	Mean reaction time (latency)	Frequency of interruptions	Percentage of interruptions	Mean duration of utterance[1]	Total talk time by interviewee	Mean reaction time (latency)	Type of S	Empathy measure
Strupp & Wallach (1965)		.30*		-.41**							outpatients	Strupp
Caracena & Vicory (1969)	.60**	.47**	.42*	-.31*							students	Truax
Truax (1970)		.56**	.44**								outpatients	Truax
Wenegrat (1976)	.10	.44**									students	Truax
Hargrove (1974)	.17†	.67**									outpatients	Listar
Pope et al. (1974)					.38**	-.32**	-.28**		.65**		students	Truax
Staples & Sloane (1976)	.45†	.11		-.69**				.63**	.57**	-.67**	outpatients	Truax

Significance levels at the .001, .01, .05, and .10 levels are shown by ***, **, *, and † respectively.

[a]Mean duration of utterance and total talk time as shown here were measured either by use of a recording instrument or by counting number of words on a typescript.

time latency before dictating what she or he would have said next, and the duration of each of these dictated responses. This latter measure was converted into total time of talk per film for each S. To derive their degree of empathy level for each S, the *content* of the same dictated responses by each S was scored *independently* by raters on a three-point empathy scale developed by Strupp.

The significant correlations between the empathy rating and each of several speech measures from their study have been reproduced in Table 1. These rs show that a therapist who is judged independently from the content of his or her verbalizations to be high in empathy (1) talks and says more words during a total therapy session (r of .30, p < .05; cross-validated on film 2 with an r of .47, p < .01), and (2) utilizes proportionally fewer times the tactic of no response of any kind when the patient completes a comment (rs of $-.41$ and $-.31$, p levels < .01 and .05, respectively). Thus, the empathic therapist, as judged by content, is the one who is more verbally active, as judged by noncontent measures.

Truax (1970) cross-validated the first of these findings in another study using real psychotherapists and their patients, although, as shown in Table 1, he used his own empathy scale and the talk measures of therapist total talk time and proportion of total talk time utilized by the interviewer (rs of .56 and .44, p < .01 in both instances). Similarly, the study of Caracena and Vicory (1969), utilizing taped segments from interviewers interviewing undergraduate Ss and also independent ratings of the degree of empathy in E's comments, reported values of rho for empathy × talk (.60, p < .01; .42, p < .05) not unlike those in the Strupp and Wallach and the Truax studies. Pope (personal communication), as a byproduct of a study by Pope, Nudler, Vonkorff, and McGhee (1974), confirmed the findings of Strupp and Wallach, Truax, and also Caracena and Vicory, by demonstrating with novice interviewers an equally highly significant r of .67 (p < .01) between the Truax empathy measure and Pope's own measure of productivity (a simple word count of an S's utterances). Interestingly, study of the Pope *et al.* second group of Es, experienced interviewers, revealed no such r between empathy and words in an utterance. Thus, *novice* interviewers who spoke more words were found to be high in empathy as judged independently, and vice versa, whereas this relationship did not hold for their sample of *professional* interviewers interviewing the same pool of student Ss.

Consistent with the finding in these four studies that interviewers who are rated to be high in empathy from the *contents* of their utterances also talk longer (or talk in longer mean durations of single utterances), Staples and Sloane (1976), utilizing short-term analytically oriented psychotherapists treating 17 patients from an outpatient psychiatry service, and Hargrove (1974), utilizing both outpatients and college student clients talking with Ph.D. and Master's level therapists, reported results in this same direction but could only confirm this same finding at much lower magnitudes of correlation (rs of .45 and .17, each of which, with their own, albeit differing, Ns, fell between the .05 and .10 level of confidence). However, in a follow-up paper, Staples, Sloane, Whipple, Cristol, and Yorkston (1976) extended this earlier N of 17 to 60 patients, choosing their additional 43 patients from among those seen by *behavior therapists* as well as by *psychotherapists*. Although reporting their findings in this follow-up paper by bar graphs rather than by correlations, they found with this larger N what appear to be even stronger relationships between speech and empathy than those shown in our Table 1 from their initial study. We shall return to this study when we discuss Table 2.

Finally, one study of the seven found by us in the literature reported results at variance with the thrust of these other six. Specifically, Wenegrat (1974), in a study utilizing 12 University of California (Berkeley) Psychology Clinic therapists employing *psychoanalytically oriented* therapy with 30 clients, reported a lack of correlation between the Truax empathy measure and each of several speech measures roughly comparable to those used by us and the other investigators shown in Table 1. However, in a replication of this study with tapes of *client-centered therapy* provided her from three settings, Wenegrat (1976) found a correlation of .44 (p of .01) between total number of words spoken by her therapists in the 4-minute segments of therapy analyzed and the Truax accurate empathy ratings independently derived from the same segments. Mean duration of utterance, measured by mean number of words per response, showed no correlation (r of .10) with empathy. These results also are shown in Table 1. Thus, in regard to these particular speech measures, Wenegrat found no speech correlates of empathy in psychoanalytically oriented therapy, but did find one such correlate in client-centered therapy.

To summarize, then, we located seven studies in the literature which have correlated the level of judged empathy in a person's speech content and the length, duration, or total talk time of that person in the same conversation or interview. Five of these studies show a moderately strong positive correlation between these two variables, one has shown a positive but more modest relation, and one found a strong relationship only in the client-centered therapy group but no relationship in psychoanalytic therapy group. Interestingly, those studies utilizing real psychotherapists and real (or simulated) outpatients (Staples & Sloane, 1976; Strupp & Wallach, 1965; Truax, 1970) did not appear to show the empathy × speech correlations to a greater extent than did the studies

TABLE 2
Speech and Silence Correlates of Ratings on Outcome of Psychotherapy

	Interviewer					Interviewee			Outcome measure
	Mean duration of utterance[a]	Total talk time[a]	Proportion of total talk time	Number of therapist speech units	Mean reaction time latency	Mean duration of utterance	Total talk time	Mean reaction time latency	
Truax (1970)			.39*						Therapist rating of global impression
			.34*						Patient rating of global impression
Staples & Sloane (1976)	.25	−.43†		−.58**	−.02	.36	.57**	−.51*	Rating by an experienced psychiatrist

Significance levels at the .01, .05, and .10 levels are shown by **, *, and †, respectively.

[a]Mean duration of utterance and total talk time were measured by use of a recording instrument.

utilizing undergraduate Ss, with the strongest correlations being found in two of these latter (the Caracena & Vicory and the Pope *et al.* studies).

It would appear from these seven studies that *interviewers who talk for longer durations than other interviewers are also the interviewers who are highest in empathy, as independently judged from listening to the tape recordings.* However, a methodological caution has been introduced in such a straightforward interpretation of these reported correlations between empathy and duration of speech by both Strupp and Wallach (1965, p. 128) and Caracena and Vicory (1969, p. 514). Each of these investigators caution that the empathy ratings, although made by judges independent from those who analyzed the speech durations, could nevertheless be spurious, because interviewers who speak little might be receiving the lowest empathy ratings primarily because of insufficient word-data upon which to base a higher rating. Thus, the positive rs shown in Table 1 merely may be reflecting the artifact that Es who speak more provide more data for judgment and, thus, more data upon which to be given a higher empathy rating.

This caution regarding a potential methodological artifact is a good one, and the problem might be studied in a number of ways. For example, as recently considered by Staples (personal communication), one could concurrently vary both utterance length and level of empathy in a factorial design. Thus, one could use predesigned interviewer utterances of 10 seconds, 20 seconds, and 30 seconds in length and vary the level of interviewer empathy (low, medium, and high) of each utterance at *each* of these three durations of utterance. Using a dependent measure such as interviewee duration of utterance or interviewee "satisfaction with" or "liking of" the interviewer should allow one to sort out the relative contribution of each of the two independently controlled interviewer variables. Staples *et al.* (1976) have made a beginning in just such studies.

An alternative approach, one that could be carried out by psychotherapy investigators on data they already have collected, would utilize a correlational design involving a series of single psychotherapist-patient pairs. By selecting out single psychotherapist tape recorded *segments* of an interview in which the therapist talked in differing mean lengths of utterance (say, means of 5, 8, 12, and 15 seconds), and having these same segments rated independently for the level of empathy exhibited, the investigator need merely compute a Pearson *r* and thereby determine to what extent, if any, ratings of empathy level increase as mean utterance length increases. In the absence of empirical data from either of these two designs, there is today no reason to believe empathy level either is or is not associated with longer therapist–interviewer utterances. It is a question, nevertheless, that should be examined.

The remainder of the interviewer data in Table 1 reveals that there have been fewer findings published on the two other speech measures, silence (or reaction time) and interruption, than those just reviewed on duration of utterance. Nevertheless, from the Strupp and Wallach (1965) and the Staples and Sloane (1976) studies the three rs ($-.41$, $-.31$, and $-.69$; two at the .01 and one at the .05 level) shown in the Total Silence column are consistent in direction and suggest that an interviewer who is rated high in empathy is one who less frequently uses *total* silence (no response) following an interviewee comment. Additionally, the single rs for the reaction time and two interruption measures in the Hargrove (1974) study suggest that an interviewer who is rated high in empathy waits longer before speaking (with a longer reaction time) when answering the interviewee, and, also, that he or she tends not to interrupt the speech of his interviewee. Clearly, further independent confirmation of the findings by other investigators is necessary before they can be reliably interpreted.

Taken as a whole, however, the interviewer–therapist data in Table 1 suggest that, relative to interviewers who are judged lower in empathy, interviewers who are rated high in level of empathy by judges who listen to randomly selected tape segments are also interviewers who: (1) talk more per utterance and per total segment; (2) use total silence (no response) less; (3) speak with a longer reaction time when they do answer their conversational partner; and (4) interrupt the latter less frequently. Given the disparate ways in which these three speech variables have been recorded from one study to another in Table 1 (actual timed duration of utterance, word count from a transcript, and so on), and the fact that three different *measures* of empathy were employed (Strupp, Truax, Lister), the consistency in these findings shown in Table 1 is even more impressive. Nevertheless, a bit of attention should be paid in future studies to the Strupp and Wallach (1965) caution that two few words in an utterance may provide too small a sample from which to ascertain a high level of empathy. A factorial or correlational study along the lines suggested above should provide a quick answer to whether or not this is in fact the case.

The *interviewee* data shown in the right half of Table 1 is much sparser, with only two of the seven studies (Pope *et al.*, 1974; Staples & Sloane, 1976) finding any such interviewee correlations. Both studies, reporting strong correlations, found that interviewees talk more (rs of .65, $p < .01$; and .57, $p < .01$) in interaction with interviewers of higher judged levels of empathy. Additionally, the single finding reported in the very last column in Table 1 indicates that higher interviewer empathy was associated with a shorter patient reaction time (r of $-.67$, $p < .01$) in the interview. These last interviewee speech and silence findings were interpreted as follows: "total speech time was greater with higher therapist empathy. . . . This again resulted from an increase in the average duration of speech units rather than more frequent speech. Patients also responded more quickly to their therapists under higher levels [of empathy]" (Staples & Sloane, 1976).

Thus, along with the suggestion from the left half of Table 1 that interviewers judged high in empathy *emit* more words when they do speak, Staples and Sloane also are suggesting (right half of Table 1) that therapists high in empathy also *elicit* following a short reaction time, more total talk and more words per utterance from their clients and patients. Parenthetically, it might be interesting to note that this last finding, one cross-validated by Pope *et al.* (1974), that patients emit more words per unit in the presence of a more empathic and inferentially better liked interviewer, is consistent with a finding (Wiens, Jackson, Manaugh, & Matarazzo, 1969) that a relatively larger total number of words in a letter of recommendation is a nonverbal mirror of the communicator's more positive underlying attitude. In any event, the Staples and Sloane and the Pope *et al.* results shown in Table 1 are very promising and suggest that further research of this type also may not go unrewarded. One example of such research is the study conducted at Harvard by Harrigan and Rosenthal (1983) who, extending the research reported here by us as well as by others, studied the influence of manipulations of the bodily movements of a filmed physician on the level of rapport established under each condition as perceived by patients. The authors conclude that the "results of this study demonstrate that *head nodding* (italics added here) and leaning forward are equally influential behaviors in the judgment of rapport" (p. 504). Extending this line of research into still another dimension, Kraut, Lewis and Swezey (1982) cross-validated another of the findings from our research by showing that in a two-person conversation involving feedback about a movie, longer or shorter utterances by the speaker providing the feedback correlated .30 (*p* of .007) with similarly longer or shorter summaries of such feedback by the conversational partner (p. 723). Finally, some of the speech variables which we began studying 30 years ago with the hope of increasing our understanding of empathy, rapport, and other dynamic processing in psychotherapy, employment interviews, and other two-person conversations also are providing insights into some of today's problems in health psychology and behavioral medicine; for example, as exemplified in the study by Dembroski, MacDougall and Musante (1984). Among their many other reported findings, these authors suggest that the noncontent (stylistic) speech behavior of the person with the Type A Behavioral Pattern (those with a greater relative risk for coronary heart disease) is different than that of the Type B person.

We were able to find only two studies in the literature that related to our other earlier suggestion that objective measures of speech might be found to correlate not only with process but also with *outcome* variables. These two are the Truax (1970) and the Staples and Sloane (1976) studies, and the results relating their several interviewer and interviewee process speech measures to total therapy outcome are shown in Table 2. The results for the interviewer in this table are far from clear-cut. The Truax (1970, p. 540) study found (*r*s of .39 and .34, both *p* < .05) that there was "a moderate but positive relationship between the . . . proportion of therapist talk and (each of two) measures of patient improvement." On the other hand, the Staples and Sloane preliminary findings with 17 patients suggest (*r* of −.43, *p* of .10) that *psychotherapists* who emit less total talk time, as well as who talk a few number of times (*r* of −.58, *p* of .01) are those whose patients achieve the better outcomes. Concurrently, Staples and Sloane found that a better therapy outcome was associated with more *patient* total talk time (*r* of .57, *p* of .01) emitted after a relatively short reaction time (*r* of −.51, *p* < .05). At best, these two sets of outcome findings in Table 2 can be considered only preliminary findings. However, the results appear even more striking, for both psychotherapists *and* behavior therapists, in the recently enlarged Staples *et al.* (1976) sample. Utilizing a larger sample than the 17 shown here in Tables 1 and 2 (i.e., 30 patients treated by short-term analytic *psychotherapy* and 30 patients treated by *behavior therapy*), they found that:

> Patients who spoke more in (psycho)therapy, that is, those who showed greater total speech time, did better in *psychotherapy* than those who spoke less. Such patients did not speak more often (no difference in number of speech units), but they spoke in longer units when they did speak (marked difference in average speech durations). Successful patients also tended to react more quickly to the therapist's comments as the difference (shown in bar graphs and not as a correlation in this later paper) between high and low reaction times approached statistical significance.

> With *behavior therapy*, differences between successful and less successful patients were not as marked. As in psychotherapy, patients who spoke in longer (mean) units showed significantly greater improvement than those who spoke in shorter units. However (in these patients being treated by behavior therapy), neither total speech time nor average reaction time was related to success. [Staples *et al.*, 1976, pp. 343–344]

The following additional finding from this enlarged Staples *et al.* (1976, p. 343) report relates both to the literature we have reviewed in Table 1 and Table 2 and also quite likely will generate considerable interest:

> Behavior therapists showed significantly higher levels of depth of interpersonal contact, empathy, and self-congruence than psychotherapists, but these differences do not appear relevant to the amount of patient improvement.

Thus, it is interesting to note, both from the Staples and Sloane (1976) preliminary publication summarized in Table 2 and their just-described extended study comparing behavior therapists with psychotherapists, that: (1) significant correlations between interviewer and interviewee speech behavior and independent ratings of therapeutic outcome do already appear in the literature, and (2) successful behavior therapists evidence empathy, and this characteristic can be assessed by simply recorded, behavioral speech measures.

We do not believe, however, that the findings reviewed and summarized in Tables 1 and 2 constitute *definitive* support for our often-stated conviction that objective speech measures easily and inexpensively obtained from a tape recording show promise of being heuristically useful indices of the rich interaction that constitutes the process, and even judged outcome, of the two-person psychotherapy or other interview transaction. We do believe, however, that the data in Tables 1 and 2 are suggestive enough of this possibility that further research along these lines is warranted. Specifically, direct applications of these findings may now be possible, inasmuch as these easily recorded speech and silence behaviors of therapists are simpler for therapists to control and modify than are the more subjective intrapsychic variables, so long the focus of earlier practitioners and investigators of psychotherapy. The published articles by Staples and Sloane and their colleagues, plus their book (Sloane, Staples, Cristol, Yorkston, & Whipple, 1975) are a significant step in this direction. However, their research, like some of our own on interview and psychotherapy process, and with the exception of the studies summarized here in Figures 1 and 2, has been naturalistic and unplanned, investigating speech, process, and outcome variables as they occur *in vivo without* planned experimental intervention specifically prescribed for the individual patient.

The possibilities of *planned* thereapeutic intervention designed to produce more effective social skills in a particular patient are clearly evident in the clinical research on behavior modification of Bellack, Eisler, Hersen, McFall, and other workers that was reviewed by Hersen and Bellack (1976). Among many other variables included in these researches have been the patient's pre- and posttest duration of reply and latency of response, measures similar to those shown in our Tables 1 and 2. For example, Hersen, Turner, Edelstein, and Pinkston (1975) examined the effects of phenothiazines and social skills training in a 27-year-old chronic withdrawn schizophrenic man. An intensive social skills training program (targeted at three behaviors—eye contact, latency of response, and requests) lasting five weeks was instituted to improve interpersonal functioning. At the end of treatment, improvements in eye contact and latency were noted, but improvement in number of requests to an interpersonal partner were correlated with changes obtained when treatment was applied to latency. Interestingly, concurrent improvements in the three untreated behaviors (overall assertiveness, voice trailing off to a whisper, and speech disruptions) also were found. In addition, the patient's verbal productivity increased in group psychotherapy throughout the five-week course of social skills training. The reader wishing a more detailed review of this literature on actual and potential use of behavior modification techniques in the individual case is referred to Hersen and Bellack (1976), as well as to the many specific studies and reviews published by them, Eisler, and their coworkers.

The first empirical glimmerings suggesting the possibility of *in vivo* therapeutic modification of speech leading to the studies that we only then were designing (the later results of which we have summarized in Figures 1 and 2) began to emanate from our own research almost two decades ago. However, even in the absence of robust data in those early days, the potential for the direct application of these early findings in modifying, through *prescribed* behavior therapy, the behavior of individual patients in the clinical setting had become apparent:

> The present results indicate that planned intra-interview changes in the interviewer's behavior have a marked, and reproducible, effect on the corresponding intra-interview behavior of interviewees from a variety of crude diagnostic groups. . . . [The present results] suggest the possibility of beginning investigations of prescribed behavior therapy. That is, if one of the characteristics of some depressed patients is that they speak infrequently, and when they do, in utterances of short durations, then one might ask what would be the effect on their duration of utterances of an interviewer, himself, using only long utterances when interviewing them? Would there be a corresponding increase in the patient's own duration of utterance and, thus, along this one dimension, at least, less "depression"? Likewise, with patients who speak in unusually long utterances, e.g., the so-called manic patient, would the effect of an interviewer using unusually brief utterances (e.g., one or two words per communication unit) be to reduce these long patient utterances? Even if such suggested interviewer-produced changes in patient-interviewee behavior could be produced within the interview situation itself, such changes would be merely a beginning, since further research would then be needed to be undertaken to study whether or not, and with what persistence, such intra-interview-produced interviewee changes do, in fact, generalize to the patient's everyday behavior in a variety of life situations.
>
> Numerous studies suggest themselves here: (1) which dimensions of interview behavior can be modified within the interview? . . ., (2) which type of patient is most amenable to non-content intra-interview behavior change, and along which interview dimensions?, (3) which intra-interview behavior changes will generalize to noninterview situations, and under which extrainterview conditions?, (4) which interviewer characteristics (age, sex, experience, interaction characteristics, etc.) are related to which interviewee changes, if any?, (5) under which conditions can content and non-content variables be manipulated simultaneously, or in varying combinations, to produce which effects?, etc. It is clear from merely the few research pos-

sibilities here suggested, and the results earlier described, that careful study of non-content (as well as content) interaction measures may make it possible for us someday to pair (for psychotherapy) an interviewer, with his own unique interaction characteristics, with a selected patient with whom this interviewer's interaction pattern might best be suited. (Matarazzo, 1962, pp. 491–492)

When these words were first put to pen twenty years ago, *prescriptive* behavior modification was a hope. The readers of this chapter now know it to be a reality. It is the hope of the writers that the behavioral data reviewed here in Tables 1 and 2 and Figures 1 and 2 will suggest additional ways in which the interpersonal processes associated with successful behavior modification can be both conceptualized theoretically and prescribed humanistically, thus fostering both our understanding of the processes involved in effective behavior modification and the application of these understandings to the individual who seeks help.

NOTE: RELATED SCALES OR CONSTRUCTS

The Speech Interaction System variables (duration of utterance, silence, and interruption) are very similar to some of the category scores used by Lennard and Bernstein (1960), particularly to the latter author's units of quantity. Some of the findings of the two groups are quite consistent.

Jaffe and Feldstein (1970) outlined their development of a completely automated technique of interaction chronography that feeds directly into a computer system. The Automatic Vocal Transaction Analyser (AVTA) is based on audio pickup of interview interaction from a two-channel tape recorder.

AVTA is a two-channel speech detector and analog to digital converter designed to bridge the gap between live and tape-recorded interviews and an on-line digital computer. As a two-channel A to D converter it has much in common with other interaction chronograph systems in which the subjects' behaviors are tracked either manually or by means of a voice-actuated relay. Its unique feature is a network which electronically cancels the unintended "spill" of each speaker's voice to one channel of the audio-tape even though ordinary microphones are used and the speakers are conversing at close range in a face-to-face situation. This particular feature eliminates the need to separate the participants bv isolation booths, or by use of throat or bone microphones, or other such solutions to the "cross-talk" problem. The goal was, of course, maintenance of as natural a dialogic content as possible.

Jaffe and Feldstein conclude that "we have completely automated the technique of interaction chronography. The complete process, from microphone input to computer generated statistical summary, is accomplished in a single operation without human intervention" (p. 123).

Since analyses of interaction processes occurring in psychotherapy have shown results having clear relevance to psychotherapy theory and other research, perhaps the day will come when all interview researchers will record their interview materials on two-channel tape recorders hooked into an AVTA system, which would permit easy comparison of interaction variables with the other measures that a particular researcher employs. Importantly, investigators wishing to do research in this area, especially graduate students, not having access to the Matarazzo Interaction Recorder or Jaffe's AVTA, can tape-record sessions and then use either a word count or stopwatch as described by Wiens, Molde, Holman, and Matarazzo (1966) and Matarazzo, Holman, and Wiens (1967), or any of a number of inexpensive recording devices costing only a few dollars. Examples of the latter have been described by Kasl and Mahl (1956), Lauver (1970), and Hargrove and Martin (1982), among others. Simple word count as a measure of utterance duration has also been used by Pope and Siegman (1966), and Ray and Webb (1966).

REFERENCES

Allen, B. V., Wiens, A. N., Weitman, M., & Saslow, G. (1965). Effects of warm-cold set on interviewee speech. *Journal of Consulting Psychology, 29,* 480–482.

Bergin, A. E., & Garfield, S. L. (1971). *Handbook of psychotherapy and behavior change: An empirical analysis.* New York: John Wiley.

Bergin, A. E., & Strupp, H. H. (1972). *Changing frontiers in the science of psychotherapy.* Chicago: Aldine.

Bierman, R. (1969). Dimensions of interpersonal facilitation in psychotherapy and child development. *Psychological Bulletin, 72,* 338–352.

Caracena, P. F., & Vicory, J. R. (1969). Correlates of phenomenological and judged empathy. *Journal of Conseling Psychology, 16,* 510–515.

Chapple, E. D. (1939). Quantative analysis of the interaction of individuals. *Proceedings of the National Academy of Science, 25,* 58–67.

Chapple, E. D. (1956). *The Interaction Chronograph manual.* Noroton, CT: E. D. Chapple Company.

Chapple, E. D., & Arensberg, C. M. (1940). Measuring human relations: An introduction to the study of the interaction of individuals. *Genetic Psychology Monographs, 22,* 3–147.

Chapple, E. D., & Donald, G., Jr. (1946). A method for evaluating supervisory personnel. *Harvard Business Review, 24,* 197–214.

Chinsky, J. M., & Rappaport, J. (1970). Brief critique of the meaning and reliability of "accurate empathy" ratings. *Psychological Bulletin, 73,* 379–382.

Craig, K. D. (1966). Incongruencies between content and temporal measures of patients' responses to confrontation with personality descriptions. *Journal of Consulting Psychology, 30,* 550–554.

Dembroski, T. M., MacDougall, J. M., & Musante, L. (1984). Desirability of control versus locus of control: Relationship of paralinguistics in the Type A interview. *Health Psychology, 3,* 15–26.

Duncan, S., Jr. (1969). Nonverbal communication. *Psychological Bulletin, 72,* 118–137.

Goldman-Eisler, F. (1968). *Psycholinguistics: Experiments in spontaneous speech.* New York: Academic Press.

Goldstein, A. P., Heller, K., & Sechrest, L. B. (1966). *Psychotherapy and the psychology of behavior change.* New York: John Wiley.

Hargrove, D. S. (1974). Verbal interaction analysis of empathic and nonempathic responses of therapists. *Journal of Consulting and Clinical Psychology, 42,* 305 (and manuscript of extended report).

Hargrove, D. S., & Martin, T. A. (1982). Development of a microcomputer system for verbal interaction analysis. *Behavioral research methods and instrumentation, 14,* 236–239.

Harrigan, J. A., & Rosenthal, R. (1983). Physicians' head and body positions as determinants of perceived rapport. *Journal of Applied Social Psychology, 13,* 496–509.

Hersen, M., & Bellack, A. S. (1976). Social Skills training for chronic psychiatric patients: Rationale, research findings, and future direction. *Comprehensive Psychiatry, 17,* 559–580.

Hersen, M., Turner, S. M., Edelstein, B. A., & Pinkston, S. G. (1975). Effects of phenothiazines and social skills training in a withdrawn schizophrenic. *Journal of Clinical Psychology, 31,* 588–594.

Jackson, R. H., Manaugh, T. S., Wiens, A. N., & Matarazzo, J. D. (1971). A method for assessing the saliency level of areas in a person's current life situation. *Journal of Clinical Psychology, 27,* 32–39.

Jackson, R. H., Wiens, A. N., Manaugh, T. S., & Matarazzo, J. D. (1972). Speech behavior under conditions of differential saliency in interview content. *Journal of Clinical Psychology, 28,* 318–327.

Jaffe, J., & Feldstein, S. (1970). *Rhythms of dialogue.* New York: Academic Press.

Johnston, G., Jansen, J., Weitman, M., Hess, H. F., Matarazzo, J. D., & Saslow, G. A. (1961, July). A punched tape data preparation system for use in psychiatric interviews. *Digest of the 1961 International Conference on Medical Electronics,* p. 17.

Kasl, S. V., & Mahl, G. F. (1956). A simple device for obtaining certain verbal activity measures during interviews. *Journal of Abnormal and Social Psychology, 53,* 388–390.

Kiesler, D. J. (1973). *The process of psychotherapy: Empirical foundations and systems of analysis.* Chicago: Aldine.

Kraut, R. E., Lewis, S. H., & Swezey, L. W. (1982). Listener responsiveness and the coordination of conversation. *Journal of Personality and Social Psychology, 43,* 718–731.

Lauver, P. J. (1970). Inexpensive apparatus for quantifying speech and silence behaviors. *Journal of Counseling Psychology, 17,* 378–389.

Lauver, P. J., Kelly, J. D., & Froehle, T. C. (1971). Client reaction time and counselor verbal behavior in an interview setting. *Journal of Counseling Psychology, 18,* 26–30.

Lennard, H. L., & Bernstein, A. (1960). *The anatomy of psychotherapy: Systems of communication and expectation.* New York: Columbia University Press.

Manaugh, T. S., Wiens, A. N., & Matarazzo, J. D. (1970). Content saliency and interviewee speech behavior. *Journal of Clinicial Psychology, 26,* 17–24.

Matarazzo, J. D. (1962). Prescribed behavior therapy: Suggestions from interview research. In A. J. Bachrach (Ed.), *Experimental foundations of clinical psychology* (pp. 471–509). New York: Basic Books.

Matarazzo, J. D. (1965a). The interview. In B. B. Wolman (Ed.), *Handbook of clinical psychology* (pp. 403–450). New York: McGraw-Hill.

Matarazzo, J. D. (1965b). Psychotherapeutic processes. In P. R. Farnsworth, O. McNemar, & Q. McNemar (Eds.), *Annual review of psychology*, (Vol. 16). Palo Alto, CA: Annual Reviews, Inc.

Matarazzo, J. D., & Wiens, A. N. (1967). Interviewer influence on duration of interviewee silence. *Journal of Experimental Research in Personality, 2*, 56–59.

Matarazzo, J. D., & Wiens, A. N. (1972). *The interview: Research on its anatomy and structure.* Chicago: Aldine.

Matarazzo, J. D., & Wiens, A. N. (1977). Speech behavior as an objective correlate of empathy and outcome in interview and psychotherapy research: A review with implications for behavior modification. *Behavior Modification, 1*, 453–480.

Matarazzo, J. D., Saslow, G., & Matarazzo, R. G. (1956). The interaction Chronograph as an instrument for objective measurement of interaction patterns during interviews. *Journal of Psychology, 41*, 347–367.

Matarazzo, J. D., Saslow, G., & Hare, A. P. (1958). Factor analysis of interview interaction behavior. *Journal of Consulting Psychology, 22*, 419–429.

Matarazzo, J. D., Weitman, M., Saslow, G., & Wiens, A. N. (1963). Interviewer influence on durations of interviewer speech. *Journal of Verbal Learning and Verbal Behavior, 1*, 451–458.

Matarazzo, J. D., Wiens, A. N., Saslow, G., Allen, B. V., & Weitman, M. (1964). Interviewer mm-hmm and interviewee speech durations. *Psychotherapy: Theory, Research and Practice, 1*, 109–114.

Matarazzo, J. D., Wiens, A. N., Saslow, G., Dunham, R. M., & Voas, R. B. (1964). Speech durations of astronaut and ground communicator. *Science, 143*, 148–150.

Matarazzo, J. D., Wiens, A. N., & Saslow, G. (1965). Studies in interview speech behavior. In L. Krasner & L. P. Ullmann (Eds.), *Research in behavior modification: New developments and clinical application* (pp. 179–210). New York: Holt, Rinehart & Winston.

Matarazzo, J. D., Wiens, A. N., Matarazzo, R. G., & Saslow, G. (1968). Speech and silence behavior in clinical psychotherapy and its laboratory correlates. In J. M. Schlien, H. F. Hunt, J. D. Matarazzo, & C. Savage (Eds.), *Research in psychotherapy* (Vol. 3, pp. 347–394). Washington, DC: American Psychological Association.

Matarazzo, J. D., Holman, D. C., & Wiens, A. N. (1967). A simple measure of interviewer and interviewee speech durations. *Journal of Psychology, 66*, 7–14.

Matarazzo, J. D., Wiens, A. N., Jackson, R. H., & Manaugh, T. S. (1970a). Interviewee speech behavior under conditions of endogenously-present and exogenously-induced motivational states. *Journal of Clinical Psychology, 26*, 141–148.

Matarazzo, J. D., Wiens, A. N., Jackson, R. H., & Manaugh, T. S. (1970b). Interviewee speech behavior under different content conditions. *Journal of Applied Psychology, 54*, 15–26.

Matarazzo, J. D., Wiens, A. N., & Manaugh, T. S. (1975). IQ correlates of speech and silence behavior under three dyadic speaking conditions. *Journal of Consulting and Clinical Psychology, 43*, 198–204.

Mehrabian, A. (1972). *Nonverbal communication.* Chicago: Aldine.

Morganstern, K. P. (1976). Behavioral interviewing: The initial stages of assessment. In M. Hersen & A. S. Bellack (Eds.), *Behavioral assessment: A practical handbook.* New York: Pergamon Press.

Morris, R. L., Johnston, G. L., Bailey, D. D., & Wiens, A. N. (1968). A twenty-four channel temporal-event digital recording system. *Medical Research Engineering, 7*, 32–37.

Phillips, J. S., Matarazzo, J. D., Matarazzo, R. G., & Saslow, G. (1957). Observer reliability of interaction patterns during interviews. *Journal of Consulting Psychology, 21*, 269–275.

Pope, B., & Siegman, A. W. (1966). Interviewer–interviewee relationship and verbal behavior of interviewee in the initial interview. *Psychotherapy: Theory, practice and research, 3*, 149–152.

Pope, B., Nudler, S., Vonkorff, M. R., & McGhee, J. P. (1974). The experienced professional interviewer versus the complete novice. *Journal of Consulting and Clinical Psychology, 42,* 680–690.

Rappaport, J., & Chinsky, J. M. (1972). Accurate empathy: Confusion of a construct. *Psychological Bulletin, 77,* 400–404.

Ray, M. L., & Webb, E. J. (1966). Speech duration effects in the Kennedy News Conferences. *Science, 153,* 899–901.

Rogers, C. R. (1957). The necessary and sufficient conditions of therapeutic personality change. *Journal of Consulting Psychology, 21,* 95–103.

Rogers, C. R., Gendlin, E. T., Kiesler, D. G., & Truax, C. B. (1967). *The therapeutic relationship and its impact: A study of psychotherapy with schizophrenics.* Madison: University of Wisconsin Press.

Sanford, F. H. (1942). Speech and personality. *Psychological Bulletin, 39,* 811–845.

Saslow, G., & Matarazzo, J. D. (1959). A technique for studying changes in interview behavior. In E. A. Rubenstein & M. B. Parloff (Eds.), *Research in psychotherapy* (Vol. 1, pp. 125–159). Washington, DC: American Psychological Association.

Siegman, A. W., & Pope, B. (1972). *Studies in dyadic communication.* New York: Pergamon Press.

Simpkins, L. (1967). The effects of utterance duration on verbal conditioning in small groups. *Journal of Social Psychology, 71,* 69–78.

Sloane, R. B., Staples, F. R., Cristol, A. H., Yorkston, N. J., & Whipple, K. (1975). *Psychotherapy versus behavior therapy.* Cambridge, MA: Harvard University Press.

Staples, F. R., & Sloane, R. B. (1976). Truax factors, speech characteristics, and therapeutic outcome. *Journal of Nervous and Mental Disease, 163,* 135–140.

Staples, F. R., Sloane, R. B., Whipple, K., Cristol, A. H., & Yorkston, N. J. (1976). Process and outcome in psychotherapy and behavior therapy. *Journal of Consulting and Clinical Psychology, 44,* 340–350.

Strupp, H. H. (1973). *Psychotherapy: Clinical, research, and theoretical issues.* New York: Jason Aronson.

Strupp, H. H., & Wallach, M. S. (1965). A further study of psychiatrists' responses in quasi-therapy situations. *Behavioral Science, 10,* 113–134.

Truax, C. B. (1970). Length of therapist response, accurate empathy, and patient improvement. *Journal of Clinical Psychology, 26,* 539–541.

Truax, C. B., & Carkhuff, R. R. (1967). *Toward effective counseling and psychotherapy.* Chicago: Aldine.

Truax, C. B., & Mitchell, K. M. (1971). Research on certain therapist interpersonal skills in relation to process and outcome. In A. E. Bergin & S. L. Garfield (Eds.), *Handbook of psychotherapy and behavior change: An empirical analysis.* New York: John Wiley.

Weitz, S. (Ed.). (1974). *Nonverbal communication: Readings with commentary.* New York: Oxford University Press.

Wenegrat, A. (1974). A factor analytic study of the Truax Accurate Empathy Scale. *Psychotherapy: Theory, Research and Practice, 11,* 48–51.

Wenegrat, A. (1976). Linguistic variables of therapist speech and accurate empathy ratings. *Psychotherapy: Theory, Research and Practice, 13,* 30–33.

Wiens, A. N., Matarazzo, J. D., & Saslow, G. (1965). The Interaction Recorder: An electronic punched paper tape unit for recording speech behavior during interviews. *Journal of Clinical Psychology, 21,* 142–145.

Wiens, A. N., Matarazzo, J. D., Saslow, G., Thompson, S. M., & Matarazzo, R. G. (1965). Interview interaction behavior of three groups of nurses: Supervisors, head nurses, and staff nurses. *Nursing Research, 14,* 322–329.

Wiens, A. N., Molde, D. A., Holman, D. C., & Matarazzo, J. D. (1966). Can interview interaction measures be taken from tape recordings? *Journal of Psychology, 63,* 249–260.

Wiens, A. N., Saslow, G., & Matarazzo, J. D. (1966). Speech interruption behavior during interviews. *Psychotherapy: Theory, Research and Practice, 3,* 153–158.

Wiens, A. N., Jackson, R. H., Manaugh, T. S., & Matarazzo, J. D. (1969). Communication length as an index of communication attitude: A replication. *Journal of Applied Psychology, 53,* 264–266.

Wiens, A. N., Manaugh, T. S., & Matarazzo, J. D. (1976). Speech and silence behavior of bilinguals conversing in each of two languages. *International Journal of Psycholinguistics, 5,* 79–94.

6

Everyday Disturbances of Speech

George F. Mahl

INTRODUCTION

Are there not very important things which can only reveal themselves, under certain conditions and at certain times, by quite feeble indications?
Sigmund Freud (1963, p. 27)

This chapter concerns one of the extralinguistic dimensions of speech, the "roughness" or "influency" or "normal disturbances" in word–word progression.

The following excerpt from the transcript of a sound-recording of a psychotherapy interview illustrates an extreme degree of such speech disturbances in the speech of the patient (P). At other times, this same patient spoke fluently. The patient is telling the therapist (T) about a pogrom that occurred in his childhood in Russia.

P: My uncle had his throat cut.
T: Mhm.
P: And my uncle . . . ah . . . he wasn't killed, but they tortured him. They took him and they slit his throat right . . . the skin . . . just cut the skin right around like this.

GEORGE F. MAHL • Departments of Psychiatry and Psychology, Yale University, New Haven, CT 06519. The research in this chapter was supported primarily by USPHS Grant M-1052, "The Patient's Language as Expressive Behavior" (G. F. Mahl, principal investigator). A Fellowship at the Center for Advanced Study in the Behavioral Sciences, 1963–1964, and indirect support by The Foundations' Fund for Research in Psychiatry also contributed to this work. Veterans Administration and NIMH Fellowship funds also supported the study to be described that Schulze conducted. Seymour Sarason contributed support from his Yale Test Anxiety Program NIMH grant to the study with Zimbardo and Barnard. The Connecticut Mental Health Center, a joint venture of Yale University and the State of Connecticut, facilitated Lassen's study.

T: Who did that? (said in a sudden manner).
P: Mmm . . . hulligan . . . holigan . . . huligans, whatever you call them.
T: The who?
P: The . . . ah . . . you know the . . . ah . . . sss . . . he was in . . . the . . . he . . . was dri . . . traveling from one town to the oth . . . next and
T: Mhm.
P: —he was stopped by a couple . . . ah . . . if you know the situation in the South . . .

Such disrupted speech also occurs in other interactions besides psychotherapy interviews, even in the speech of very articulate people.

We developed a measure of the degree of such speech disturbance and have investigated aspects of variations in this measure during verbal interaction. In the remainder of this chapter, I shall, first, describe the initial context of our work. That context largely determined my choice of this particular extralinguistic dimension for study and influenced the direction of our subsequent work. Secondly, I shall discuss the nature of the measure, and, thirdly, certain of our findings about it.

THE INITIAL CONTEXT

Preceding the onset of this work, my research interests were mainly in physiological psychology. My concerns had evolved from the experimental production of increased gastric (HC1) acid secretion in dogs, monkeys, and humans via the instigation of chronic anxiety in the laboratory to a desire to study variations in HC1 secretion in humans during spontaneously occurring, "real life" fluctuations in anxiety (Mahl, 1949, 1950, 1952; Mahl & Brody, 1954; Mahl & Karpe, 1953). The intensive psychotherapeutic interview promised to be a fruitful situation for such research. Variations in the patient's anxiety regularly occur there, and that situation provides more information about the meaning of such variations than is usually the case for laboratory or life stress studies. To achieve my research goal, I needed a measure that would be *unobtrusive* to make and that would portray the *immediate, fluctuating* intensities in the patient's anxiety as they occurred in the course of a therapeutic interview. Ideally, moreover, the measure should be a nonphysiological one: it should be a "psychic" one, for the study of the psychosomatics of anxiety and HC1 secretion, as well as for the future study of other somatic correlates of anxiety in this situation.

I had another, nascent research interest when I started this work. I had become interested in the objective studies of the *process* of psychotherapy, which were flourishing at that time, due largely to the influence of Carl Rogers and his students (to cite only a few examples: Carnes

& Robinson, 1948; Gillespie, 1953; Page, 1953; Porter, 1943; Raimy, 1948; Snyder, 1945; Tindall & Robinson, 1947). Since the patient's anxiety is at the heart of the psychotherapeutic process, it was clear that significant research on the therapeutic process must include the study of the patient's anxiety. A review of the literature showed that only a few objective studies of therapy had tried to measure concurrent anxiety during interviews. Thus, the development of such a measure promised to be useful to psychotherapy research, as well as in psychosomatic investigation.

What could be developed into the desired measure? The then rapid development of high fidelity sound recording techniques made available a very convenient method for recording the ongoing vocal-verbal interchange of the patient and therapist. This constitutes a major, very important portion of the therapeutic interaction. Thus, the sound-recorded behavior of the patient could be the source of the desired measure of anxiety.

The *manifest verbal content, what* is said, is an obvious part of the sound recording, and is of special interest to most therapists. It was also of special interest to nearly all objective investigators of the therapeutic process: *manifest verbal content measures were the order of the day*. One could conceive of developing such a measure of the patient's anxiety. It would be a measure of the extent to which the patient's utterances dealt explicitly with "anxiety," "fear," "conflict," "nervousness," and so forth, and with situations that seemed to clearly involve such emotions. My clinical experience, however, as well as theoretical reasoning, had convinced me that the *most generally applicable valid measure* of the patient's anxiety would be one based on the "expressive" aspects of his speech, on *"how"* he spoke rather than *"what"* he said (e.g., Reich, 1948; Sullivan, 1954). Space restriction does not permit me to discuss adequately here the background for this decision. I have done so elsewhere (e.g., Mahl, 1959, 1961), and I shall discuss matters related to it later in this chapter.

The "expressive," extralinguistic dimensions of speech are varied and, thus, offered many potential content-free measures of anxiety and conflict. I chose to begin with the dimension of normal "disturbances" of the word–word progression. I based that decision on two considerations. First, when one encounters instances of disturbed or flustered speech, one immediately assumes that the speaker is anxious about something related to the content or to the situation or whatever. That assumption is based upon everyday, as well as clinical, experience. Secondly, that experientially based assumption was consistent with a theoretical bias of mine: that one effect of anxiety, regardless of its source, is to disrupt all complex ongoing behavior. Speech is an instance *par excel-*

lence of complex, skilled behavior, involving a peculiar blend of the execution of integrated motoric and cognitive processes. These considerations dictated our initial task: the quantification of "rough," "disturbed," "flustered" speech. I shall turn to the discussion of that task in the next section.

Before doing so, however, I shall complete the preceding account of the context for the origin of this work. What I have said so far describes all the *conscious, rational factors* that led me to choose *an aspect of speech* for intensive study. In retrospect, I have realized that an *unconscious, emotional factor* also contributed significantly to that particular choice. This purely personal factor was a complex one involving: (1) an undergraduate exposure, some 15 years earlier, to the science of phonetics as taught by Professor R. H. Stetson (Oberlin College), who was a world-renowned scholar of phonetics; (2) a subsequent strong intellectual-emotional attachment to Professor Stetson unrelated to any interest in phonetics, however, on my part; (2) his death only a few years before I ventured into this heretofore, for me, largely foreign territory; (4) an unconscious, partial identification with Professor Stetson (following the loss of him) that influenced my conscious, perfectly reasonable programmatic research decisions. Professor Stetson would turn over in his grave if he knew how I blended his indirect influences into my own evolving scientific career. What he cannot know will not disturb his peace, however, and it enables me to give a more complete description of what would otherwise be understood as an episode in the supposedly impersonal, rational scientific process.

While my interest in psychosomatics and psychotherapy played a major role in the onset of this work, you will see that my ensuing research was concerned almost entirely with the speech measure itself. I behaved like parents whose reasons for wanting and having children give way to a consuming interest in the children themselves.

THE MEASURE

Speech Disturbance Categories and Ratios

We first tried to quantify the degree of speech disturbance by identifying clinically perceived episodes of flustered speech by the patient in tape recordings of therapy interviews. That attempt was based on the (mistaken) assumption that ordinarily a patient's speech proceeds smoothly, but episodically becomes "flustered." We learned that the reliability with which independent observers identified such episodes was poor. And we learned that the concept of "flustered" speech is too crude. Such episodes consist of various discrete types of disturbances. We empirically developed, from the study of many tape recordings, a set of such speech disturbance categories that promised to be generally useful for our purposes. Our final set is presented in Table 1, where the categories are defined and illustrated.

We have used the category set in studying the speech of some 500 English-speaking individuals representing both sexes, a wide range of ages, social backgrounds, educational levels, personality structures, and speaking situations. The preceding includes patients in psychotherapy, interviewers in intial and therapy interviews, schizophrenic patients in research interviews, college students during role-playing and in investigative interviews, children during research interviews, university faculty members in seminar discussions, and various normal adults in various situations. We have not found it necessary to modify the present set for any particular individuals, samples of subjects, or speaking situations. Several other investigators have also used the set without reporting a need to modify it (Feldstein, 1962; Boomer & Goodrich, 1961; Siegman & Pope, 1965; and Blumenthal, 1964, for example). Thus, the set is a useful one for describing and measuring commonly found, everyday disturbances of speech.[1]

Hesitations and silent pauses, for example those not filled with "ah," do not appear in the category set, although they too often disrupt verbalization. Initially, their omission resulted from a methodological decision to measure them separately by quantitative techniques (Kasl & Mahl, 1956). Subsequently, we had sufficient doubt about the functional equivalence of hesitations to the categories of the present set that we did not intensively pursue their investigation. It is possible, of course, that the present set could be usefully expanded by the addition of a suitable category for these phenomena. Anyone contemplating such a step, however, must contend with a variety of problems. One of these is distinguishing between pauses that disrupt speech and those that do

---

[1]Richard Karpe, M.D., and I collaborated in the development of the present set of speech-disturbance categories. That was exacting, but exciting, work. I am grateful to him for the time, energy, and clinical experience which he contributed, often at a sacrifice of his limited leisure time.

In the beginning I was aware only that Freud (1960) had worked with tongue-slips. Since then, of course, I have discovered that others had been interested, to some extent, in phenomena similar to the speech disturbance categories: for example, Meringer and Mayer (1895), Froschels and Jellinek (1941), Davis (1940), Sanford (1942), and Baker (1948, 1951). Dibner (1956) developed a similar category set quite independently, and later workers proposed other sets derived in part from, or related to, ours and Dibner's: among them, Krause and Pilisuk (1961), Maclay and Osgood (1959), and Boomer (1963).

TABLE 1
Definitions and Illustrations of the Speech Disturbance Categories[a]

Category	Examples
(1) "Ah." Wherever the "ah" sound occurs it is scored. Less frequent variants are "eh", "uh," "uhm."	Well . . . ah . . . when I first came home.
(2) Sentence change (SC). A correction in the form or content of the expression while the word-word progression occurs. To be scored, these changes must be sensed by the listener as interruptions in the flow of the sentence.	Well she's . . . already she's lonesome. That was . . . it will be two years ago in the fall.
(3) Repetition (R). The serial, superfluous repetition of one or more words— usually of one or two words.	'Cause they . . . they get along pretty well together. He was . . . he was sharing the office.
(4) Stutter (St.)	It sort of well l . . l . . leaves a memory.
(5) Omission (O). Parts of words, or rarely entire words, may be omitted. Contractions not counted. Most omissions are of final one or two parts of words and are associated with sentence change and repetition.	She mour . . . was in mourning for about two years before. Then their anni . . . wedding anniversary comes around.
(6) Sentence incompletion (Inc.) An expression is interrupted, clearly left incomplete, and the communication proceeds without correction.	Well I'm sorry I couldn't get here last week so I could . . . ah . . . I was getting a child ready for camp and finishing up swimming lessons.
(7) Tongue slips (TS). Includes neologisms, the transposition of entire words from their "correct" serial position in sentence, and the substitution of an "unintended" for an intended word.	We spleat the bitches (for "split the beaches"). He was born in their hou(se) . . hospital and came to their house. The reason that I don't . . . didn't seem to feel the love for him (son) that I felt for J . . (daughter).
(8) Intruding incoherent sound (IS). A sound which is absolutely incoherent to the listener. It intrudes without itself altering the form of the expression and cannot be clearly conceived of as a stutter, omission, or neologism (though some may be such in reality).	If I see a girl now I'd like to take out I just . . . dh . . . ask her.

[a]From Kasl and Mahl, 1965.

not. Another is distinguishing "anxious" silence from other kinds (e.g., hostile).[2]

Speech may be peppered with the various disturbances, but most of them escape the awareness of both speaker and listener. Only when they occur at relatively rapid rates and are "bunched" does the listener perceive them, sensing an episode of flustered speech. Independent observers may have different thresholds for perceiving the disturbances and different criteria for that rate which constitutes "flustered" speech. If so, their reliability in judging speech as "flustered" suffers. The use of the categories shown in Table 1 minimizes such problems of observer judgment.

A useful measure of the general level of speech disturbance can be obtained by identifying the various disturbances in a verbatim transcript and then computing the following ratio for any given language sample:

$$\text{General speech disturbance ratio} = \frac{N \text{ speech disturbances}}{N \text{ words in sample}}$$

(The time spent talking can be used instead of N words in the denominator, if that measure is more convenient. We found the correlation between these two ratios to be .91, on the one occasion we compared them.)

I shall show that the "ah" category should be omitted from the ratio if it is to be used for anxiety measurement. In this case, all the remaining ("Non-ah") categories are used in determining the following ratio:

$$\text{Non-ah Ratio} = \frac{N \text{ Non-ah disturbances}}{N \text{ words in sample}}$$

One can, of course, compute comparable Ah Ratios. I shall occasionally refer to them.

[2]Other vocal phenomena come to mind as possibly related to the categories presented here, and thus as candidates for inclusion in the category set. These include such things as "nervous" laughs, sighs, lip-smacking, the characteristic use of intruding idiosyncratic expressions such as "you see," "see what I mean," "I don't know," "you know what I mean," "understand"?, and so forth. Such phenomena have been studied as expressive behavior by others and ourselves but are not included in our set of speech-disturbance categories. We intended the category set to cover the majority of syntactical and lexical disruptions and distortions in spontaneous speech that result in confused messages when they occur at a rapid rate, not to include all possible expressive behavior accompanying the act of speaking. Nervous laughs, sighs, lip-smacking, and so on may accompany speech, but they are not uniquely involved in it. They may occur when a person is not speaking or even when he is alone. And neither they nor intruding characteristic expressions regularly, or necessarily, contribute to episodes of confused speech.

Scoring Speech Disturbances

This is easy and interesting for anyone curious about the details of the speech process. The essential features of our procedure may be summarized as follows:

1. *High quality equipment and verbatim transcriptions.* The sound recordings, verbatim transcripts, and sound playback equipment were of generally superior quality (Mahl, Dollard, & Redlich, 1954). Wherever we had to sacrifice fidelity of the sound recording or playback, the ease and quality with which the speech was transcribed or scored decreased. The speech disturbances are more difficult to perceive even as one moves from a tape speed of 7½ to 3¾ inches per second. We obtained as accurate transcripts as possible so as to reduce to a minimum the wasting of time and effort correcting the typescript when scoring the disturbances. The typist, of course, must be trained to transcribe verbatim and not "edit out" speech disturbances.

2. *The scorers.* Seven different people scored the speech disturbances in our research. All were bright college students or graduates. No person who ever attempted to score failed to do so successfully. Since we have not investigated the matter, we cannot say what minimal intellectual or educational level, or what degree of sensitivity to patterns of spontaneous speech, are required for this task.

3. *Learning to score.* Our coworkers learned to score satisfactorily by studying a simple manual and practicing scoring the speech of about a half-dozen recorded psychotherapy interviews, each with a different patient.[3] The first two practice interviews were for people with relatively few disturbances and thus easy to score; the subsequent interviews were of higher disturbance levels and thus more difficult. After scoring each interview, the learner compared his scored transcripts with those previously scored by an experienced person. Conferences then occurred for clarification of scoring questions. We found that requiring the learner to actually tabulate successive instances of agreement and disagreement with the criterion scoring, and to account for all the disagreements, facilitated the development of scoring skill and brought into focus questions requiring discussion.

4. *The actual scoring.* All of this was done with the simultaneous use of the verbatim transcripts and the tape recordings. Actual hearing of the speech is essential for the most accurate scoring, which sometimes

[3]The essential parts of the scoring manual consisted of category definitions, illustrations, and scored interview excerpts similar to those presented in the first part of this chapter.

The scorers included Jack Austin, Sue Cohen, Stanislav V. Kasl, Katherine McGraw, Sally Green Risberg, Gene Schulze and myself. I am grateful to the others for their interest and diligent collaboration.

depends upon cues of intonation. The simultaneous use of a transcript makes for more accurate hearing. With it, the listener can keep track of what is being said better than without it. Since the transcript has been prepared by another listener, it also provides the scorer with a check for his speech perception. He must, of course, guard against being unduly influenced by what has been typed. The transcript is essential if one wishes, as we did, to study such questions as the distribution of the disturbances within sentences, the interrelationship of various disturbances within sentences, the frequency of disturbances in sentences differing in verbal content, and so forth.

When scoring, the incidence and category of the disturbances are marked directly on the transcript, as is illustrated in the following scored excerpt from a psychotherapy interview. The abbreviations are those cited in Table 1. Since the scoring was done when listening and reading, some of it may not be completely clear from this written material alone. Poor grammar, inaudibility of the recording, and interruptions by the other person are not grounds for scoring a disturbance. (Only the patient's, (P) disturbances have been scored.)

P: My impression of my relation to D_____ (son) have always been that the reason
              TS, SC
      that I don't . . . didn't seem to feel the love for him that I felt for J_____
      (daughter) was that during the first sixteen months of his life I was away. I
      didn't grow up with him. If there was any jealousy of D_____ it was in relation
      to his in-laws. Now that is very possible. Although it's something which I also
      suppressed. [Ah] . . . and the reason I say it's possible 'cause it sort of well
      St   St   *R*
      le . . le . . leaves a . . . [ah] . . . a sort of memory. When (?) I . . .
T: You're jealous of his in-laws?
                                                                     SC
P: Of his in-laws, yeah. Because he was brought up with them till . . . until I came
      TS, O, SC
      home. He was born in their hou . . . hospital and came to their house, and my
      wife lived with her parents.
T: Ho . . . how do you mean you're jealous of his in-laws?
P: Well . . . [ah] . . . when I first came home, and for the first year or so, or more
      than a year . . . [ah] . . . D_____ was more prone to turn to his grandfather and
      grandmother than he was to me.
T: Mhm.
P: And although I understood it, there was certain amount of . . . [ah] . . . well not
                                                     SC
      bitterness, I wasn't bitter about it, but a certain amount of . . . a sort of
      resentment, a mild type of resentment.
T: You make this sound so . . . [ah]
P: Well
T: So diluted.
P: Well it was diluted. I mean it wasn't something which I felt keenly enough to be

angry at his grandparents, let's say, or with D_____ himself. I mean I realized that he had grown up with them.

T: Mhm.

                                                                    Inc.
P: And therefore, it was more natural for him to . . . until he
                        SC   *St*
        became . . . completely o . . overcame his . . . [ah] . . . strangeness to me, and it
                                                                    R
        took quite a long time. [Ah] . . . then there was . . . there was a certain amount
        of resentment. It wasn't directed against the parents or
        IS, (O?)   *IS   St*
        dec . . . was . . . den . . . ac . . actually directed against a circumstance which
                                                    O, SC
        kept me away. And it was a resentment which re . . . in a
                        SC
        certain . . . [ah] . . . to a certain extent reflected itself also in the (clears throat)
        feeling I had toward people who had remained and had made money.

T: Mmm. Your in-laws make money?

P: Yes. My father-in-law made a lot of money from the war.

The method of marking the disturbances on the transcript provides for various types of analyses. The frequency can be readily counted, and this can be done for various time intervals (successive 2 minutes, for example) or language samples (successive 200 words of a person's speech, for example) which can be readily noted on the transcript. Also, all of the problems stated at the end of the preceding paragraph that require a transcript can be readily studied by scoring directly on the transcript.[4]

Reliability of Speech Disturbance Scoring

Our reliability data deal largely with the frequency of speech disturbances, since nearly all of our research has concerned questions involving that parameter. In our first studies, we combined all the categories into one frequency measure. The interobserver reliability of that measure was determined by correlating the total N of disturbances scored by independent judges in unselected samples of psychotherapy interview transcript pages ($N = 28$–65) for several different patients ($N = 3$–5). The average product–moment intercorrelation was .94. The interobserver reliabilities of the Ah and Non-ah Ratios obtained in our subsequent work are shown in Table 2. As might be expected, the agreement is higher for the Ah than for the Non-ah measure; the perception of Ah is a relatively simple matter. The correlations for the Non-ah measure range

[4]Feldstein and his colleagues devised methods for scoring the disturbances directly from the tape onto IBM cards for use with programmed computers (e.g., Feldstein & Jaffe, 1963).

TABLE 2
Inter-Observer Correlations (Pearson r) of Speech Disturbance Frequencies[a]

Item	Scorers	Nature of speakers and situation	Nature of Reliability Sample (N)	Ah	Non-ah
1.	A-B	Psychoneurotics in psychotherapy interviews	65 transcript pages of 3 patients. (65)		.90
2.	A-C	Undergraduates in role-playing	Total speech sample of 10 subjects (10)	.99	.98
3.	A-D	Undergraduates in personal interviews (Kasl and Mahl, 1965)	36 pages of 5 subjects (36)	.99	.96 (SC .87) R .97)
4.	A-E	Hospitalized schizophrenic and orthopedic patients telling stories about pictures (Schulze, Mahl, and Holzberg, 1959)	12 means of 3 stories from 6 subjects (12)	.97	.99
5.	A-F	Undergraduates in personal interviews under varying auditory and visual feedback conditions	27 pages from 3 subjects (27)		.85
6.	A-F	Undergraduates in personal interviews under varying visual feedback conditions	32 pages from 16 subjects (16)	.96	.90
7.	A-G	Secondary school children giving open-ended responses to questions. (Zimbardo, Mahl, and Barnard, 1963)	Responses to two questions of 16 subjects (16)		.89
8.	B-C	Psychoneurotics in psychotherapy interviews	56 transcript pages 6 patients (56)		.91
9.	E-F	Undergraduates in personal interviews under varying auditory and visual feedback conditions	69 pages of 9 subjects (69)		.88
10.	E-F	Adult twins in personal views	59 pages from 16 subjects (59)		.86
11.	E-F	Undergraduates responding to TAT inquiries and describing motion-pictures (Schulze, 1964)	(a) Speech of 5 subjects during one-minute intervals ($\overline{X}$ per S=81)		.89[b]
			(b) 25 means of 5 conditions for 5 subjects (25)		.96

[a]From Mahl, 1987.
[b]Average r.

from .85 to .99. In one sample, we determined the reliabilities of Sentence Change and Repetition scores, which were .87 and .97 respectively. Workers in other laboratories have used our categories, definitions, and examples with reliability results that are in substantial agreement with ours, even though scoring often was done directly from the tapes (Blumenthal, 1964; Boomer & Goodrich, 1961; Feldstein, 1962; Feldstein, Brenner, & Jaffe, 1963; Feldstein & Jaffe, 1963; Panek & Martin, 1959).

The preceding data concern the reliability for scoring speech disturbances *frequencies*. Those data do not reflect the reliability of *exact* scoring of the individual disturbances making up the frequency measures. We explored the degree of exact agreement in scoring, defined as degree of agreement in the incidence or placement of a disturbance in the transcript *and* in the categorization of it. Three scorers participated in this study; one (A) was considerably more experienced than the other two (B and C), who were about equally experienced. Since "ah" is very easy to score, and its inclusion is misleading, we will omit reference to it. One study compared the exact agreement of A and C in scoring the Non-ah categories in 34 transcript pages of four psychotherapy interviews of two patients. They agreed exactly in 60% of all the disturbances they both scored. B and C also agreed exactly in 60% of all the disturbances they both scored in 44 transcript pages of five interviews from five different patients. These percentages represent the agreement in "positive scoring"; they do not reflect the fact that the judges were in very high exact agreement in *not* scoring. This "negative" agreement was not determined, for what the unit should be in doing so is not at all clear to us. No matter what it might be—for example, the word, the clause,—it is obvious that even the degree of exact agreement is better than chance and adequate for investigations concerned with individual disturbances within sentences, such as I shall mention occasionally. Actually, a great deal of our speech disturbance scoring has been done by one person and then carefully checked in entirety by another person.

SOME GENERAL PROPERTIES OF "NORMAL" SPEECH DISTURBANCES[5]

Frequency of Occurrence

Judged against the background of everyday speech perception, the frequency of speech disturbances in our materials turns out to be surprisingly high. Table 3 shows just how frequent they are.

[5]Most of the quantitative data presented in this section were previously presented at the Annual Meeting of the American Psychological Association, 1956 (Mahl, 1956a).

TABLE 3
Seconds of Talking per 1 Speech Disturbance[a]

Sample	N	Mdn	Q₁–Q₃
Patients in initial interviews	31	4.7	3.5– 5.4
Interviewers			
A	11	3.8	3.5– 4.3
B	10	6.5	5.9– 8.8
C	10	11.9	8.9–15.6
Undergraduate men role playing	26	3.9	2.5– 5.2
Undergraduate men			
personal investigative interviews	25	4.0	3.0– 4.9
University faculty	12	5.1	4.1– 6.4

[a]From Mahl, 1987.

The samples cited in Table 3 are: (1) a sample of initial interviews of 20 women and 11 men who were applying for psychiatric outpatient treatment; (2) male interviewers who participated in the initial interviews; (3) Yale undergraduates who played the role of a student suspected of cheating on examinations who was appearing before a faculty committee (also played by undergraduates) which was "unsympathetic" in half the cases but "sympathetic" in the other half; (4) Yale undergraduates who were the subjects of "control," "anxiety," and "anger"-provoking interviewing and (5) faculty members who were engaged in two rather heated seminar discussions on the validity of Rorschach test interpretations.

The data of Table 3 were obtained for each language sample by totaling the number of seconds of talk by the individual and dividing by the total number of speech disturbances in that time. The medians and quartiles of this frequency measure are very similar for the patients, the undergraduates, and the faculty members. The median of their medians gives an estimate of the general frequency of the speech disturbances: *one disturbance for every 4.4 seconds of spontaneous speech.* Even the data for two of the three interviewers, who, because of their roles, were much more constrained and less voluble, show a comparable rate.

We do not know for sure just how representative these rates are of more "relaxed" speaking situations, but it is our impression that even that rate would be surprising.

Awareness of Speech Disturbances

The vast majority of the disturbances in spontaneous speech occur outside the awareness of either the speaker or the listener. This is probably the basis for our surprise at the frequency data just presented.

Our evidence about the speaker's and listener's awareness consists of informal observations only, but they are so clear-cut that any reader can readily repeat them. We have never known an interviewer who was not surprised, upon seeing an interview transcription and hearing the tape recording, at the many speech disturbances contained in the speech of both himself and the patient. Subjects, assistants, secretaries, and friends have all reacted with similar surprise when just seeing or working with typescripts and tapes. Beyond surprise, these people have reacted with interest and sudden awareness of disturbances in the speech they subsequently hear. Sudden confrontation with their own speech, in the form of transcripts with the disturbances scored in red pencil, has caused some people to react with disbelief in the accuracy of the typing, disowning their own speech, and with despair, shame and anger. All of these responses testify to the lack of awareness of the vast majority of speech disturbances and to the wish not to know of them.

Knowing that they do occur in his or her speech, the speaker is able to observe them actually taking place. The speaker may then notice that the disturbances *happen* to him or her, so to speak, as if he or she is passive and they are produced by processes occurring outside his or her conscious control. If the speaker deliberately commits the speech disturbances, they will not sound or feel the same as those occurring spontaneously. The subjective experiences are very similar to those accompanying the self-observation of motor tics and the voluntary imitation of them.

Individual Differences in Frequency of Speech Disturbances

The use of the speech disturbance ratios defined earlier reveals these differences. The latter are readily illustrated by Figure 1, which contains the distributions of the 11 different General Speech-Disturbance Ratios of Interviewer A in the 11 different initial interviews conducted by him and comparable distributions for B and C in their 10 interviews each. By analysis of variance, the differences between the three interviewers are highly significant, $p < .001$. These interviewers also differed significantly from one another in their Ah Ratios ($p < .001$) and their Non-ah Ratios ($p < .001$), as determined by simple analyses of variance.

The ratios of the 31 patients taking part in the interviews were also subjected to an analysis of variance to test for individual differences. Each interview was divided into successive 2-minute intervals and the ratios for each patient's speech computed for each two-minute interval. We then determined if the variance in all such 2-minute ratios due to individual patients was greater than the variance within interviews. It

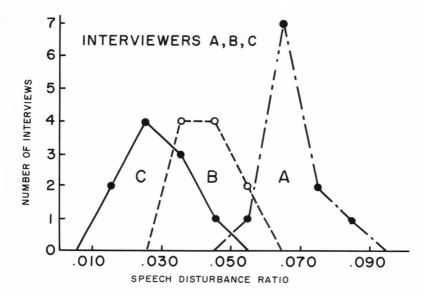

FIGURE 1. Frequency distributions of general speech disturbance ratios of three interviewers in initial interviews (From Mahl, 1987).

was, for the General Ratio, the Ah Ratio, and the Non-ah Ratio (p
< .001), in each instance.

The reader might wonder if the differences among the interviewers
and among the patients represent true individual differences or merely
reflect correlations between speech disturbance levels of the interviewers and the patients. The latter does not appear to be the case, for
the average ratios are practically identical for the patients interviewed by
the three different interviewers, as Table 4 shows. One cannot conclude
from these data, however, that there may never be a relationship between the speech-disturbance levels of people talking with one another.

Another method of testing for individual differences is to correlate
peoples' speech-disturbance measures obtained at various times and see
if the individuals maintain their relative ranks upon these various occasions. Two such studies (Blumenthal, 1964; Kasl & Mahl, 1965) have
demonstrated stable individual differences.

Intraindividual Variations in Speech-Disturbance Frequency

The speech disturbance level of a person varies from time to time
around his characteristic level. For example, patients' speech during
interviews shows two kinds of such intraindividual variations: their

TABLE 4
Speech Disturbances of Patients Seen by
Three Different Therapists[a]

	Interviewer		
Patients	A	B	C
X̄ Gen. Ratio	.055	.058	.057
X̄ Non-ah Ratio	.037	.037	.037
X̄ Ah Ratio	.018	.021	.020

[a]From Mahl, 1987.

average level of disturbance varies from interview to interview, and their level changes in a *nonrandom manner* with interviews.

Table 5 illustrates intraindividual variation from interview to interview for two patients in psychotherapy. The table summarizes the 2-minute General Speech Disturbance Ratios for eight interviews for each patient. The relevant question is whether or not the variations in the interview averages of these 2-minute ratios are significant. To answer this question we used Bartlett's test and a simple analysis of variance to test for the between-hour differences in variability and means. The results in Table 6 show that there are significant between-hour differences in both variability and means for both measures. Since the variances and the sample Ns meet the conditions for which no appreciable error is made in interpreting the F test (Jones, 1955), it can be concluded that the

TABLE 5
Summary of Two-Minute General Speech Disturbance Ratios
for Two Patients in Psychotherapy[a]

	Mrs. Y				Mr. Z		
Interview no.	N 2' ratios	Mean	SD	Interview no.	N 2' ratios	Mean	SD
1	24	.037	.019	2	30	.057	.021
2	25	.041	.014	15	30	.068	.023
5	30	.038	.015	17	31	.060	.040
10	33	.052	.018	20	29	.062	.026
13	28	.042	.015	26	32	.064	.034
17	28	.049	.026	67	30	.055	.029
20	26	.036	.013	83	30	.075	.024
26	29	.048	.024	88	30	.050	.027
Mean =		.043	.018	Mean =		.061	.028

[a]From Mahl, 1956b.

TABLE 6
Intraindividual Variation in Speech Disturbances of Two Patients across Eight Interviews[a]

Patient	Bartlett's test		Analysis of variance	
	χ^2	p	F	p
Mrs. Y	24.39	<.001	2.7	<.02
Mr. Z	16.14	<.05	2.19	<.05

[a]From Mahl, 1956b.

differences in means are true differences and not due to the within-interview heterogeneity of variance. Similar intraindividual interview–interview variations in the Non-ah Ratios have regularly been found in the studies of anxiety to be cited below. We have not tested statistically for the presence of comparable interview variations in Ah ratio, but inspection of them indicates that they also occur.

The representative graphs of the General Speech-Disturbance Ratios in Figure 2 illustrate the variations *within* interviews. Here the reader can see how the disturbance level varies in successive 2-minute intervals of some of the initial interviews. The inspection of many such graphs strongly suggests that the within-interview variations are systematic instead of "chance" oscillations.

One way to test for the presence of systematic variations is by means of the Wald–Wolfowitz run test (Moses, 1952). Defining a run as one or more successive measures falling either below or above the median of an interview, one determines the statistical significance of the difference between the obtained number of runs and the number expected as a result of chance factors alone. The median and runs are indicated on the first graph of Figure 2. In this instance, there are eight runs, in contrast to 15 that would be expected by chance. In pooling the results from a sample of interviews, one transforms the difference between the number of observed runs and that expected by chance into standard error units and then sums these transformed values. Under the null hypothesis, in a given sample of interviews, the sum of the deviate scores would be zero. The standard error of the sampling distribution of such sums would be $\sqrt{N}$. The significance of the departure of the obtained sum from zero is then evaluated with the normal probability table.[6]

[6]The writer is grateful to Professor Robert Abelson for advice on this application of the Wald-Wolfowitz test.

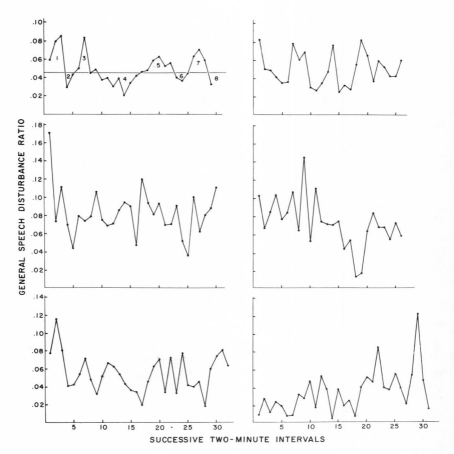

FIGURE 2. General speech disturbance ratios in successive 2-minute intervals of initial interviews of six psychiatric outpatient clinic patients. The speech disturbance level varies from moment to moment *within* interviews in nonrandom fashion (From Mahl, 1987).

The Wald–Wolfowitz test was applied according to the procedure just described to 2-minute speech disturbance measures for the 31 initial interviews. Separate analyses were done for the 2-minute General Ratios, Ah Ratios, and Non-ah Ratios of the 31 initial interviews; fewer runs than would be expected by chance occurred in each case, $p < .08$, $< .001$, $< .04$ respectively.[7] Our research has regularly revealed such within-interview variation.

---

[7]A "fewer-than-chance" number of runs in these interviews is to be expected from the general mode of interaction between therapist and patient. Usually, the interviewer "fol-

TABLE 7
Speech Disturbance Category Percentages[a]

Speech disturbance category	Average percentage of all disturbances	Cumulative percentage
'Ah'	40.5	40.5
Sentence-change	25.3	65.8
Repetition	19.2	85.0
Stutter	7.8	92.8
Omission	4.5	97.3
Sentence-incompletion	1.2	98.5
Incoherent sound	1.2	99.7
Tongue-slip	.7	100.4

[a]From Mahl, 1987.

Relative Frequencies of Individual Speech-Disturbance Categories

There is a great range in the frequency of the individual categories, with ah being the most prevalent and tongue-slips being relatively rare. Table 7 summarizes the relative frequencies in the speech of the 31 patients and the three interviewers in the initial interviews, the speech of the 12 faculty members and of the 26 role-playing undergraduates, and the speech of six psychoneurotic patients in a total of 25 psychotherapy interviews. The average percentages of Table 7 are the averages of the averages for these different groups.

Speech-Disturbance Profiles

Individuals not only differ from one another in the general frequency of speech disturbances, but also in their relative predilection for "ah," sentence changes, and repetitions—the categories making up about 85% of all speech disturbances. Speech-disturbance profiles, illustrated in Figures 3 and 4, demonstrate this phenomenon. Interviewer A is an "ah-er" and a "repeater," while Mrs. Y is a "sentence-changer."

Inspection of the category profiles revealed that as the ah-percent increases the sentence-change and repetition percents decrease, yet this kind of relationship does not exist between the sentence-change and repetition categories. Table 8 shows that these results are quite con-

---

lows" the patient, and the patient's psychological state usually changes at a much slower rate than every 2 minutes, the basic time unit used in the quantitative analyses reported here. It is quite possible that other types of interaction, and/or the choice of different time units, could produce a "greater-than-chance" number of runs.

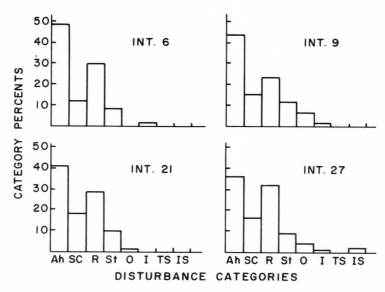

FIGURE 3. Category percentages of Interviewer A's speech disturbances in four initial interviews (From Mahl, 1987). SC = sentence change, R = repetition, O = omission, I = incomplete sentence, TS = tongue slip, IS = incoherent sound.

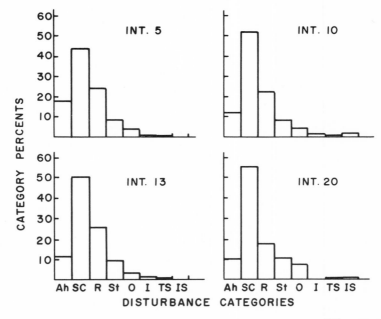

FIGURE 4. Category percentages of Mrs. Y's speech disturbances in four psychotherapy interviews (Mahl, 1987). SC = sentence change, I = incomplete sentence, TS = tongue-slip, R = repetition, O = omission, IS = incoherent sound.

TABLE 8
Intercorrelations between Ah, Sentence Change, and Repetition Percentages[a]

Sample	Ah-sentence change	Ah-repetition	Sentence change-repetition
31 Outpatients	−.81	−.54	.09
26 Undergraduates	−.57	−.65	−.01
6 Therapy patients	−.75	−.21	−.04
X̄ Ah% = 35%	X̄ Sentence change % = 28%	X̄ Repetition % = 21%	

[a]From Mahl, 1987.

sistent, holding true for the three samples of speakers analysed for such trends.

Summary

Starting with the attempt to identify episodes of flustered speech that might be used to identify transitory increases in the patient's anxiety during psychotherapy, we came upon the speech-disturbance categories. They promised a useful approach to the measurement of disruption in the flow of spontaneous speech. Speech disturbances can be reliably scored. After scoring considerable material, some of their general properties emerged.

They are surprisingly frequent in spontaneous speech uttered under a variety of conditions by a variety of individuals. Yet, the vast majority escape the awareness of both speaker and listener.

Speech disturbances are not merely "random noise," but variations in them manifest regularities of various kinds. People differ from one another in the frequency with which disturbances occur in their speech. And, for a given person, the level of disturbance may change from time to time, even within minutes, in a nonrandom fashion. People differ in the type of speech-disturbance most characteristic of them, some showing a striking degree of consistency in this regard. There also appear to be certain regularities in the relationships between the disturbances themselves.

Speech disturbances are not part of the linguistic code of English; they have no semantic function. They are not subject to tight restraint by the rules of the language. If they were, they would not be so frequent, and speech would become incomprehensible as their frequency increased. The latter happens only rarely. Being without linguistic function and "free" to vary over a wide range, the frequency and type of speech disturbances may perhaps be functionally related to a variety of extralinguistic variables—such as personality processes and structure, situational factors, and biological states of the speakers.[8]

The speech-disturbance level of patients in psychotherapy was seen to vary from interview to interview, yet this was not true for the three initial interviewers. This discrepancy suggests that intraindividual variations in the speech-disturbance level reflects changes in the psychological state of the speaker, for patients obviously change over a series of 26 or 86 interviews, the time spans covered in our samples. The psychological state of skilled interviewers, however, is not supposed to be markedly different as they talk to different patients.

Having outlined several quantitative aspects of normal speech disturbances, I shall now summarize some of our research concerning variables that might influence, or be related to, those quantitative characteristics.

ANXIETY

Naturally, we were most interested in the relationship between concurrent anxiety of speakers and the frequency of their speech disturbances. We conducted six studies of this relationship, which I shall now discuss briefly.

Speech Disturbances during Defensive and Conflictful Phases of Psychotherapy Interviews

We saw that the level of speech disturbance typically rises and falls in phasic fashion during interviews. Our first investigation (Mahl, 1956b) concerned the relationship between such variations and concurrent changes in the patient's anxiety level. We wanted to determine if these variations validly reflect variability in the immediate anxiety of the patient.

Psychotherapy interviews often appear to be divisible into natural phases, each of which can be assigned to a single theme of content or

[8]Mark Twain, generally acknowledged to be a master of dialect, made frequent use of our speech-disturbance categories in the dialogue of *The Adventures of Tom Sawyer* (Mahl, 1980). (He used Ah, sentence changes, sentence incompletions, repetitions, and stutters.) Rural Missourians of the last century committed speech disturbances, too. This indicates that these phenomena are relatively time and culture free, for American English. Verón *et al.* (1966) developed analogous categories for Spanish. Bond and his coworkers (Bond & Iwata, 1976; Bond & Ho, 1978) did so for Japanese. We cited related observations of Freud and Meringer and Mayer; those pertained to German. Nosenko *et al.* (1977) applied our General Speech Disturbance Ratio to Russian speech. Thus, the speech disturbance phenomena are relatively free from *linguistic*, as well as cultural, influence. (See Mahl, 1987.)

interaction, and the patient seems to become anxious and conflictful in some, but less anxious in others. In some of the latter, one can often observe that the patient has changed the topic or begun a new line of interaction with the therapist, in such a way that one interprets the behavior to be a relatively successful defensive maneuver. One might observe, for example, that a young man becomes anxious as he expresses affectionate thoughts about his older male therapist, and that he relaxes when he spontaneously shifts to angry statements about his therapist. Or, another male patient might seem to show just the opposite behavior.

During actual interviews or when listening to recordings, judgments of the just-mentioned changes in the patient's anxiety are based to a large degree upon changes in expressive speech properties. The assumption underlying the validation test of this study was that, given adequate context for interpretation, it would be possible to judge such phases in typescripts only (i.e., not recordings). We assumed, for example, that if a judge had learned enough about the patients cited above, he would know which patient would be likely to become anxious with the expression of affectionate feelings and relaxed with angry statements, and vice versa. If such judgments were made correctly, and if the frequency of speech disturbances is a valid index of concurrent patient anxiety, then that frequency should be higher in the phases judged to be anxiety-arousing and conflictful than in the phases judged to be low in anxiety or successfully defensive.

Procedure

We tested this prediction in the case of Mrs. Y (referred to earlier), using her interviews 5, 10, 13, 17, 20, and 26 as the critical "test" hours. We did so after pretesting our procedures with interviews from Mr. Z (Mahl, 1955a) and other patients.

With Mrs. Y, the first major problem was to prevent contaminated judgments. (Judgments could be contaminated for various reasons. If the judge were her therapist and the interviews were recent ones, for example, he might remember when she had become visibly anxious or relaxed on certain occasions. Or, if the judge based his observations on hearing tape recordings of her interviews, he might inadvertently base his judgments, to some unknown degree, on hearing the speech disturbances themselves, as was noted above.) I had, in fact, been Mrs. Y's therapist, but the test interviews had occurred slightly over two and one-half years before this validation test was made. I had not replayed the recordings or studied the transcripts of them. After practicing with other materials, a secretary edited verbatim transcripts of the test inter-

views, preparing clean scripts that did not contain any speech disturbances or any annotations or references about pauses and silences. Of
course, these edited scripts were no longer exactly verbatim. With these
precautions—the long period of elapsed time since the test interviews
occurred, the lack of replaying the tapes or studying their transcripts,
and the removal of all indications of speech disruption from the transcripts—we believed we prevented contamination of the phase judgments.

The judgment of the proper anxiety category for phases requires
intimate knowledge of the context of the interviews. One of the main
reasons for this is that the judgment cannot be based on manifest content alone. The meaning of manifest content depends in part upon context. Knowledge of the context includes both general knowledge of the
patient and knowledge of the dynamic setting of a given therapeutic
session. The development of an understanding of the context was another major problem. I knew a good deal about Mrs. Y since we had had
over 100 interviews. I obtained the more immediate context of the test
interviews by listening to the recordings of the first 29 sessions, *excepting
the test interviews*. I then reviewed in sequence notes I made of each of
the nontest interviews and the complete edited typescripts of the test
interviews. Before making the final judgment of phases in any given test
interview, I wrote a rough clinical description of the therapeutic situation at the time of the interview.

After I had divided the interviews into phases and judged them as
to anxiety type, I marked off the beginning and end of the phases in the
original verbatim typescripts. I did not, however, record the judgment
as to anxiety type in the latter. A second person then scored the speech
disturbances in the verbatim typescripts and determined the disturbance ratios for the phases. Just as I had no prior knowledge of the
speech disturbances when judging the phases, the scorer of the speech
disturbances had no knowledge as to the identity or meaning of the
phases.

A total of 19 defensive and/or low anxiety and 19 anxious or conflictful phases were judged in the six test hours. For any given interview, however, I had not always judged an equal number of each type
of phase. Therefore, equal numbers of the phase types were randomly
selected for each interview, in order to control for the confounding of
the "hour effects" demonstrated earlier. This process yielded a sample
of 15 phases in each group.

Results

The interjudge reliability of the person scoring the speech disturbances had been determined on several occasions, with two other judges. Her average intercorrelation was .94.

Figure 5a shows that Mrs. Y's Non-ah Ratio was significantly greater in the phases judged as conflictful-high anxiety than in those judged
as defensive-low anxiety. Her Ah Ratio was also higher in the former,
but not as statistically significantly so.[9] Generally, she did not use "Ah"
often. The original report of this study (Mahl, 1956b) presents a detailed
illustration of phases and associated speech-disturbance levels. Shortly,
I shall present a brief illustration of this basic phenomenon from materials concerning another patient.

Speech Disturbances and Rated Anxiety of Patients During Initial Psychiatric Interviews

The preceding study used the *within-individual method*. The primary
question of the study to be reported now was whether or not the use of a
between-individuals method with a larger sample of speakers would yield
similar results. In addition, we also studied, as secondary questions, the
role of various additional factors in the occurrence of speech disturbances.

Procedure

We obtained the materials of this study for quite different purposes
several years before our present use of them. Thus, they are probably
free from subtle, unconscious biases that might arise when materials are
obtained for predetermined ends. It is highly unlikely, for example, that
the interviewers involved unwittingly influenced the patients' speech
disturbance levels in ways that could account for the results to be
presented.

The primary data derive from the initial interviews of 31 representative patients applying for treatment at a psychiatric out-patient clinic.
The sample consisted of 20 women and 11 men. Their recorded diag-
noses were: 18 psychoneuroses, eight character disorders, and five
schizophrenics. Their ages ranged from 19 to 49. Their educational levels
ranged from completion of the eighth grade through one or more years
of college, but no one had graduated from college.

Two male psychiatric residents and myself conducted and observed
the interviews in rotation.[10] One of us interviewed every third patient in

---

[9]The original report of this study (Mahl, 1956b) contained only the results concerning the
General Speech Disturbance Ratio. We had not yet learned that the Non-ah Ratio is
generally the truly sensitive indicator of anxiety.

[10]George Andrews, M.D., and Louis Micheels, M.D., now well-established senior psychiatrists, were my friendly collaborators in this study. Andrews, in fact, was the instigator
of the basic plan of interviewer rotation, instituted for purposes quite remote from my
eventual use of the materials.

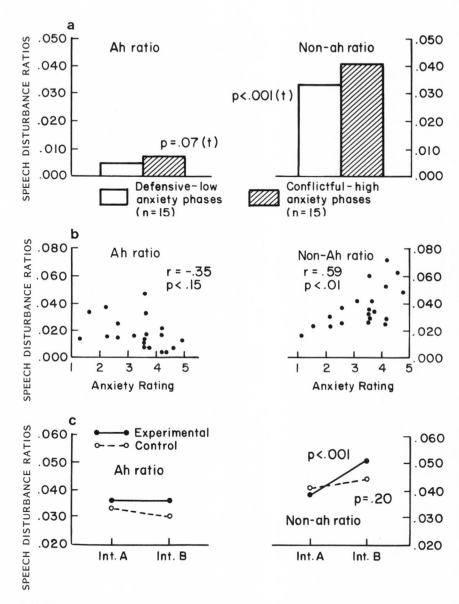

FIGURE 5. (a) Mean speech disturbance ratios of a patient during successful defensive phases and conflictful phases of therapeutic interviews (derived from data of Mahl, 1956b). (b) Scattergram of speech disturbance ratios and anxiety ratings of 20 women patients, initial interviews (Mahl, 1956c). (c) Mean speech disturbance ratios of male undergraduates during two interviews. Interview B is an anxiety interview for experimental group (Kasl and Mahl, 1958). (From Mahl, 1987).

the series, while the other two observed the interview through a one-way mirror and heard the verbal interchange over a monitoring system. Immediately after each interview, we independently rated on 5-point scales the degree of anxiety and of hostility manifested by the patient during the interview.

Two of us turned out to be notably more reliable raters of both anxiety and hostility than the third person was. Consequently, the means of these two raters were taken as the anxiety and the hostility measures for each patient. The reliability coefficients for these mean ratings are .83 for anxiety, and .73 for hostility.

We found a marked difference in the reliability of the anxiety ratings for the men and for the women. The reliability coefficient of the anxiety rationgs for the 11 men was only .57, contrasted with .86 for the 20 women. Because of the geometric nature of the correlation scale, these coefficients mean that the high reliability for the women was over twice as great as the low reliability for the men.

The interviews had also been tape recorded and the tapes preserved. These were transcribed for the present study. Speech-disturbance ratios were scored from the typescripts and tapes. All three ratios—General, Ah, and Non-ah—were determined, taking the entire interview as the language sample for each patient.

Results

Speech Disturbances and Rated Anxiety. We first correlated the three speech-disturbance ratios with the mean anxiety ratings for all 31 patients. The three product–moment correlations were: Non-ah Ratio-Anxiety Rating $r = .36$ ($p < .06$); Ah Ratio-Anxiety Rating $r = -.30$ ($p < .10$); and General Ratio-Anxiety Rating $r = .08$. These findings indicated that neither the Ah Ratios nor the General Ratio increased with rated anxiety. Therefore, the remaining results shall focus on the Non-ah Ratio.

We next correlated the Non-ah Ratios and the anxiety ratings separately for the male and for the female patients, in view of the difference in the reliability of these ratings for the men and the women. For the women, there was a significant positive product-moment correlation of .59 ($p < .01$) between the anxiety ratings and the Non-ah Ratios. For the men, however, the correlation was $-.47$ and was insignificant ($p < .16$). The most parsimonious explanation of the difference in these correlations is that it is due to the difference in the reliabilities of the anxiety ratings. Since we did not investigate the reasons for this difference, we cannot explain it. Figure 5b presents the scattergram of the Non-ah Ratio data for the women. It also presents the scattergram of their Ah Ratio data, which reveals that this measure was negatively, but insignificantly, correlated with their anxiety ratings.

Were the raters in this study basing their anxiety ratings on the speech disturbance levels of the patients? The correlation for the men indicates the raters were not doing this. So do the different correlations between the anxiety ratings and the Ah Ratios and Non-ah Ratios. Prior to this study, no one had ever demonstrated such a difference. And, very importantly, it was most unlikely that the observers of the live interviews could have computed the different frequencies of the Ahs and the Non-ahs in the flow of the patients' speech.

Speech Disturbances and Other Variables. The three interviewers spoke with significantly different degrees of speech disturbance. (They are the three interviewers of Figure 1.) The speech disturbance levels of their interviewees, however, were identical. This suggests that the patients' speech disturbance levels were determined by factors within the patients themselves. Anxiety was shown to be one such determinant in the women, accounting as it did for over one-third of the variance in their Non-ah Ratios.

The product-moment correlations between the other patient variables studied—hostility ratings, years of education, age, and speech rate—and the Non-ah Ratios, for both the men and women, did not differ from zero correlations.

Speech Disturbances and Experimentally Induced Anxiety

The methodology of the preceding two studies was correlational. In both, we compared variations in the frequency of speech disturbances with variations in measures (judgments) of spontaneously varying anxiety. Correlational research is never completely convincing. Wherever possible, we aim to supplement it (or even supplant it) with data obtained with the experimental method. This was the goal underlying the next three studies to be described. In them, we attempted to experimentally induce anxiety in people speaking under controlled conditions and to observe changes in the frequency of their speech disturbances when we did so.

The First Experiment

Procedure

In this experiment, which is reported in more detail elsewhere (Kasl & Mahl, 1958, 1965), there were 25 experimental and 20 control subjects, all male college students who were paid volunteers. In general, the procedure used a two-session interview sequence conducted in a room equipped for sound recording and observations. The subject's palmar perspiration was measured at discrete points during the experiment, according to the procedure described by Mowrer, Light, Luria and Zeleny (1953).

The details of the experimental procedure were as follows. The subject was brought to the interview room and his palm moisture measured. Then he was seated in an upholstered armchair and donned a set of earphones. Then ensued the "neutral" interview (Interview A), which lasted about 30 minutes. During one-half of this interview, the male experimenter was in the interview room with the subject. During the other half, the experimenter was in the monitor room, separated from the interview room by a wall and a one-way mirror and containing the recording apparatus. Throughout the interview, the subject heard the experimenter through the earphones, although they were required in reality only when the experimenter was in the monitor room. When he was in the monitor room, the experimenter heard the subject over a monitoring speaker, via a microphone placed in a lamp on a table next to the subject's armchair. The subject knew the interview was being recorded and the location of the microphone. Throughout Interview A, the subject was put at ease and encouraged to talk freely, as he saw fit, about school, extracurricular activities, and so forth. Direct, probing or "searching" questions were avoided. When Interview A ended, the experimenter again measured the subject's palm moisture. Then, the subject took the individual form of the MMPI a personality inventory. The subject then left.

He returned for the second session after at least 24 hours had elapsed. His palm moisture was measured. Then he completed several intellectual tasks, judged irrelevant in the present context, and his palm moisture was again measured. At this point, the experimenter went into the monitor room, while the subject remained in the interview room. This was the setting for Interview B, throughout which the interviewer and the subject communicated by means of the microphone-headphones or speaker arrangement.

For the experimental subjects, Interview B was an "anxiety" interview. The experimenter attempted to induce anxiety in two ways: (1) presenting each subject with the same set of anxiety stimuli and (2) raising anxiety-provoking topics for discussion, which were "tailor-made" for each subject, and asking probing questions about them. The standard set of anxiety stimuli included: revealing to the subject, at that point, the presence of the one-way mirror through which the experimenter was observing him, as well as asserting that the long test (the MMPI) he had taken was an "adjustment inventory" and asking what he recalled about it; announcing that certain topics of the experimenter's choice would now be probed; and interspersing the ensuing discussion with silences at points where the subject might have reasonably expected some comment from the experimenter. Now the subject was in the "tailor-made" part of the interview. Using his knowledge about each subject gained from Interview A and from the subject's MMPI answers, the experimenter raised topics for discussion which he believed would be anxiety-provoking to the particular subject. And he asked probing questions about them. Interview B lasted about 30 minutes, whereupon the subject's palm moisture was measured, for the last time. The experimenter then "debriefed" each subject. For the *control subjects,* Interview B was again a "neutral" interview. In it they were given the same freedom of choice of conversation topics as in their first interview and were not subjected to any of the anxiety stimuli. Ten of the control subjects were given the palm moisture tests before and after Interviews A and B. The control subjects were not given any of the psychological tests.

The interviews were all tape recorded and transcribed. The speech disturbances were then scored, using both tapes and typescripts. Speech disturbance ratios were then determined: the Ah Ratio, Non-ah Ratio, and the ratios for the individual Non-ah categories.

Results

Reliabilities. High reliability of the palmar sweat measures was indicated by high stability of individual differences during the repeated palmar sweat measures. The average intercorrelation on these repeated measurements was .74.

The interjudge reliabilities of the scoring of the speech disturbance ratios are reported in Table 2. (Item 3.)

Validation of the Experimental Manipulation. We assumed this would be demonstrated if (a) the palm moisture of the experimental subjects increased in Interview B, but not in the neutral Interview A, and (b) if the control subjects showed no differences in palm moisture between their first and second interviews. The data supported these expectations. During Interview A, 17 of the 25 experimental subjects decreased in their palmar sweat ($p < .06$), but 18 of the 25 increased during Interview B ($p = .02$). The difference between the decrease in Interview A and the increase in Interview B was also significant ($\chi^2 = 6.5$, $p < .02$). The 10 control subjects on whom palmar sweat data were collected showed only random fluctuations in the changes during and between their two interviews.

Changes in Speech Disturbance Ratios. The Non-ah Ratios of 24 of the 25 experimental subjects were higher in the anxiety Interview B than in the neutral Interview A ($p < .0001$). Only 12 of the 20 control subjects showed such an increase from their first to their second interview (*ns*). The difference between the experimental and control groups was significant at the .004 level, using Fisher's exact test. The average increase in the Non-ah Ratios of the experimental subjects, going from Interview A to B, was a sizeable 34%. Furthermore, all seven of the Non-ah categories of the experimental subjects were higher in their anxiety Interview B than in the neutral Interview A ($p<$ .01, using t-tests).

The Ah Ratios showed no significant change among either the experimental or the control subjects between the first and the second interviews.

Figure 5c illustrates the findings for the Non-ah and Ah Ratios, presenting as it does the data for the 25 experimental subjects and those 10 control subjects for whom both speech and palmar sweat data were obtained.

The changes in the Non-ah Ratios were positively associated with changes in palmar sweat during Interview B, compared with Interview A. Thus, subjects who showed a relatively large increase in sweat during Interview B, as compared with their change in sweat during Interview A, had a larger increase in the Non-ah Ratio than subjects who showed a relatively small increase in sweat. This association was mild, however, and suggests that some subjects may react to anxiety mainly in the somatic channel, while other may react mainly in the speech channel.

A serendipitous finding concerning the use of "Ah" emerged as we analyzed the data so as to compare the effects of the presence versus the absence of the interviewer within Interview A, that is, of the face–face versus the "telephone" interview situations. This difference left the Non-ah Ratio unchanged, but had a strong effect on the Ah Ratio. Thirty-two of the 45 subjects had higher Ah Ratios when the interviewer was off in the monitor room, two subjects showed no changes, and only 11 subjects had higher Ah Ratios when the interviewer was present together with the subject in the interview room ($p <$ .001). All 45 subjects were used in this analysis, because the first interview was the same for both experimental and control subjects. Of course, the order of the two speaking situations of this interview was counterbalanced.

The Second Experiment

This experiment was Schulze's (1964). It was a two-part study. In the first part, he used probing questions to arouse anxiety in his subjects. In the second part, he presented the same subjects with a presumably anxiety-inducing film and asked them to describe aloud its proceedings. His principal dependent measures were the Non-ah Ratios and a variety of autonomic measures generally regarded as sensitive to stress.

In the following description of the procedures and results, I shall focus on the main features most relevant in the present context. The reader interested in further details will find them discussed by Schulze (1964). (See also Mahl, 1987.)

Procedures

The subjects were 24 male undergraduate students who volunteered for the study with the inducement of gaining credits to fulfill a psychology course requirment for minimal participation in experiments, and pay for overtime. The precise purpose of the study was not revealed to the subjects until the "debriefing" phase at the very end.

Schulze met with the subjects twice. At the first meeting, from two to eight of the subjects met on campus as a group and responded with written stories to nine pictures of the Thematic Apperception Test (TAT). The pictures used were the nine highest in Stimulatory Value (number of different themes) as rated by Eron (1950). The second meeting took place several days later in the laboratory. During it, the subjects underwent the two parts of the study.

The First Part of the Laboratory Study. An interview organized about questions concerning each subject's TAT stories constituted this part of the study. Schulze had formulated these questions, tailor-made for each subject, by carefully studying the TAT stories between the first and second meeting. He had designed and now asked each subject two kinds of questions.

One kind, *High Anxiety Probes,* was used to arouse the subject's anxiety by asking him about ideas in their TAT stories which seemed to be anxiety-laden, conflicted, and avoided. Illustrative indicators of such ideas included instances where subjects crossed out part of their story, started to write something but left it hanging, hinted at something and then changed the subject, and failed to mention feelings or thoughts which were conspicuous by their absence (for example, a victim of assault feeling no emotion).

The second kind of questions, *Low Anxiety Probes,* was used to elicit talking by the subjects without arousing anxiety in them. These questions were about TAT story content that did not seem to be involved in conflict and thus avoided. They included questions about ideas consistent with the expressed or implied point of the story, along with irrelevant details and themes that served a defensive function by contradicting or supplanting anxiety-arousing ideas.

During this interview, the subject sat in a comfortable reclining chair. The TAT cards were placed on a viewing board before him and remained there while he heard and responded to the probes dealing with them. Three cards with four questions per card were used in each of the anxiety probe conditions. Half the subjects had the *Low Anxiety Probes* first, and then the *High Anxiety Probes*. The other half followed the reversed sequence of *High* and then *Low* Anxiety Probes. Subjects were randomly assigned to their sequences.

The TAT interview was tape recorded and later transcribed verbatim. The speech disturbances were scored later by the experimenter and, for a reliability sample, by an independent judge. Continuous physiological recordings that yielded five autonomic indices were made during the interview: volume pulse, heart rate, skin temperature, galvanic skin potential level, and galvanic skin potential positive deflections. Unobtrusive sensors picked up the relevant physiological data, which were recorded on a multichannel polygraph.

At the end of the interview, the subjects rated each probing condition with respect to the strongest intensity of anxiety experienced during that condition. The anxiety ratings were preceded by ratings of anger intensity and followed by ratings of effort, to assist subjects in discriminating anxiety from those emotional experiences.

The Second Part of the Laboratory Study. Upon completing the TAT interview self-ratings, the subject remained seated in his chair, with the physiological sensors still attached, and participated in the second part of the laboratory study following a "rest" period. In this part, each subject viewed two 8-minute segments of silent black-and-white pictures portraying various activities of the Arunta tribesmen. One film segment was intended to provide the subject with a *Low Stress* experience, while the other segment was intended to provide a *High Stress* experience.

The *High Stress* film segment showed a close range subincision of the penis of adolescent Arunta tribesmen. (Subincisiion is one particular form of circumcision.) The *Low Stress* film segment showed the Arunta engaged in less dramatic activities (practicing hunting, for example) and included no scenes of bodily mutilation.

The subject was asked to describe aloud what he was seeing in the motion pictures. The verbal descriptions of the films were tape recorded and later transcribed verbatim. The Non-ah speech disturbances were scored as for the TAT interview, and continuous physiological measures were recorded during both film descriptions.

The subjects were randomly assigned to two groups of 12 subjects each. One group received the *Low Stress–High Stress* film sequence and the other the *High Stress–Low Stress* sequence. A 5-minute recovery period followed each film.

The subjects made self-ratings of anxiety intensity, anger intensity, and degree of effort experienced during the film presentations.

Results

I shall discuss together the results of the two parts of this experiment.

Reliabilities. The average interscorer reliability coefficient of the Non-ah speech disturbance ratios are reported in Table 2, Item 11.

The interscorer reliability coefficients of the various physiological measures were also very high, ranging from .92 to .99.

Validation of the Experimental Manipulations. Let us assume that changes in the Anxiety Self-Ratings and in the autonomic-measures validity reflect variations in the subject's anxiety levels, and see if the experimental manipulations seemed to have achieved their intended effects.

TAT Interviews. The Anxiety Self-Ratings were significantly higher during the High-Anxiety Probe TAT interview than during the Low-Anxiety Probe interview ($p < .03$). This was a special effect, since the Hostility and Effort Self-Ratings did not differ for the two TAT interviews.

Considered individually, none of the physiological measures was significantly higher during the High Anxiety than during the Low Anxiety Probe interview. However, the average heart rate, galvanic skin potential level, number of galvanic responses, and (inverted) skin temperature were all higher during the High Anxiety Probe interview. In combination, they were significantly higher in that interview than in the Low Anxiety Probe interview ($p = .003$). The use of tailor-made probes designed to increase the subjects' anxiety did seem to have achieved the intended effect.

Film Descriptions. The Anxiety Self-Ratings were significantly higher during the High Stress than during the Low Stress film ($p < .001$). The self-ratings of Hostility and Effort, however, were also significantly higher during the High Stress film. Thus, the effect of the film manipulation was not specific to anxiety.

The averages of all the physiological measures were higher during the High Stress than during the Low Stress film. These increases were statistically significant for the galvanic skin potential level ($p < .04$) and for the number of galvanic responses ($p < .02$). These results and the self-ratings suggest that the subincision film created a general state of stress, rather than a specific state of only increased anxiety.

Changes in the Non-ah Speech Disturbance Ratios. These were significantly greater in the High Anxiety than in the Low Anxiety Probe TAT interviews ($p < .03$). There was not, however, any difference in the speech disturbance ratios for the Low and High Stress films. Figure 6 portrays these results.

The failure to obtain a difference in speech disturbances with the film manipulation may be due to various factors. First, it may be an actual instance where increased anxiety in the speaker is not accompanied by increased speech disturbances. Secondly, it may be due to the fact that the subincision film created higher stress, rather than creating a relatively pure increase in anxiety. Thirdly, the verbal behavior of the subjects during both film presentations consisted mainly of description of external scenes, rather than revelation of (projected) internal, personal matters, as occurred in the TAT interviews. Figure 6 shows that the speech disturbance levels during the description of both the Low and High Stress films were markedly lower than during both the Low and High-Anxiety Probe interviews. This suggests that description of external scenes results in a generally lowered level of speech disturbances and may prevent that level from changing as a result of changes in the emotional state of the speaker. One possible reason for these effects is that description may involve fewer choice points in the process of verbalizing than does spontaneous self-revelation. Hopefully, future research will decide which of these possibilities, or another, was responsible for the lack of change with the film manipulation.

What about the relationship of variations in speech disturbances with variations in the physiological measures? Schulze computed many

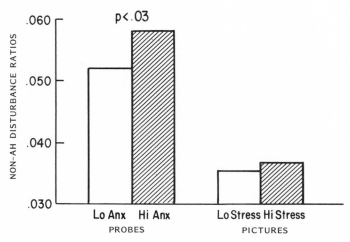

FIGURE 6. (a) Mean non-ah ratios of 24 male undergraduates under different degrees of anxiety probing about TAT scores (based on Schulze, 1964). (b) Mean non-ah ratios of 24 male undergraduates when describing orally control film and Arunta subincision film (based on Schulze, 1964; from Mahl, 1987).

kinds of correlations between these two classes of measures. Some significant positive correlations were obtained, but no more than would be expected to occur by chance when so many correlations are computed. These results are similar to those in the first experiment (Kasl & Mahl, 1958, 1965), where palmar sweat and speech disturbances both increased during the anxiety interview, and yet the two measures were only modestly correlated with each other.

The Third Experiment

The experiment proper was originally conducted (Zimbardo, Barnard, & Berkowitz, 1963) as part of the pioneering program of research on *test anxiety* in school children that Seymour Sarason and his colleagues conducted over many years. Sarason, Zimbardo, and colleagues generously placed at our disposal the materials of their study. We jumped at the opportunity to use them and thus investigate the effect of still a third experimental manipulation of anxiety on speech disturbances, especially since this one dealt with children, rather than adults. In this study, we can see the interactive effect of both characterological and (mild) situational anxiety on the level of speech disturbances in grade-school children. The interested reader will find other aspects of this study reported in greater detail elsewhere (Zimbardo, Mahl, & Barnard, 1963). (See also Mahl, 1987.)

Procedure

The *subjects* were 40 boys, selected from a population of over 500 third-grade children tested in 11 elementary schools in a Connecticut city. Eighteen months before the present study, the entire population had received the Test Anxiety Scale for Children, developed by Sarason and his colleagues (Sarason *et al.*, 1960). The scale is a 30-item questionnaire that elicits self-reports by a child of the degree of anxiety he or she feels in a wide variety of testing situations and when anticipating them. Twenty of the subjects of the present study were in the highest 15% of the anxiety scale distribution and are called here "High-Anxious." Twenty "Low-Anxious" subjects were in the lowest 15% of the distribution. The subjects in the two groups were matched individually in IQ.

These boys participated in an interview that consisted of a series of nine standardized questions and relevant probes and the responses to them. The interview was conducted by one of two male interviewers who did not know the anxiety categories of the subjects. The interviews were tape-recorded, and verbatim transcripts were prepared for later use in scoring the Non-ah speech disturbances.

Although the same questions were used in every interview, they were presented to half the boys in the context of an Evaluative Interview and to the other half in the context of a Permissive Interview. In turn, each of these two groups of boys included 10 High Anxious and 10 Low Anxious subjects.

The Evaluative Interview was designed to lead the boys experiencing it to believe that the interviewer was evaluating them and that they would be given a test following the interview. These expectations were induced by the adoption of a distant and authoritative manner and by relevant instructions. When the interview was over, the interviewer told the boys there was not time for the test, but that it was not necessary since they had talked enough. He was then friendly, supportive and encouraging to every boy.

In the Permissive Interview the instructions, the interviewer's manner, and his frequent use of the boy's first name were conducive to creating a permissive and nonevaluative situation. And the boys did not expect to be tested afterwards.

Results

Validation of the Experimental Manipulation. Were the differences in instructions and in the interviewer's manner in the two interviews successful in creating differential expectations of the threatening testing situation? This question was investigated by determining if the boys experiencing the *Evaluative Interviews* were more likely to expect a test and to feel that other people in addition to the interviewer would know what they talked about than were the boys experiencing the *Permissive Interview*. On both open-ended and forced choice questions, significantly more of the evaluative boys expected to get a test, while the permissively treated children expected a game, more talk, or something other than a test ($p < .01$). Additionally, 35% of the evaluative boys believed others ("parents, peers, or everyone") would know what was said in the interviews, but only 15% of the permissively treated boys had this expectation. This difference, however, was not statistically significant.

In their own investigation, Zimbardo, Barnard, and Berkowitz (1963) had already demonstrated that the interview manipulation was effective, in interaction with the test anxiety grouping of the subjects. This was demonstrated by the fact that they attained significant, predicted effects on a variety of attributes of the boys' verbal behavior during the interviews. Needless to say, those attributes did not include speech disturbances.

Reliability of Speech Disturbance Scoring. This is reported in Table 2, Item 7. All scoring was done without knowledge of the anxiety group of the subjects.

Effect of Test Anxiety and Interviews on Non-ah Speech Disturbances. Naturally, we expected that boys with High Test Anxiety would speak with more speech disturbances in the Evaluative Interview than would similar boys in the Permissive Interview. That is exactly what happened, as Figure 7 shows. We also expected that boys with Low Test Anxiety would have more speech disturbances in a Permissive Interview than would similar boys in the Evaluative Interview. And that is exactly what happened, as Figure 7 shows. This surprising expectation about the Low Anxious boys was based primarily on the empirical fact that two previous studies, one of which was the experiment yielding the raw interview tapes used in the present study, had shown that, on a variety of verbal behavior measures, Low Anxious boys spoke in the Permissive Interview the way High Anxious boys spoke in the Evaluative Interview (Barnard, Zimbardo, & Sarason, 1961; Zimbardo, Barnard, & Berkowitz, 1963).

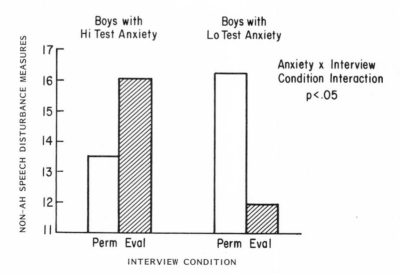

FIGURE 7. Mean non-ah speech disturbance measures (arc sine transforms of ratios) of 40 third-grade boys during interviews conducted under permissive (Perm) and evaluative (Eval) conditions (based on Zimbardo, Mahl, & Barnard, 1963, from Mahl, 1987).

The reason for this reversal is not firmly established, but those observing it have proposed the following, interesting hypothesis about it (see especially Zimbardo, Barnard, & Berkowitz, 1963). Perhaps, they suggest, the Low Anxious group includes a fair number of boys who are basically quite frightened by testing situations and self-revelation, but who have developed successful defenses that enable them to conceal their test anxiety and all other personal concerns and feelings and to cope with testing situations. (The utilization of these defenses when responding to the test-anxiety questionnaire results in them falling in the Low Anxiety group.) These defenses are elicited in a testing situation, but not in a nontesting one. Thus, the Permissive Interview aroused their anxiety about self-revelation, but did not elicit their successful defense against such anxiety.

Summary of the Studies of Anxiety and Speech Disturbances

We have reported six studies that used a variety of subjects and a variety of speaking situations. In five of the studies, the speaker's anxiety was positively associated with the Non-ah speech disturbances. The speaking situations of those five studies had one thing in common: they called for self-revelation by the speaker, either in psychotherapeutic or in personal investigative interviews. In the one negative instance (Schulze's film study), the speaker's task was to describe pictorial scenes involving others. The data strongly suggested that description lowers the level of speech disturbance. Additionally, that study involved a general stress effect rather than a "pure" anxiety effect.

Three of the studies also investigated the relationship between the Ah Ratio and anxiety. In none was there any significant relationship.

Work of Others

In the last 30 years, many investigators have contributed to the growth of a substantial literature concerned with the relationship between transient anxiety and nonfluency. This growth started with the simultaneous and independent work of Dibner (1956, 1958) and ourselves (Mahl, 1956) on nonfluencies in the speech of patients in interviews and that of Lerea (1956) on nonfluencies during public speaking.

Our Non-ah Ratio is the single most researched measure of nonfluency in the literature we have located. Sixteen studies have concerned the relationship of this measure and transient anxiety in the speaker. Twelve of them confirmed our findings, either as main or interaction effects (Blass & Siegman, 1975; Blumenthal, 1964; Boomer, 1963; Bradac, Konsky, & Elliott, 1976; Brady & Walker, 1978 [2 experiments]; Cook, 1969; Feldstein, Brenner, & Jaffe, 1963; Musumeci, 1975; Pope, Blass, Siegman, & Raher, 1970; Pope, Siegman, & Blass, 1970; Siegman & Pope, 1965). One study was inconclusive (Boomer & Goodrich, 1961), and three failed to obtain positive results (Geer, 1966; Meisels, 1967; Reynolds & Paivio, 1968).

Fifteen additional studies of transient anxiety and nonfluency have involved the General Speech Disturbance Ratio, analogues of it, or explicitly made modified versions of it. Thirteen of these have yielded positive results (Dibner, 1958; Edelmann & Hampson, 1979, 1981; Eldred & Price, 1958; Horowitz, Sampson, Siegelman, Wolfson, & Weiss, 1975 [2 studies]; Horowitz, Weckler, Saxon, Livaudais, & Boutacoff, 1977; Krause & Pilisuk, 1961; Lerea, 1956; Levin, Baldwin, Gallwey, & Paivio, 1960; Nosenko, Yelchaninov, Krylova, & Petrukhin, 1977 [2 experiments]; Panek & Martin, 1959). Two studies failed to obtain positive results (Levin & Silverman, 1965; Paivio, 1963).

I have discussed all the preceding studies in detail elsewhere (Mahl, 1987). Suffice it to say here that they involved a variety of methods, speakers, and situations, just as our work did. The combination of our studies with those of others provides a corpus of 37 studies of the relationship between nonfluency and transient anxiety. Thirty gave positive results, despite the psychological complexities involved in such research. The evidence is overwhelming that measures of nonfluency are valid indicators of transient anxiety.

Seven of the studies by others (cited two paragraphs above) examined the relationship between the Ah-Ratio, as well as the Non-ah Ratio, and concurrent anxiety. Six of them confirmed our findings that the Ah-Ratios did not increase with the speakers' anxiety, while the Non-ah Ratio did.

We also noted (cf. fn. 8) that the speech disturbance categories are applicable to English, German, Japanese, Spanish, and Russian. Now we can state that there is some evidence that the relationship between the speech disturbances and transient anxiety is a cross-cultural one. Thus it has been demonstrated in Russians (Nosenko *et al.* 1977), in English speaking Australian college students (Brady & Walker, 1978), and in English college students (Cook, 1969; Endelmann & Hampson, 1979, 1981) as well English speaking subjects of the United States. We commented above on the significance of freedom from linguistic restraint for the vocal-verbal measurement of anxiety. It will be very interesting to see the extensions of and limits to the cross-cultural dimensions that might emerge in future research.

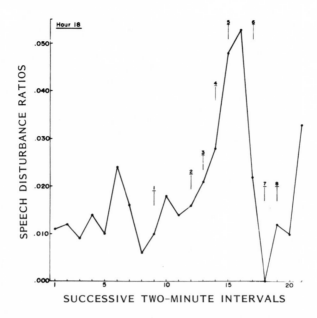

FIGURE 8. Variation in the patient's 2-minute non-ah speech disturbance ratios during a psychotherapy interview (from Mahl, 1961).

CLINICAL ILLUSTRATIONS

I shall now present three clinical illustrations to acquaint you further with speech disturbances *in vivo*.

The first example concerns the graph in Figure 8, which shows the course of a patient's Non-ah Ratio during successive 2-minute intervals of his 18th psychotherapy interview.[11] It is apparent that from the 18th to the 36th minute of the interview the patient's speech disturbance level progressively rises. Then it abruptly falls. Why? In answering, we can show how the disturbance ratio may sensitively reflect the therapist–patient interaction, and also illustrate how speech disturbances vary with the types of phases judged clinically in the first study we presented concerning anxiety and speech disturbances. The latter is the case because the first 18 minutes was a low anxiety phase, the segment from the

---

[11]Dr. Alberto DiMascio provided me with this interview, to use in my contribution to a symposium on the program of the 1959 New York Divisional Meetings of the New York State District Branches, American Psychiatric Association. The entire symposium, including detailed analyses of two interviews of this patient by various investigators, is reported in Gottschalk (1961).

18th to the 36th minute was a high anxiety or conflicted phase, and the segment covering the abrupt drop right after the 36th minute was another low anxiety phase.

The patient was a young professional worker in the behavioral sciences whose obsessive-compulsive character disorder had manifested itself partly in work inhibition including procrastination. The therapist's notes about the earlier interviews were available to us and showed that being on time for his interviews was an emotionally charged matter, as one might expect from his history of procrastination in life. The patient was often late and in the past had failed to notify the therapist adequately of absences. His handling of time had all the signs of symptomatic behavior and resistance to therapy. He started this interview by being late. He referred to his lateness at the outset of the interview, but then avoided talking further about it for the first 18 minutes. The therapist was quiet during this time. Thus, the patient was successful in avoiding a currently active, emotionally charged issue during this segment of the interview. His speech disturbance level remained at a relatively low level.

The therapist actively intervened, however, at point 1 in the graph, by stating "You seem not to want to talk about the motivation for your being late today," and "I wonder if we could go into it." Throughout the subsequent minutes when the disturbance curve was rising the therapist maintained a steady, active pressure on the patient to explore his lateness. He did this by commenting at points 2, 3, 4, and 5 in ways that focused on his lateness and factors that seemed to be related to it. In doing this he was energetically and persistently preventing the patient from defensively avoiding his lateness and the reasons for it. This type of activity by a therapist typically arouses the patient's anxiety. We can reasonably presume this happened in this instance and was manifested in the progressive rise of the speech disturbance curve.

The ensuing decline in the speech disturbance curve was associated with a marked turn of events at point 6. First, the patient became briefly angry. The therapist then offered a lengthy interpretation of the patient's lateness, and the patient then experienced an insight and wept as though with cathartic relief. At points 7 and 8 the therapist responded empathically to the patient's tears. This type of interaction is typically reassuring and comforting to patients. Thus, it is fitting that the speech disturbance level reached zero at one point and remained low for several minutes.

The next two clinical examples are ones in which such "feeble indications" as a sentence incompletion, or an omission and a sentence change, resulted from conflicts over very important matters. The speaker is a successful young professional man who was in psychoanalysis with me, where these examples occurred. In each of them, I asked about the speech disturbances, a practice not followed in the research described in this chapter.

One day, when he was speaking about an upcoming vacation trip, I asked him where he was going. He said:

> Oh, to B. I have a friend . . . well I planned first to go to A. Then I got the idea of making a circuit by going to B, C, D, and then to A. But when I started to plan the days, I realized it would take two weeks to go to all those places. So we'll just go to B.

I then commented: "You said, 'I have a friend . . .' and broke off." He replied:

> Well, I was referring to L_____, a woman at Z (where he worked the previous year). We bedded together and became close friends. She is from B.
> L_____ was older than me [about 10 years older]. When I first started at Z she seemed prudish, stern, remote. I decided to make her a challenge—to see if I could succeed in getting her into bed and sticking it to her. I did. We did it several times. She became quite fond of me. She was like a mother to me. She used to cook meals for me.

The preceding interchange occurred at a period in his analysis when the patient, with considerable surprise and conflict, was discovering what a significant role his attachment to his mother played in his choice of women as lovers and friends. This conflict, operating with unconscious anticipatory precision, had caused the sentence incompletion. The latter was so "innocent" that one would ordinarily attach no significance to it whatsoever. Since the vast majority of speech disturbances are just as "innocent" in external appearance, many people hesitate to attribute deep, inner significance to them. Our example illustrates how ill-founded this hesitancy is.

The same young man committed the disturbances in the following example. These disturbances are less "innocent" because they were less anticipatory—that is, they occurred as conflicted thoughts were on the verge of being spoken, not well in advance of them as in the preceding example. The disturbances may have been more numerous for the same reason.

The young man was lying on his back on the analytic couch, with legs raised, flexed at the knees so that the soles of his feet were flat on the surface of the couch. Lying thus he said:

> I feel like a wo . . . this position. . . . (Here he left the sentence incomplete. He lowered and straightened his legs and shifted to another line of thought, which he followed for some time.)

Eventually I drew his attention to the omission, sentence change, and incompletion by saying: "You said, 'I feel like a wo . . .' and then veered off to what you've just been talking about. What occurs to you about your phrase, 'I feel like a wo . . .'?"

> (His associations led to thinking about his previous leg position, and to wondering what a woman feels during intercourse.) Believe me, I don't feel like a woman in relation to you. . . . Do you think each of us men has a little of a woman in us; and each woman, a little of a man in her? I do.

It is obvious that these less "innocent" disturbances were indicative of anxiety over thoughts not completely camouflaged by the disturbances. But even these more transparent disturbances did not reveal just how conflicted the nature of the related thoughts was.

These three clinical examples illustrate some of the lasting impressions I have as a result of my immersion in studying the normal disturbances of spontaneous speech: (a) their exquisite sensitivity to changes in the speaker's anxiety—whether reflected in measures like 2-minute ratios or in discrete occurrences of isolated disturbances, (b) their range in apparent "innocence"—with most of them appearing to be quite "innocent," and (c) their derivation from personally very significant psychological materials and conflicts—no matter how "innocent" or "blameful" they seem to be.

THE RELATIONSHIP BETWEEN SPEECH DISTURBANCES AND MANIFEST VERBAL CONTENT

The two preceding examples also illustrate the impression I formed early in my work that there is little relationship between the incidence of the speech disturbances and the emotions expressed in the concurrent manifest verbal content. In neither example did the manifest content refer to any emotional state. Moreover, only in the second example could a judge reasonably have inferred that some negative affect might have been present. And, if the judge were ignorant of what we have shown about the significance of speech disturbances, that influence would have to be based on general psychodynamic knowledge, rather than on the manifest content. For example, the content makes no reference to anxiety or conflict, but the judge might infer that uttering, or perhaps even thinking about, what appear to be references of having experiences of resembling a woman would probably be anxiety-arousing and thus conflicted for this masculine young man.

Naturally, we were interested in systematically investigating our early impression to see if it would be substantiated, or invalidated. The answer would add to our knowledge about speech disturbances. And it would have implications for the use of manifest verbal content to measure anxiety and conflict. We have conducted two such studies, which I shall now mention.

Speech Disturbances and Discomfort-Relief: Verbal Content in Initial Inteviews

Procedure

This study (Mahl, 1957) involved further work with the 31 initial psychiatric interviews mentioned previously. This further work started with unitizing the typescripts of the patients' speech in the interviews into sentence units, according to rules developed by Frank Auld (Auld & White, 1956). Then each of these sentence units was categorized as a Discomfort, Relief, or Neutral unit, according to the method of manifest verbal-content analysis developed by Dollard and Mowrer (1947). In this method, a sentence is classified as a Discomfort unit if its manifest verbal content refers to mounting drive tension or various forms of distress (anxiety, for example). A sentence is classified as a Relief unit if its manifest verbal content refers to decreased drive tension or decreased distress. A Neutral unit is one in which the manifest verbal content refers to neither discomfort-distress nor relief.

One judge unitized and scored the content of all 31 typescripts. His scores were used in obtaining the results presented below. An independent judge unitized and scored 21 typescripts. A secretary independently unitized 10. The first judge scored the speech disturbances as well.

For this study, we used 25% unbiased samples of the discomfort and the neutral sentences in each interview, and all of the much less frequent relief sentences.[12] The frequency of the Non-ah speech disturbances was then determined for each patient's sample of discomfort sentences, of relief sentences, and of neutral sentences.

Results

Reliabilities of the various operations were as follows. The reliability of the sentence unitizing was determined by comparing the secretary's unitizing with that of the two judges. There was agreement on placement of more than 95% of the unit markings. The reliability of scoring the verbal content was determined by comparing the scoring of the two

[12]The resulting samples are portions of the material used for other purposes by Auld and Mahl (1956).

judges of all the material in 10 interviews. These interviews contained 5,660 sentence units. The judges agreed exactly in 75% of them. In only 3% of the units had one judge scored a unit in the discomfort category that the other had scored as a relief unit. Twenty-two percent of the units had been scored as neutral by one judge, but as either a discomfort or a relief unit by the other judge. The reliability of the speech disturbance scoring was not determined for the interview material used here. The reliability of this judge's scoring, however, had been found repeatedly high. He was Scorer A of Table 2.

The relationship between the speech disturbances and the content categories was found to be zero. Table 9 contains the relevant data. The mean Non-ah Ratios of the women is the same for the utterances in the three content categories. The variations of the ratios of the men is greater, but no one of the ratios differs significantly from the others.

One could argue that the meaning of this "negative" finding is uncertain, because the "discomfort" category is not specifically an anxiety category. It includes utterances referring to any kind of discomfort or distress (increased anger, sexuality, frustration, guilt, as well as anxiety, for example). Since speech disturbances appear to be highly related to anxiety, it would be of greater interest and significance to see how they would be related to manifest content scored specifically for anxiety. The following study addresses this question. (I shall return to the previous results after describing the next study.)

Speech Disturbances and Manifest Verbal Content in Psychotherapy Interviews

We investigated the question by determining how the frequency of speech disturbances varied with the more fine-grained verbal content

TABLE 9
Summary of Sentence Analysis of Initial Interviews[a]

		Discomfort sentences	Relief sentences	Neutral sentences
Mean speech				
disturbance ratio	20 Women	.038	.036	.038
(Non-Ah)	11 Men	.041	.044	.035
Mean N				
sentences	20 Women	90	51	74
analyzed	11 Men	65	40	70

[a]From Mahl, 1987.

categories developed by Murray for the study of psychotherapy (Murray, 1956; Schulze, Mahl, & Murray, 1960; Mahl, 1987).

Procedure

Wishing to have an "objective" system, Murray devised verbal-content categories that required relatively little inference by the scorer. Thus, the categories reflected chiefly manifest verbal content. He chose categories influenced by psychoanalytic concepts and Neal Miller's Approach–Avoidance Conflict Theory (Dollard & Miller, 1950). His system included categories for statements expressing a need (Approach categories), for statements expressing anxiety about a need (Anxiety categories), and for statements expressing hostility because of frustration of a need (Hostility categories). The needs included were: sex, affection, dependence, independence, and "unspecified" drive. Thus the total array of Murray's categories for patient utterances included Sex, Sex Anxiety, Sex Hostility, Affection, Affection Anxiety, Affection Hostility, and so forth.

Murray scored the verbatim transcripts of 17 recorded psychotherapy interviews from the tape recorded treatments of three psychoneurotic patients. Eight interviews were from Mr. Z, who entered psychotherapy for relief from anxiety attacks and duodenal ulcer. Four interviews were from Mrs. T, who sought treatment for anxiety, depression, and frigidity. Five interviews were from Mr. S, who suffered from impotence and depression. All three treatments included many more interviews. The interviews Murray used was determined solely by the availability of the typescripts at the time of his study.

Multiple copies of the verbatim typescripts had been prepared for the interviews involved. Using one set of the copies, Murray divided the patient's speech into sentence units and scored their manifest content according to his categories. His scoring was independent of the speech disturbance scoring. He did his scoring while we were developing our speech disturbance categories and doing our first studies of them. He had no knowledge of the speech disturbance categories, nor of their scoring in any of the interviews.

A completely independent judge, a research assistant of mine who had no knowledge of Murray's system of scoring, scored the Non-ah speech disturbances while reading a second copy of the typescripts and listening to the tapes.

Results

Reliability of Scoring. Murray found that his scoring of all but two of the content categories was reliable. (The exceptions were Dependence

Hostility and Independence Hostility.) The reliabilities of the scores for the combined Approach categories was .89; that for the combined Anxiety categories was .77. The reliability of the speech-disturbance scorer in this study had been found to be .86, .88, and .90 on three previous occasions.

The relationship of manifest-anxiety verbal content and the Non-ah speech disturbance ratios was found to be zero, for all practical purposes. I shall report two of the ways we assayed this relationship. In the first, we grouped together the various Anxiety content units and the Approach content units in each interview, and computed the Non-ah Ratios for each sample of units. From these interview measures we then computed each patient's average Non-ah Ratios for these two broad verbal-content groups. Table 10 contains the results. The Non-ah Ratio is no higher in the Anxiety than in the Approach categories. In fact, Mr. Z's average ratio was significantly lower when he uttered manifest Anxiety content. I shall comment on this later.

In the second assay, we determined the average Non-ah Ratios for each of the content categories for the three individual patients. Table 11 contains these data, which reveal two general findings.

The average Non-ah Ratios for each of the content categories used by the patients are presented in rank order in Table 11. You can see that the various specific Anxiety categories tend to accumulate in the lower rankings for each of the three patients. This is the first general finding.

The second general finding revealed by Table 11 is the striking fact that open utterance by each of these patients of Dependence needs is associated with the greatest disturbance of speech. This ranking is prominent. For each patient, the difference between the Non-ah Ratio of the Dependence category and that of the next ranking category considerably exceeds all remaining ratio differences between adjacent content-categories. Thus, Dependent manifest verbal content, rather than Anxiety content, is associated with the highest levels of speech disturbance in these samples.

TABLE 10
Mean Non-Ah Speech Disturbance Ratios for Approach and Anxiety Content Categories[a]

	Approach	Anxiety	t	p
Mr. Z	.0545	.0416	2.97	<.01
Mrs. T	.0539	.0618	0.87	N.S.
Mr. S	.0529	.0489	0.67	N.S.

[a]From Mahl, 1987.

TABLE 11
Verbal Content Category Profiles of Non-Ah Ratios for Individual Psychotherapy Patients[a]

Mr. Z		Mrs. T		Mr. S	
.0686	Dependence	(.0922)	Dependence	.0711	Dependence
(0.535)	Dependence-hostility	.0793	Sex-hostility	.0583	Unspecified anxiety
.0477	Affection	(0.701)	Independence-hostility	.0575	Unspecified hostility
.0473	Dependence-anxiety	.0698	Unspecified hostility	.0499	Independence
(.0466)	Independence-hostility	(.0693)	Independence-anxiety	.0463	Affection
.0448	Sex	(.0671)	Dependence-hostility	.0459	Affection-hostility
(.0447)	Sex-hostility	.0661	Affection	.0452	Affection-anxiety
.0440	Unspecified anxiety	.0626	Affection-hostility	.0382	Sex-Anxiety
.0435	Unspecified hostility	.0625	Sex-Anxiety	(.0357)	Independence-hostility
.0421	Affection-anxiety	.0611	Affection-anxiety	(.0336)	Independence-anxiety
.0410	Sex-anxiety	(.0576)	Unspecified anxiety		
.0363	Independence-anxiety	(.0512)	Sex		
(.0334)	Affection-hostility	.0406	Independence		

[a]Parentheses indicate Mean Non-Ah Ratios with low reliability due to small samples of sentence units in the verbal content categories or to unreliability of content scoring for Dependence Hostility and Independence Hostility. Categories not listed for a given patient were completely lacking in the hours scored. (From Mahl, 1987).

Comment on the Lack of Relationship between Manifest Verbal Content and Speech Disturbances

Why is it that the Non-ah speech disturbances do not, in general, occur with concurrent verbal content manifestly referring to distress-discomfort or to anxiety? And why might Dependence content have been associated with the highest levels of speech disturbances? I do not believe I know the complete answers to these questions, but I do think the following observations about anxiety and verbal behavior concern some of the important factors involved:

1. Sometimes, some people do utter "anxious" content when they are in fact anxious. (One frightened child might say "I'm scared."

2. But just as often, I believe, frightened people may utter verbal content of quite a different kind, depending upon their particular development of defenses and coping mechanisms. (Another frightened child might speak with anger; another might, in effect, say "Help"; still another might simply say "Mom! Mom!")

3. Sometimes people utter "anxious" content when they are not frightened, but are in fact feeling quite comfortable and are trying to maintain that state. (A child might say "I'm scared, Mom" simply so that his mother will hold him or continue to do so.)

4. Sometimes people will become anxious as they utter "non-anxious" content because of the personal, private meaning of that content. (A child might become anxious as he tells his mother how "good" he has been, if he is afraid his mother will discover how "bad" he really was.)

The veridical relationship between anxiety and verbal content referred to in the first instance certainly does operate at times in psychiatric and psychotherapy interviews. There are times when mounting anxiety (which would be indicated by increased speech disturbances) causes the patient to directly and explicitly refer to that anxiety or to indirectly utter displaced anxiety content. But the veridical relationship of the first instance may be overshadowed by the operation of the varied, discrepant relationships of the other instances. It seems quite likely that this happens in situations like psychiatric or psychotherapy interviews, where people are free to express themselves spontaneously in their preferred ways.

The following observations about the use of Discomfort and Relief or Neutral content in the initial interviews suggest that this happened in them and one reason why. In executing that study, I would often listen to the tape recording of the particular interviews after scoring the corresponding typescripts for the verbal content categories. Often the vocal signs of the emotional state of a patient and the manifest content in the typescript were markedly discrepant. For example, a patient might sound relaxed while uttering a long run of Discomfort sentences pertaining to his or her symptoms, or a patient might sound quite distraught while uttering such Neutral manifest content as where he or she lived and worked. An examination of the distribution of scores of the prevalence of Discomfort sentences in the interviews (the Discomfort–Relief Quotient of Dollard & Mower, 1947) suggests one reason for my impression of this discrepancy. Those scores could have ranged from .000 to 1.000. Yet they were restricted to the high end of the scale, ranging from .77 to .97. (By contrast, the anxiety ratings ranged over the entire 5-point scale used, and the speech-disturbance ratios were quite widely distributed. See Figure 5.) I believe the restriction of the Discomfort scores to the high end of the scale is the result of a process analogous to the third instance cited above. Verbal "distress" messages are entirely appropriate to the initial psychiatric interview situation. First, the interview is usually aimed at eliciting a description of his suffering. Second, the patient has come to obtain help with his psychic distress. He must (reasonably) assume, consciously or preconsciously, that the utterance of Discomfort units will maximize the likelihood of obtaining that help. He wants help and, in effect, cries "help." Yet, right at that moment he may feel comfortable and relieved, because he is being heard, tended to, and feels future relief lies ahead.

The following observation about the use of "anxious content" by Mr. Z, one of the three patients in the second study, illustrates how the veridical relationship between anxiety and verbal content might have been overshadowed in that study, and how his Non-ah Ratio might have come to be significantly lower in his Anxiety units than in his Approach units. I had been his therapist and I still remember the following interaction. In one phase of his therapy, Mr. Z spoke in detail about many frightening experiences in his life. I finally said to him that he must have felt anxious as he recounted his frightening experiences. Not at all, he answered. He had felt comfortable, believing he had aroused my interest, sympathy, and concern. Such observations strongly suggest that for some people anxiety content may serve interpersonal and intrapersonal functions that render it nonveridical to the state of being anxious.

Conversely, the utterance of nonanxious content may be associated with increased anxiety, and of increases in such indicators of it as the speech disturbances. The second instance cited above might apply to the utterance of Dependence content by the three psychotherapy patients when their speech disturbances were at the highest levels. Increased anxiety might have caused them to speak of Dependence because their anxiety aroused a sense of helplessness in them. Or perhaps, as in the fourth instance, speaking of Dependence was most anxiety-provoking for them. One of these possibilities might have applied to one or two of the patients, and the other to the remaining patient or patients. Our clinical example of "I have a friend . . . and so forth" clearly illustrates the occurrence of the fourth instance in psychotherapy.

ASSORTED SUGGESTIVE FINDINGS ABOUT SPEECH DISTURBANCES

In isolated studies, I and my colleagues have investigated the relationship of the speech disturbances to additional variables. The results of these studies are very interesting, but they have not yet been confirmed by replications or closely related investigations. Therefore, I am presenting them here briefly, and as "suggestions" for further research. This further research should be aimed both at replication and at elucidating relevant mechanisms involved.

Lassen (1973) studied the impact of varying the proximity of the client and interviewer in initial psychiatric interviews. She determined the effect of this variation on many dimensions of the client's behavior and experience, including the effect on the Non-ah speech disturbance level. That effect was marked. As the distance between the client and interviewer varied from 3 to 6 to 9 feet, the clients' Non-ah Ratios increased in linear fashion ($p < .01$).

We (Mahl & Kasl, 1958) studied the relationships between the speech disturbance levels of the young adult males of our anxiety study and the time and condition of their having been weaned in childhood, as well as the age of onset of their talking. Both kinds of childhood data were obtained by questionnaires answered by their mothers. The most significant results concerned the relationship between weaning and the speech disturbances. These included the findings: (1) that the earlier-weaned subjects used "ah" more frequently under neutral conditions of speech than did the later-weaned, (2) that early weaning was related to a much greater increase in the Non-ah Ratio upon anxiety induction, and (3) that this latter effect was considerably enhanced by the virtual absence of breast feeding.

In the first part of this chapter you saw that the speech disturbance category profiles revealed some people to be mainly "Ah-ers," others to be "Sentence-changers," and so forth. In a preliminary study, (1958) I found that "Ah-ers" report having had strict parents and being ruminative in thinking, while "Sentence-changers" have difficulty in concentrating and in speaking publicly. I used an "arm-chair" item-analysis of responses to The Minnesota Multiphasic Personality Inventory to obtain these findings.

A study of the association of the various speech disturbance categories within individual sentences (Mahl, 1955b) revealed that the utterance of "Ah" in a sentence was associated with fewer of each of the Non-ah categories in the sentence, and that this negative relationship was stronger if "Ah" occurred at the outset of the sentence than if it occurred elsewhere in the sentence.

We found that the speech disturbance categories we have studied in normal and neurotic speakers were also characteristic of the speech of paranoid schizophrenics (Schulze, Mahl, & Holzberg, 1959). The fact that others have used our speech disturbance ratios to investigate various aspects of schizophrenia indicates that they, too, have found this to be so (Blumenthal, 1964; Feldstein, 1962).

CONCLUDING COMMENT

My quest for an objective indicator of transitory anxiety that could be applied to patients' speech in psychotherapy led me to the normal disturbances of spontaneous speech. This encounter resulted in the development of a method for studying them: the speech disturbance categories and ratios. In turn, we investigated the purely quantitative aspects of the phenonema. We presented these results and have already summarized and discussed them in the early part of this chapter.

Naturally, our research also concerned the validity of the speech-disturbance measure as an index of the speaker's transitory anxiety during spontaneous speech. I believe our research has substantially demonstrated that validity.

Our research into the relationship of the speech disturbances to relevant manifest verbal content is less extensive. But it strongly suggests that this relationship is essentially zero. I discussed my ideas why this might be so.

I have just mentioned some additional "suggestive" findings concerning thenormal speech disturbances.

This is a fascinating dimension of speech. Our own work has barely scratched the surface of all the research concerning it that remains to be done.

ACKNOWLEDGMENTS

I am grateful for the dedicated, invaluable help of Carmel Lepore in the preparation of this manuscript.

REFERENCES

Auld, F., & Mahl, G. F. (1956). A comparison of the DRQ with ratings of emotions. *Journal of Abnormal and Social Psychology, 53,* 386–388.

Auld, F., & White, A. M. (1956). Rules for dividing interviews into sentences. *Journal of Psychology, 42,* 273–281.

Baker, S. J. (1948). Speech disturbances: A case for a wider view of paraphasias. *Psychiatry, 11,* 359–366.

Baker, S. J. (1951). Autonomic resistances in word association tests. *Psychoanalytic Quarterly, 20,* 275–283.

Bernard, J. W., Zimbardo, P. G., & Sarason, S. (1961). Anxiety and verbal behavior in children. *Child Development 32,* 379–392.

Blass, T., & Siegman, A. W. (1975). A psycholinguistic comparison of speech, dictation and writing. *Language and Speech, 18,* 20–34.

Blumenthal, R. L. (1964). The effects of level of mental health, premorbid history, and interpersonal stress upon the speech disruption of chronic schizophrenic subjects. *Journal of Nervous and Mental Disease, 139,* 313–323.

Bond, M. H., & Ho, Y. H. (1978). The effect of relative status and the sex composition of a dyad on cognitive responses and non-verbal behavior of Japanese interviewees. *Psychologia: An international journal of psychology in the Orient, 21,* 128–136.

Bond, M. H., & Iwata, Y. (1976). Proxemics and observation anxiety in Japan: Non-verbal and cognitive responses. *Psychologia: An international journal of psychology in the Orient, 19,* 119–126.

Boomer, D. S. (1963). Speech disturbances and body movement in interviews. *Journal of Nervous and Mental Disease, 136,* 263–266.

Boomer, D. S., & Goodrich, D. W. (1961). Speech disturbance and judged anxiety. *Journal of Consulting Psychology, 25,* 160–164.

Bradac, J. J., Konsky, C. W., & Elliott, N. D. (1976). Verbal behavior of interviewees: The effects of several situational variables on verbal productivity, disfluency, and lexical diversity. *Journal of Communication Disorders, 9,* 211–225.

Brady, A. T., & Walker, M. B. (1978). Interpersonal distance as a function of situationally induced anxiety. *British Journal of Social and Clinical Psychology, 17,* 127–133.

Cook, M. (1969). Anxiety, speech disturbances, and speech rate. *British Journal of Social and Clinical Psychology, 8,* 13–21.

Carnes, E. F., & Robinson, F. P. (1948). The role of client talk in the counseling interview. *Educational & Psychological Measurement, 8,* 635–644.

Davis, D. M. (1940). The relation of repetitions in the speech of young children to certain measures of language maturity and situational factors. *Journal of Speech Disorders, 5,* 235–246.

Dibner, A. S. (1956). Cue-counting: A measure of anxiety in interviews. *Journal of Consulting Psychology, 20,* 475–478.

Dibner, A. S. (1958). Ambiguity and anxiety. *Journal of Abnormal and Social Psychology, 56,* 165–174.

Dollard, J., & Miller, N. E. (1950). *Personality and Psychotherapy.* New York: McGraw-Hill.

Dollard, J., & Mowrer, O. H. (1947). A method of measuring tension in written documents. *Journal of Abnormal and Social Psychology, 42,* 3–32.

Edelmann, R. J., & Hampson, S. E. (1979). Changes in non-verbal behaviour during embarrassment. *British Journal of Social and Clinical Psychology, 18,* 385–390.

Edelmann, R. J., & Hampson, S. E. (1981). Embarrassment in dyadic interaction. *Social Behavior and Personality, 9,* 171–177.

Eldred, S. H., & Price, D. B. (1958). A linguistic evaluation of feeling states in psychotherapy. *Psychiatry, 21,* 115–121.

Eron, L. D. (1950). A normative study of the TAT. *Psychological Monographs, 64,* No. 9.

Feldstein, S. (1962). The relationship of interpersonal involvement and affectiveness of content to the verbal communication of schizophrenic patients. *Journal of Abnormal and Social Psychology, 64,* 39–45.

Feldstein, S., & Jaffe, J. (1962). The relationship of speech disruption to the experience of anger. *Journal of Consulting Psychology, 26,* 505–509.

Feldstein, S., & Jaffe, J. (1963). An IBM 650 program written in SOAP for the computation of speech disturbances per time, speaker, and group. *Behavioral Science, 8,* 86–87.

Feldstein, S., Brenner, M., & Jaffe, J. (1963). The effect of subject sex, verbal interaction and topical focus on speech disruption. *Language and Speech, 6,* 229–239.

Freud, S. (1960). The psychopathology of everyday life. In J. Strachey (Ed.), *The standard edition of the complete psychological works of Sigmund Freud* (Vol. 6). London: Hogarth Press.

Freud, S. (1963). Introductory lectures on psychoanalysis. In J. Strachey (Ed.), *The standard edition of the complete psychological works of Sigmund Freud* (Vols. 15 and 16). London: Hogarth Press.

Froschels, E., & Jellinck, A. (1941). *Practice of voice and speech therapy.* Boston: Expression Co.

Geer, J. H. (1966). Effect of fear arousal upon task performance and verbal behavior. *Journal of Abnormal Psychology, 71,* 119–123.

Gillespie, J. F., Jr. (1953). Verbal signs of resistance in client-centered therapy. In *Group report of a program of research in psychotherapy.* Pennsylavnia State College.

Gottschalk, L. A. (1961). *Comparative psycholinguistic analysis of two psychotherapeutic interviews.* New York: International Universities Press.

Horowitz, L. M., Sampson, H., Siegelman, E. Y., Wolfson, A., & Weiss, J. (1975). On the identification of warded-off mental contents: An empirical and methodological contribution. *Journal of Abnormal Psychology, 84,* 545–558.

Horowitz, L. M., Weckler, D., Saxon, A., Livaudais, J. D., & Boutacoff, L. I. (1977). Discomforting talk and speech disruptions. *Journal of Consulting and Clinical Psychology, 45,* 1036–1042.

Jones, L. V. (1955). Statistical theory and research design. *Annual Review of Psychology, 6,* 405–430.

Kasl, S. V., & Mahl, G. F. (1956). A simple device for obtaining certain verbal activity measures during interviews. *Journal of Abnormal and Social Psychology, 53,* 388–390.

Kasl, S. V., & Mahl, G. F. (1958). Experimentally induced anxiety and speech disturbances. *American Psychologist, 13,* 349. (Abstract)

Kasl, S. V., & Mahl, G. F. (1965). The relationship of disturbances and hestiations in spontaneous speech to anxiety. *Journal of Personality and Social Psychology, 1,* 425–433.

Krause, M. S., & Pilisuk, M. (1961). Anxiety in verbal behavior: A validation study. *Journal of Consulting Psychology, 25,* 414–419.

Lassen, Carol L. (1973). Effect of proximity on anxiety and communication in the initial psychiatric interview. *Journal of Abnormal Psychology, 81,* 226–232.

Lerea, L. (1956). A preliminary study of the verbal behavior of speech fright. *Speech Monographs, 23,* 229–233.

Levin, H., Baldwin, A. L., Gallwey, M., & Paivio, A. (1960). Audience stress, personality, and speech. *Journal of Abnormal and Social Psychology, 61,* 469–473.

Levin, H., & Silverman, I. (1965). Hesitation phenomena in children's speech. *Language and Speech, 8,* 67–85.

Maclay, H., & Osgood, C. E. (1959). Hesitation phenomena in spontaneous English speech. *Word, 15,* 19–44.

Mahl, G. F. (1949). Effect of chronic fear on the gastric secretion of HC1 in dogs. *Psychosomatic Medicine, 11,* 30–44.

Mahl, G. F. (1950). Anxiety, HC1 secretion, and peptic ulcer etiology. *Psychosomatic Medicine, 12,* 158–169.

Mahl, G. F. (1952). Relationship between acute and chronic fear and the gastric acidity and blood sugar levels in *Macaca mulatta* monkeys. *Psychosomatic Medicine, 14,* 183–210.

Mahl, G. F. (1955a). *Disturbances and silences in the patient's speech in psychotherapy.* Unpublished progress report, January.

Mahl, G. F. (1955b). *The use of 'Ah' in spontaneous speech.* Paper presented at The Annual Meeting of The Eastern Psychological Association.

Mahl, G. F. (1956a). Normal disturbances in spontaneous speech: General quantitative aspects. *American Psychologist, 11,* 390. (Abstract).

Mahl, G. F. (1956b). Disturbances and silences in the patient's speech in psychotherapy. *Journal of Abnormal Social Psychology, 53,* 1–15.

Mahl, G. F. (1956c). *Disturbances in the patient's speech as a function of anxiety.* Paper presented at Annual Meeting of The Eastern Psychological Association.

Mahl, G. F. (1957). *Speech disturbances and emotional verbal content in interviews.* Paper presented at Annual Meeting of The Eastern Psychological Association.

Mahl, G. F. (1958). On the use of 'Ah' in spontaneous speech: Quantitative, developmental, characterological, situational, and linguistic aspects. *American Psychologist, 13,* 349. (Abstract).

Mahl, G. F. (1959). Exploring emotional states by content analysis. In I. deSola Pool (Ed.), *Trends in content analysis* (pp. 89–130). Urbana: University of Illinois Press.

Mahl, G. F. (1961). Measures of two expressive aspects of a patient's speech in two psychotherapeutic interviews. In L. A. Gottschalk (Ed.), *Comparative psycholinguistic analysis of two psychotherapeutic interviews* (pp. 91–114; 174–188). New York: International Universities Press.

Mahl, G. F. (1980). *Mark Twain's use of speech disturbances in the dialogue of Tom Sawyer.* Unpublished manuscript.

Mahl, G. F., & Brody, E. B. (1954). Chronic anxiety symptomatology, experimental stress, and HC1 secretion. *Archives of Neurology & Psychiatry, 71,* 314–325.

Mahl, G. F., & Karpe, R. (1953). Emotions and HC1 secretion during psychoanalytic hours. *Psychosomatic Medicine, 15,* 312–327.

Mahl, G. F., & Kasl, S. V. (1958). *Weaning, infantile speech development and "normal" speech disturbances in young adult life.* Paper presented at The Annual Meeting of The Eastern Psychological Association.

Mahl, G. F., Dollard, J., & Redlich, F. C. (1954). Facilities for the sound recording and observation of interviews. *Science, 120,* 235–239.

Mahl, G. F. (1987). *Explorations in nonverbal and vocal-behavior.* Hillsdale, NJ: Erlbaum.

Meisels, M. (1967). Test anxiety, stress, and verbal behavior. *Journal of Consulting Psychology, 31,* 577–582.

Meringer, R., & Meyer, K. (1895). *Versprechen und Verlesen [Misspeaking and Misreading].* Stuttgart.

Moses, L. E. (1952). Non-parametric statistics for psychological research. *Psychological Bulletin, 49,* 122–143.

Mowrer, O. H., Light, B. H., Luria, Z., & Zeleny, M. P. (1953). Tension changes during psychotherapy, with special reference to resistance. In O. H. Mowrer (Ed.), *Psychotherapy, theory and research* (pp. 546–640). New York: Ronald Press.

Murray, E. J. (1956). A content-analysis method for studying psychotherapy. *Psychological Monographs, 70*(13, Whole No. 420).

Musumeci, M. (1975). *Speech disturbances as a function of stress induced anxiety in children.* Unpublished doctoral dissertation, Fordham University, New York.

Nosenko, E. L., Ylchaninov, P. E., Krylova, N. V., & Petrukhin, E. V. (1977). On the possibility of assessing emotional stability using speech characteristics. *Voprosy Psikhologii,* 46–56.

Page, H. A. (1953). An assessment of the predictive value of certain language measures in psychotherapeutic counseling. In *Group report of a program of research in psychotherapy.* Pennsylvania State College. Chapter VII.

Paivio, A. (1963). Audience influence, social isolation, and speech. *Journal of Abnormal and Social Psychology, 67,* 247–253.

Panek, D. M., & Martin, B. (1959). The relationship between GSR and speech disturbance in psychotherapy. *Journal of Abnormal Social Psychology, 58,* 402–405.

Pope, B., Blass, T., Siegman, A. W., & Raher, J. (1970). Anxiety and depression in speech. *Journal of Consulting and Clinical Psychology, 35,* 128–133.

Pope, B., Siegman, A. W., & Blass, T. (1970). Anxiety and speech in the initial interview. *Journal of Consulting and Clinical Psychology, 35,* 233–238.

Porter, E. H. (1943). The development and evaluation of a measure of counseling interview procedures. Part II. The evaluation. *Educational & Psychological Measurement, 3,* 215–238.

Raimy, V. C. (1948). Self reference in counseling interviews. *Journal of Consulting Psychology, 12,* 153–163.

Reich, W. (1948). On character analysis. In R. Fliess (Ed.), *The psychoanalytic reader.* (Vol. 1). New York: International Universities Press.

Reynolds, A., & Paivio, A. (1968). Cognitive and emotional determinants of speech. *Canadian Journal of Psychology, 22,* 164–175.

Sanford, F. H., (1942). Speech and personality. *Psychological Bulletin, 39,* 811–845.

Sarason, S. B., Davidson, K. S., Lighthall, F. F., Waite, R. R., & Ruebush, B. K. (1960). *Anxiety in elementary school children.* New York: Wiley.

Schulze, G. (1964). *Speech disturbances, verbal productivity, self-ratings, and autonomic responses during psychological stress.* Unpublished doctoral dissertation, Yale University (New Haven).

Schulze, G., Mahl, G. F., & Holzberg, J. D. (1959). A comparison of speech disturbance levels of paranoid schizophrenics and control subjects prior to and during exposure to an erotic stimulus. *American Psychologist, 14,* 403. (Abstract).

Schulze, G., Mahl, G. F., & Murray, E. J. (1960). Speech disturbances and content analysis categories as indices of emotional states of patients in psychotherapy. *American Psychologist, 15,* 405. (Abstract).

Siegman, A. W., & Pope, B. (1965). Effects of question specificity and anxiety producing messages on verbal fluency in the initial interview. *Journal of Personality and Social Psychology, 4,* 188–192.

Snyder, W. U. (1945). An investigation of the nature of non-directive psychotherapy. *Journal of General Psychology, 33,* 193–223.

Sullivan, H. S. (1954). *The psychiatric interview.* New York: Norton.

Tindall, R. H., & Robinson, F. P. (1947). The use of silence as a technique in counseling. *Journal of Clinical Psychology, 3,* 136–141.

Verón, E., Korn, F., Malfé, R., & Sluzki, C. E. (1966). Perturbación lingüística en la comunicación neurótica. [Linguistic Disturbance in Neurotic Communication]. *Acta Psiquiátrica y Psicológia de America Latina, 12,* 129–143.

Zimbardo, P. G., Barnard, J. W., & Berkowitz, L. (1963). The role of anxiety and defensiveness in children's verbal behavior. *Journal of Personality, 31,* 79–96.

Zimbardo, P. G., Mahl, G. F., & Barnard, J. W. (1963). The measurement of speech disturbance in anxious children. *Journal of Speech & Hearing Disorders, 28,* 362–370.

IV
Linguistic Strategies

7

The Analysis of Natural Language in Psychological Treatment

Michael J. Patton and Naomi M. Meara

INTRODUCTION

For a number of years, we have conducted research designed to promote increased understanding of psychological treatment through an analysis of the language used by those who are participating in such treatment. Although our assumptions, conceptual work, and method have been shaped by work in several areas such a linguistics, psychology, and sociology, the research itself is a direct development from theorizing and earlier empirical investigations conducted by Pepinsky and his colleagues (cf. Pepinsky, 1970; Pepinsky & Karst, 1964; Pepinsky & Patton, 1971). This early work developed an interactive definition of psychological treatment (Pepinsky & Patton, 1971) which subsequently became the basis for a still developing model of counselor–client interaction and change (Patton, Fuhriman & Bieber, 1977; Pepinsky, 1974, 1984; Pepinsky & DeStefano, 1983; Rush, Pepinsky, Landry, Meara, Strong, Valley, & Young, 1974).

Our problem in this chapter is, therefore, to illustrate how the analysis of natural language in counseling and psychotherapy promotes our understanding of the psychological treatment process. We have attempted to accomplish our task with the aid of a comprehensive analytic scheme that incorporates (1) a set of propositions about how meaning is conveyed through language use (after Pepinsky, 1984), (2) a correspond-

MICHAEL J. PATTON • Department of Educational and Counseling Psychology, University of Tennessee, Knoxville, TN 37996.   NAOMI M. MEARA • Department of Psychology, University of Notre Dame, Notre Dame, IN 46556.

ing model of the psychological treatment process, (3) a matrix model of case grammar (Cook, 1979), and (4) a Computer-Assisted Language-Analysis System (CALAS) (Rush *et al.*, 1974). We have combined these analytic tools to account for certain classes of observable language phenomena. Our contention is that the many varieties of psychological treatment (Meara & Patton, 1984; Pepinsky & Patton, 1971) have in common the use of natural language as the primary vehicle, both for the organization of counselor and client experience generally, and then, more specifically, for the formulation of desired treatment outcomes (Meara, Pepinsky, Shannon & Murray, 1981). A comprehensive scheme for the analysis of natural language has permitted us to examine and describe the linguistic configurations and their grammatical, semantic, and stylistic properties used by counselors and clients. It has permitted us, as well, to show how the configurations of both participants are related (or unrelated) to each other, and how they change over time (Bieber, Patton & Fuhriman, 1977).

We will first present some of the assumptions that provide the foundation for our work, and then some propositions related to how language use conveys meaning. These propositions provide grounds for our developing theory of language use. Next, we will define counseling and psychotherapy as occasions for the communication of social influence via natural language. We will then present a modified matrix model of case grammar (after Cook, 1979), and then the components of CALAS (Meara, 1976). Finally, we will review several empirical studies, to illustrate what our analyses of the natural language in several different treatment encounters have revealed thus far.

ASSUMPTIONS

Pepinsky and Patton (1971) have defined psychological treatment as "any encounter between persons in which one or more participants are inferred to be acting so as to elicit in—or through—one or more other participants a change in state (e.g., belief, attitude, behavior, resources)" (p. 4). In referring to the earlier work of Pepinsky, Weick, and Riner (1965), these authors go on to explain that, at least in the view of one other person (be it participant or spectator), the activities of psychological treatment are directed toward reducing what the changers define as discrepancy between an "existing and a desired state of affairs" (p. 4). The majority of the research we will present here refers to data related to interactive discourse in counseling, although we believe the work we are doing applies equally well to other forms of psychological treatment and spoken interaction (cf. De-Stefano, Pepinsky & Saunders, 1982; Pepinsky & DeStefano, 1983).

Psychological treatments have natural language as a primary resource, both for organizing counselor and client experience generally (Patton, *et al.*, 1977) and, more specifically, for formulating desired psychotherapeutic policies and outcomes (Meara *et al.*, 1981). By natural language use, we mean "patterns of sounds spoken by a collection of individuals where the sounds are commonly understood by the members" (Patton *et al.*, 1977). In spite of the increasing abundance and excellence of the research literature on counseling and psychotherapy, the language of psychological treatment is often an unanalyzed resource in studying what occurs in therapy (Kiesler, 1973; cf. Zimmerman & Pollner, 1970).

We have assumed that language, as a system of signals and rules for coding those signals (cf. Schutz, 1967a, 1967b), conveys meaning if and only if intended to do so by a user of language in a situated, social occasion. Persons' understandings of the social occasions in which they find themselves are provided, in large part, by the language they use and how they use it to create and maintain those occasions. We are persuaded by Brentano (1955) and others that the phenomenon of meaning in language resides in the act of using it. It is a matter of the signals being presented to an experiencing person who then acts to cognitively work them into a re-presentation. In this way, persons use language to perform several functions or convey different kinds of meanings.

Thus, our attempts at an empirical statement of these processes rely upon a more general "representational theory of mind" (Chafe, 1970; Patton & Sullivan, 1980) characteristic of most contemporary cognitive psychologies. The research rests, therefore, on a commitment to the existence of both cognitive processes and structures, but the former are assumed to be central to the conveying of meaning in language. Meaning inheres in the act of using language. This construction of events ultimately directs our attention to the practices of language use exhibited by counselors and clients.

PROPOSITIONS ABOUT HOW MEANING IS CONVEYED BY LANGUAGE USE

One of the most obvious things to be said about psychological treatment is that counselors and clients somehow put words together to convey understandings that facilitate a change in state for one or both members of a therapeutic dyad. In our research, we have been interested in understanding how counselors and clients put words together such that they are recognizable to the participants as linguistic units of informative display, and how they proceed to further use and interpret these structures to convey meaning (Pepinsky & Patton, 1971). To build refutable and empirically derived explanations of these phenomena, we have had recourse to conceptions of how meaning is conveyed by the use of a language (after Pepinsky, 1984), the psychology of social influence (cf. Goldstein, 1962; 1966; Strong, 1968), and a matrix model of case grammar (Cook, 1979).

Our own approach has been to try to distinguish among the ways meaning is conveyed by using language. We are attempting to make explicit how speakers and observers interpret or make sensible what is happening in discourse. Our general question has been: How are persons using language such that they understand what each is talking about? With Garfinkel (1967), we regard common understanding between persons to be a contingent, ongoing accomplishment that is produced by persons' knowledge and use of recognizable methods of speaking. The achievement of common understanding via language use entails ongoing interpretive work by persons.

Three dimensions of language use that convey meaning are of concern to us: naming, relating, and formulating. In short, the first dimension of meaning in language use is the naming of things. The second dimension of meaning is the relating of things that have been named. The third dimension of meaning is the formulating of what has been named and related, as a way of talking about something in a specific conversation among persons (cf. Garfinkel, 1967; Patton, 1984). In each case, we infer a process of interpretive work that occurs as either antecedent to, or consequent of, the actual appearance of an utterance.

For example, the first dimension of meaning in language use is the operation of naming or identifying things (cf. Schutz, 1967a). Our definition of naming is as follows:

> Naming is a method of interpreting talk whose use enables a person to assign to an utterance its meaning as the name for something. The person's recognition of a word as the name for something entails the use of some intersubjective, interpretive scheme, which, for the sake of definition, we have called naming. Thus, naming as a method for analyzing talk provides persons with a standardizing method for achieving common understanding on the meaning of terms in a language, and thereby, the identification of objects in the world.

Understanding that, when speaking, a person is naming things is a method of achieving common understanding in discourse. Naming as a method of speaking, and thereby of common understanding, has an operational structure (cf. Garfinkel, 1967). The elements of this structure are a *sign*, a *significate*, and a person as *interpretant* (cf. Percy, 1972). A sign is an utterance or word; a significate is the thing named; and the interpretant is the person who recognizes a word as the name for the thing. As we learned to typify objects in our world, we learned how to relate, for example, the word WATER to the cool liquid found, among other places, in a glass on our high chair tray.

Theories about connecting one element with another, for example, associationism, are sufficient to provide a simple explanation of how names are connected to things. It is not, however, sufficient to account for the person's use of words in discourse. Our definition above mentions naming as a way of using language and thereby extends beyond a word in itself. Naming is a fundamental and pervasive method of using words in speaking. It is a form of the process of typifying our experience and thereby making it familiar and accountable to ourselves and others. We take it for granted that the adult competent member of society can and will, when speaking, convey some of his or her experience by naming objects and events.

The second dimension of meaning in language use, and the one we have studied most often in our research to date, is the operation of relating named things. Our definition of relating is as follows:

> Relating is a method of interpreting talk whose use enables a person to assign to two or more names their meaning in relation to each other. A person's recognition of the meaning of names in relation to each other entails the use of an intersubjective scheme that contains knowledge of how certain words (e.g., verbs) function to relate names. Meaning is conveyed in this dimension of language when a string of terms is recognized as a more or less grammatically correct string of terms in some language known to the user.

The elements of this operational structure in language are *name*, *name*, and *relator*. In this case, the relator may be a verb phrase; the names may be noun phrases; and the unit of meaning can be identified grammatically as a clause (for example, name relator name, or Sarah drank the water). Again, the unit becomes recognizable as a method of expressing relations among names if intended so by one person and interpreted as such by another. Patton *et al.* (1977), in specifying the process of combining named things, have identified the verb phrase as an "interpretive relator"; that is, one uses words as verbs in order to impute relations among other words used as names. The verb interprets how one name is to be used in relation to another. When we say, "water is wet" (name relator name), we are instructed to understand that wetness *is* a state that water possesses, and intend it to be so. We assume with Cook (1979) that verb phrases have inherent semantic properties and are therefore critical for the comprehension of language in use. In this way, words used as verbs are not names; instead we use such words to inform us how to further understand what is named. The clues to our recognition that, in speaking, a person intends a relation among names reside in his or her use of words that are recognizable as relators.

The operations of naming and relating provide for standardized, intersubjective schemes of analysis, whereby a speaker and auditor may analyze each other's talk for its recognizable grammatical features. They provide, as well, for the study of language qua language. With such schemes, we are able to recognize that something is said in standard English, for example. Yet such recognition does not guarantee our further understanding of *what* was said, or what was being talked about. Still another dimension of meaning in the use of language is necessary for our comprehension of ongoing discourse.

The third dimension of meaning in language use is the operation of formulating:

> Formulating is a method of interpreting talk whose use enables a person to assign to an utterance its meaning as a way of speaking about something. A person's recognition of how another person is speaking entails the use of an intersubjective scheme for analyzing talk for its understandable character. The clues to what a person is talking about reside in our recognition of how a speaker is using words. Therefore, our recognition of what is being talked about is identical with our recognition of how the other person is talking.

For example, imagine that a student is in conversation with a college English professor when at a point in the discourse the latter says, "Stay varlot! Never darken my door again!" To understand what the professor is talking about, we recognize that either he or she is speaking jokingly, or narratively, or metaphorically, or cryptically, or instructively, or is being silly, or in any other of the countless ways persons speak. For the student and professor the recognizable character of their conversation does not come about because each knows what the other "has in mind"; rather, each knows what the other has in mind by formulating each other's talk, that is, by seeing how the other is using words (cf. Garfinkel, 1967). Formulating relates the syntactical and semantic features of language to their use as situated events of occasioned talk (cf. Garfinkel, Lynch & Livingston, 1981; Patton, 1984; Pepinsky, 1984). Unless we recognize how a person is using words, we do not know what he or she is talking about. Thus, to formulate a conversation (cf. Garfinkel & Sacks, 1971), persons use commonly understand methods of speaking which they assume will accord with, or will create, the situation they intend. Meaning in this dimension of language use is, therefore, entirely a matter of our recognizing, first, *that* a person is speaking, and second, *how* he or she is speaking.

The elements of the operational structure of formulating are *names and relations among names,* the *discourse* (i.e., prior, present, and antici-pated elements of the conversation), and the person as *formulator.* In conversation, naming and relating names are intended by persons as informative communicative displays with which the meaning of their discourse is to be formulated. For example, as students we may recog-nize that when a mathematics teacher says, "the answer is 12," she is speaking informatively. On the other hand, when the English teacher is commenting on the significance of Lady Macbeth's handwashing, he is speaking interpretively. Our recognition or formulation of each other's method of speaking informs us of what is being talked about.

Two further comments may be made about our propositions con-cerning meaning in language. First, the interpretive operations of nam-ing, relating, and formulating are reflexive, that is, taken for granted, practices of communication. The reflexive character of these practices permits participants in a conversation to use language to say what they mean without fear of being called upon to explain how they are doing it. To make the reflexivity of these practices available to speakers is to invite confusion and to risk destabilizing otherwise concerted discourse. It is little wonder, then, that when persons talk to each other in everyday life, they are not usually talking about talking. Language for them is, and must be, an unanalyzed resource, a background of seen but un-noticed schemes for making out what is being said in so many words (cf. Schutz, 1967a). The "objective," common sense character of language and its obstinate familiarity are guaranteed as long as events do not call into serious question persons' methods of speaking, for those methods are devices for achieving a taken for granted sense of common understanding.

Second, our propositions about language use make it possible, in principle, to inquire about their empirical referents in each dimension of meaning. We have concentrated our work thus far at the second dimen-sion, the relating of names with other names. In doing so, we have used a case grammar scheme (Cook, 1979) to aid us in making elements of this operational structure evident. We have learned a great deal about the way counselors and clients signal each other to interpret how one name is to be seen in relation to another. The verb phrase as an interpretive relator has become for us a clue to how the counselor and client are also formulating their discourse. We will have more to say about this later.

LANGUAGE AND PSYCHOLOGICAL TREATMENT: A MODEL

Based on our theory of meaning in language and prior work, we constructed a model of the psychological treatment process (Meara &

Patton, 1984; Patton *et al.*, 1977; Pepinsky, 1974; Pepinsky, 1984; Pepinsky & DeStefano, 1983; Rush *et al.*, 1974). In the model, psychological treatment is construed as a process of social influence that is interactively persuasive. Our generic definition of psychological treatment as a form of social influence (see below) has permitted us over the years to examine manifestly different treatment encounters in order to reveal their common properties (Pepinsky & Patton, 1971).

Language is the primary medium through which attempts at social influence occur. The model (see Figure 1) specifies the contribution of both the interpretive work involved in language use and the elements of language itself to the production of cohesive discourse and change in counseling.

In the model, we assume that counselor and client possess knowledge about language use that consists not only of typifications about the world of objects and events, but also of typical ways to use language to convey meaning in connected discourse. For us, the structural units of names, relations and formulations serve as "informative displays" (Pepinsky & Patton, 1971) with which participants signal to each other their understanding of what is being said or done in their conversation. Following informative display, space is provided in the model for our inferred interpretive operations of naming, relating, and formulating. One observable outcome of the successful communication of social influence thus informatively displayed and interpreted as names, relations, and formulations is likely to be common understanding. Common understanding or cohesive discourse between the participants is observable to the extent that each displays, by the words he or she uses, a grasp of what the other is saying. Not all matters that the pair understands in common need be, nor can be, mentioned by them. For our purposes, however, we may regard as evidence of common understanding the following features of conversation:

1. *Convergence* (Pepinsky & Karst, 1964) and *tracking* between the participants in the similar frequency of their use of grammatical structures (Bieber, 1978; Edwards, 1978; May, 1977; Meara *et al.*, 1981; Oster, 1979);
2. counselor and client preference for the same *discussion topics* (Patton, 1969);
3. the probability that one participant's remarks will follow, or *sequence*, the topic of the other participant's remarks (Friedlander & Phillips, 1984); and
4. the extent to which one or both participants find it necessary to *comment* or otherwise talk about their talk (Garfinkel & Sacks, 1971; Patton, 1984). In this case, comments on the conversation

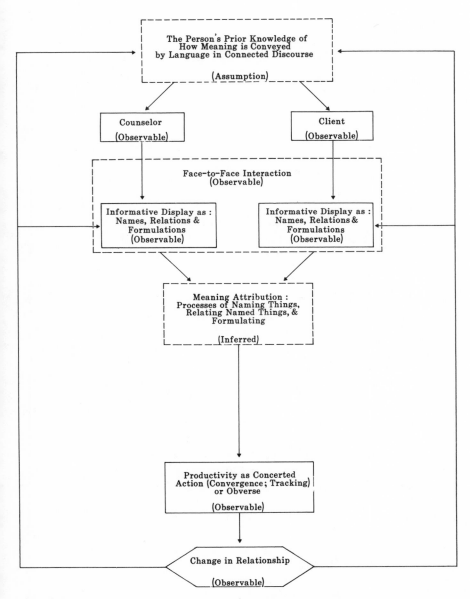

FIGURE 1. Model of counselor–client interaction and change via natural language (Adapted from Patton, Fuhriman, & Bieber, 1977; Pepinsky, 1974; cf. Pepinsky & DeStefano, 1983; Rush *et al.*, 1974).

itself are attempts to remedy the indefiniteness or alter the sense of each other's talk, that is, attempts to establish common understanding.

The model specifies, following common understanding, that a change in the relationship of interaction can occur. This change may occur in either the knowledge each participant uses to interpret language, or in the informatively displayed names, relations, and formulations.

CASE GRAMMAR AS INFORMATIVE DISPLAY

Our conceptualization of language and psychological treatment could not be empirically examined without some paradigm of language that could yield observable units of measure. One of the classic problems in psychology is choosing an appropriate unit of measure for studying the phenomenon in question. Units of measure seem particularly difficult to specify when investigating something like the discourse of counseling or other forms of spoken interaction in natural settings. One or more of several levels of analysis may be appropriate (cf. Pepinsky, 1974). As we struggled with our conceptualizations about counseling, we also struggled with problems related to choosing appropriate units of measure. To transform our work from the theoretical to the empirical realm, a means of operationalizing our linguistic informative displays was needed. The paradigm we adopted and adapted to our work, the Matrix Model of Case Grammar, was developed by Cook (1979) and relies heavily on the scholarship of Chafe (1970) and Filmore (1968) as well as other pioneers in the area of linguistics (e.g., Anderson, 1971). Case grammar classifies the structures of natural language according to the semantic relationship between what are traditionally called nouns and verbs (Reed, 1983).

The Matrix Model of Case Grammar postulates that there are essential and inherent semantic relations (such as state, process, or action) in the deep structure of English language. It is the person's use of these standardizing relations that render language meaningful in the first two dimensions. The use of these relations allows participants to form grammatically recognizable utterances and also permits, therefore, participants to interpret those utterances as something-said-according-to-a-rule. In particular, the Matrix Model of Case Grammar provides an excellent tool to investigate our second dimension of language use, that of relating named things. Simply, from a case grammar perspective, the *named things* are noun phrases and the *relators* are verb phrases, conjunctions, and prepositional or adverbial phrases. For the most part, the essential relations in utterances (e.g., state or action) are determined by the inherent semantic features of verb phrases. The verb phrase then becomes the major "interpretive relator," and its inherent semantic features determine the relationships of the noun phrases (or named things) to it and to each other. The named things (the noun phrases) and the relators (verb phrases, etc.) are designated case grammar descriptions which characterize the functions of each in the utterance. These descriptions constitute a metalanguage that we use to characterize and measure semantic attributes of informative displays. For example: *The hunter killed the bear*. *Killed* is an *action relator*, *hunter* is assigned a case role of *agent*, and *bear* a case role of object. Any competent interpretor of the language knows the difference in meaning between *The hunter killed the bear* and *The bear killed the hunter*.

Competent interpretors understand the relationships among the case role assignments that provide the basis for our inferences about what is happening in therapeutic interactions and other kinds of interactive discourse. These relationships are essential and peripheral. The essential relations are based upon the inherent semantic features of the central relators or verb phrases. The peripheral relations are based upon the semantic features of the central relators in connection with minor relations such as conjunctions, prepositions, and single word adverbials.

The verb classifications and case role assignments used in this research are derived from Cook's (1979) Matrix Model of Case Grammar, and specifically rest on two propositions:

1. Language can be characterized as having semantic structures whose essential properties are postulated to exist as "named things," or noun phrases, and "relations" between them, notably verb phrases that define "essential relations" involving noun phrases. "Peripheral relations" in a language are also postulated to exist, represented by grammatical forms such as conjunctions, and prepositional and adverbial phrases.
2. By definition, the clause exists as a structural unit of semantic information which contains one and only one verb phrase as "essential relator" (Meara *et al.*, 1981).

Three types of verb phrases, which Cook considers primary or fundamental, are postulated to exist. The three categories, with our adapted definitions and examples, are as follows:

1. *State* verbs define a particular, noncausal relation between persons or things, or state or property of such an object.
   Examples: I am happy. The wood is dry.

2. *Process* verbs define a causal relation, without specification of an agent, in which something is happening to a person or a thing. *Examples:* I was burned. The wood is dried.
3. *Action* verbs define a causal relation, with specification of an agent, in which a person or thing does something (optionally, to somebody or something). *Examples:* Mary hit John. The boy ran.

When any of the three inherent semantic features of state, process, or action is present in simple form, the verb phrase is termed *basic*.

In addition to these basic types, Cook (1979) proposed three other categories of verbs, which only exist interactively with the fundamental or basic types, forming compounds of them. This second set of interactive types includes *experiential, benefactive,* and *locative*.

Experiential verbs define relations in which states of feeling, sensing, or knowing are attributed, or acts of consciousness or awareness are imputed, to a person or thing. *Benefactive* verbs define a relation in which persons or things are identified as beneficiaries of a state, an action, or a process. The latter verbs connote ownership or possession, or that someone or something has benefitted from somebody or something.

We have excluded from our consideration Cook's third interactive category of *locative* verbs, formed by affixing prepositions to verb phrases. In our adaptation of Cook's (1979) model, this condition defines what we call nonessential, hence peripheral, relations between named persons or things. These are discussed elsewhere (Meara, 1976; Rush *et al.*, 1974; Young, 1973). Our adapted definitions and examples of the interactive verb-types are as follows:

1. *State-Experiential* verbs define cognitive or affective states. *Examples:* I know the answer. I wanted a drink.
2. *State-Benefactive* verbs define states of ownership. *Examples:* I have four daffodils. I now own the house.
3. *Process-Experiential* verbs define the experiencing of a sensory/perceptual activity. *Examples:* I heard a cat. I felt the pain.
4. *Process-Benefactive* verbs define an activity that is of benefit to someone or something. *Examples:* I received a new job. The forest is reclaiming the land.
5. *Action-Experiential* verbs define an action that provides an experience to a person or other thing. *Examples:* I spoke to them. She tells me everything.
6. *Action-Benefactive* verbs define an action that benefits someone or something. *Examples:* I gave him some money. He willed the farm to his wife.

The modified matrix has nine specific verb types: state basic, process basic, action basic, state experiential, process experiential, action experiential, state benefactive, process benefactive, and action benefactive. In addition, the types in each category can be summed to determine the total in that category. One must be aware of the interactive nature of the compound verbs when counting the totals. For instance, a *state-experiential* verb contributes to both the total *state* verb count and *experiential* verb count.

The case role designations that are related to each of the verb types, and their definitions, are presented below.

Essential Cases:

(A) Agentive—the doer of some action (Action verbs)

(E) Experiencer—the one who is affected by states of feeling, sensing, or knowing, or to whom acts of consciousness and awareness are attributed (Experiential verbs)

(B) Benefactive—the one who benefits from a state or action or a process; typically the possesser of some object (Benefactive verbs)

(O) Object—semantically the most neutral case; the neutral underlying theme of the state, action, or process described by the verb (all verbs: state verbs take 0 in both "subject" and "object" slots)

Peripheral Cases:

(L) Locative—the place where the event described by the verb occurs.

(T) Time—the time when the event described by the verb occurs

(M) Manner—the way in which the event described by the verb occurs

(P) Purpose—the reason *for,* or the goal of the event described by, the verb

(C) Cause—the motive or origin of the event described by the verb

Case grammarians believe that these semantic features describe the "deep structure" of language utterances. Analyses of these semantic features allow for descriptions and comparisons of the discourse across speakers, topics, or segments.

A second attribute of language that can be inferred from a case grammar analysis is that of "stylistics." A speaker's style is concerned more with the grammatical form with which something is said than with what may be intended. It is thought to be representative of "surface structure." As Wyman (1983) notes, it is virtually impossible to separate the semantic from the stylistic at the pragmatic level since both contribute to meaning. However, we have found it useful to measure and to talk about stylistics and semantics separately.

To operationalize the notion of stylistics, we began with the clause. By definition, the clause exists as the basic structural unit of semantic information, as it contains one and only one verb phrase or "essential relator" (Meara *et al.*, 1981). Clauses can be classified as main or subordinate and contain phrases and words. As noted above, each of the phrases, except for the verb phrase, carries a case role assignment. Such grammatical units and various configurations of them provide the basic units of measure for computing or describing the stylistics of our linguistic informative displays. The measures we have typically used are verbal productivity (e.g., number of clauses) and stylistic complexity (e.g., the number of clauses in relation to the number of main clauses). The stylistics of the discourse can also be described and compared across speaker, topic or segment.

THE COMPUTER-ASSISTED LANGUAGE-ANALYSIS SYSTEM

To assist us in testing our conceptualizations and in implementing the case grammar paradigm in our work, we sought out computer technology. What was intended as a slight digression from our task became a seven-year labor that resulted in the development of the Computer-Assisted Language-Analysis System, known as CALAS (Meara, 1976; Pepinsky *et al.*, 1977; Rush *et al.*, 1974; Young, 1973). CALAS is based on our adaptation of the Matrix Model of Case Grammar.

Briefly, CALAS includes a set of computer programs and an algorithm for translating texts in the English language into structural equivalents. The system analyzes verbatim text or discourse in three distinct sequential operations (e.g., see Meara, Shannon, & Pepinsky, 1979). It is conducted through two computer languages, SPITBALL and PL/I. Although originally designed to be run on an IBM System Model 370/168 computer using punch cards, CALAS has been adapted for use with the IBM 370/3031, using a series of interface programs with the DEC system 10 for data file storage and off-line editing with SOS editing language. CALAS has further been adapted for direct use with the IBM 370/3031 using the Conversation Monitor System (CMS).

Whatever the system, the essential operations remain the same. Text, punctuated in sentences, is transferred verbatim to computer storage discs according to simple format rules (e.g., each speaker's discourse is coded by a four digit number, and, each time there is a change of speakers, that four digit number appears on a line by itself (see Pepinsky *et al.*, 1977; Rush *et al.*, 1974). Once the text is prepared, there are three distinct sequential operations: (a) Eyeball, translation of the text into grammatical counterparts (e.g., noun, verb, adjective, adverb); (b) Phraser, aggregation of grammatical class assignments into phrases (e.g., noun phrase, verb phrase, prepositional phrase); (c) Clause and Case, grouping the phrases into clauses (e.g., main and subordinate), and assigning labels derived from case grammar to each phrase in the clause (e.g., agentive or experiential). The output from one operation provides the input to the next. And after each operation, the system provides for human editing which is to increase the accuracy of input into the next phrase. If the human editing is omitted, the errors become cumulative. Careful editing after Eyeball greatly reduces the amount of editing that is required after Phraser and Clause and Case.

In the first phase of the CALAS sequence, Eyeball, each word in the text is given a grammatical class assignment. The algorithm for accomplishing these assignments was implemented in SPITBALL and is based upon (1) the function words (e.g., prepositions, articles, auxiliary verbs) and the punctuation in a sentence, and (2) the position of each word in a sentence and the position of each word relative to the surrounding function words.

Only a very small dictionary of 400 to 600 words is used, which reduces both the time needed for processing and the space needed for storage. The algorithm for this operation allows for the isolation of assignment errors; a mistake in the classification of one word does not mean failure in the rest of the sentence. Eyeball never rejects a sentence, as long as the presentation of text adheres to the simple format rules. At worst, the sentence will be analyzed by a series of defaults. Since the assignment process relies more on context than word by word dictionary comparisons, lexical ambiguities are more likely to receive accurate assignment.

For each class of function words, a set of rules has been developed which accounts for the majority of patterns in which each function word occurs. Function-word rules are applied in a linear fashion as each function word is encountered.

Below we present an illustration of the various types of rules contained in Eyeball. The sample sentence follows:

The daffodil was in the old brass pitcher.

The first pass through the sentence results in the assignment of the grammatical class of each function word found in the dictionary. So, at the end of this pass, the Eyeball would replace the sentence by the following array of elements:

D   V   P   D
The daffodil was in the old brass pitcher.

Since the first unidentified element follows a determiner (D), it is either a noun or an adjective. Since this first unidentified element stands alone (i.e., is followed by another assignment, in this case a verb), it must be a noun (N). The three blank elements remaining are recognized on the basis of the following rule:

- *If a determiner is followed by several consecutive blank elements, the last of the series is identified as a noun and the other elements in the series as adjectives (J).*

Hence, at the end of the second pass the array has the form:

D   N   V   P   D   J   J   N   EOS (end of sentence)

The daffodil was in the old brass pitcher.

The second phase of CALAS, Phraser, is the phrase-grouping process. Definitions for each type of phrase were developed using accepted rules of English grammar (e.g., prepositional phrases, noun phrases, verb phrases and the like). A complete discussion of the definitions is found in Rush *et al.*, 1974. Based on these definitions an algorithm was developed and then implemented in PL/I. This algorithm portions each sentence into phrases, using as markers the grammatical class assignments produced by EYEBALL, and edited by hand, if necessary, before being put into Phraser. We continue with the example above to illustrate the process.

D   N   V P   D J   J   N   EOS

The daffodil was in the old brass pitcher.

After processing by Phraser, the array is: noun phrase, verb phrase, prepositional phrase.

N   V   P

The daffodil   was   in the old brass pitcher.

The final phase of CALAS is Clause and Case. This operation separates the text into clauses and assigns a verb type to each verb phrase and a case role to every other phrase in the text. The verb type and case role assignments are based on our modifications of case grammar, as discussed above. Our sample text would be assigned as follows:

O (Object)   S (Stative)   L (Locative)
       The daffodil   was   in the old brass pitcher.

The semantic and stylistic measures used in the research are computed from these linguistic displays produced by CALAS. Measures other than those we have used to date can also be constructed.

This technological tool enables us to analyze, reliably and relatively rapidly, the natural language of client and counselor across different theoretical approaches to psychological treatment. From such analyses, we have been able to describe: (a) the relative frequencies with which clients and counselors use semantically different types of verbs during an interview or series of interviews, (b) the extent to which such verb type usage differs between the participants, (c) the change in frequency of usage over time, and (d) the extent to which certain stylistic features of each participant's language are related to the other's and to measures of cognitive complexity.

To summarize our principal argument, we have said that certain structural features of language are minimum units of informative display, that is, they have semantic and stylistic attributes that convey meaning beyond their literal grammatical components. These attributes provide a means for characterizing how the participants are speaking, and for investigating such phenomena as intentionality, social influence, and concerted action. The CALAS enables us to analyze the discourse more efficiently and reliably and test hypotheses related to psychology treatment.

EMPIRICAL INVESTIGATIONS

As we were developing our model and the CALAS, it became clear that empirical work was needed to test the utility of our theorizing and conceptualizations. The empirical work that has since been generated can be divided into two categories. The first describes selected psychological treatment encounters in terms of semantic and stylistic properties of counselor and client language. From these linguistic descriptions, inferences are made related to events in the interaction, based on our model of psychological treatment. For example, Meara et al. (1979), have surmised that linguistic concerted action, when accomplished by client and counselor, may reflect more substantive kinds of concerted action, such as changes in attitudes, beliefs, and/or behavior. Likewise, Pepinsky and DeStefano (1983) termed the activities of a teacher "unilateral policy making," based on her linguistic interactions with pupils in a desegregated first grade classroom. The second category of empirical work is characterized by attempts to forge conceptual links between "established phenomena" of psychological treatment and the linguistic displays of those phenomena. For instance, Wycoff, Davis, Hector, and Meara (1982) found that counselors judged to be high-empathic responders use language that was less complex, less action oriented, and that contained fewer questions than the language used by counselors who were judged to be low-empathic responders. Davis, Meara, and Moore (1984) found that a counselor trainee coached to display resistance in a supervision session demonstrated high verbal productivity and few self-references when making statements that were judged to be high resistance.

The first category of research to be reviewed includes the following studies: Bieber, 1978; Bieber et al., 1977; DeStefano et al., 1982; Friedlander & Phillips, 1984; May, 1977; Meara et al., 1979; Meara et al., 1981; and Patton et al., 1977.

DESCRIPTIVE ANALYSIS OF NAMES AND RELATIONS IN PSYCHOLOGICAL TREATMENT

Studies conducted by Bieber (1978), Bieber et al. (1977), May (1977), and Patton et al. (1977) drew from a common data set. This set consisted of three different counselor–client pairs, two of whom were engaged in psychological treatment in a university counseling center, and the third pair of whom were in a large comprehensive community mental health center. The 1st, 11th, and 25th interviews in these three series were audio-recorded; typescripts were prepared, and the data analyzed by an early version of the CALAS.

In the first study, Patton et al. (1977) focused exclusively on the verb phrase as the central interpretive relator, as used by one of the client–counselor pairs described above. In this pair, the counselor's stated theoretical preference was client-centered. At that time, our method of verb classification was less developed, and all verbs were classified into one of four types: (a) stative, any form of the verb "to be"; (b) "experiencer," any verb expressing feeling, sensing, knowing, and so forth; (c) benefactive, any verb denoting possession; and (d) "agentive," all other verbs. The verbs from the three selected interviews were classified by hand into one of the four verb types. Results indicated that, across time, the counselor and client increased their use of stative verbs and decreased their use of agentive verbs. Moreover, the variations in the frequency of verb types in the three interviews were similar for both participants in amount and direction of change. This similarity was interpreted as evidence for a "tracking phenomenon" (Jaffe, 1964) that could be construed as evidence of concerted action. The increased usage of stative verbs was seen as representing tacit agreement or common understanding between the pair about a conversational focus on the client's inner states or conditions.

In a second study (Bieber *et al.*, 1977), a more complete analysis of this counselor–client pair was conducted. In addition to verb usage, the case roles of those noun phrases that were direct references to the client were also analyzed. Moreover, each of the three interviews were analyzed by thirds. Again, a hand analysis was used, and for the first time the clause was designated as the unit of informative display. The most noteworthy finding of this analysis was the client's increased reference to herself as experiencer in the last third of her 25th and final hour of counseling. Such talk is precisely what the counselor exhibited about himself in the first third of this final hour. It was suggested that this tracking of and convergence with the counselor's language patterns might indicate that the client had learned how to talk about herself, using the counselor's methods of speaking to form a set of cognitive premises about "treatment policy" (cf. Pepinsky & DeStefano, 1983).

In a third study using this data set, Bieber (1978) examined the spoken language of all three counselor–client pairs. In two of the pairs, the counselors identified their orientation as client-centered, and, in the other pair, the counselor orientation was psychoanalytic. An 11-cell verb matrix, similar to the current 9-cell matrix described above, was used in the analysis. In this 11-verb matrix, the stative experiencer category was divided into stative experiencer affective (SEA) and stative experiencer cognitive (SEC). The SEA verbs were characterized as describing states of emotional experiencing (e.g., love, hate, feel) and the SEC verbs as describing states of cognitive experiencing (e.g., think, know, understand).

The results indicated that initial differences in verb-type usage between counselor–client pairs decreased over time, suggesting tracking and convergence between participants in each counseling series. In addition, particular verb types were used consistently within particular discussion topics. Bieber concluded that the two pairs with the client-centered counselors had a different pattern of language usage than the pair with the psychoanalytically oriented counselor. For discussion purposes, he labelled the patterns Type I and Type II. The Type I language pattern of the two client-centered counselors appeared to be a form of communication encouraging the expression of general feelings, while not raising questions or doubting the meaning of such expression. Type I language use appeared to emphasize the reporting of the client's perception and awareness of phenomenal events, and was characterized by frequent use of stative and stative-affective experiencer verbs. Type II language, characteristic of the counselor–client pair with the psychoanalytically oriented counselor, suggested a general attitude of doubt and the expression of thoughts rather than feelings. It seemed to be a form of communication that promoted understanding, rather than a strictly perceptual awareness of one's immediate experiencing. Type II language was characterized by the counselor's use of process and process-experiencer verbs and indicated more concern about the course of events and the client's reactions to them, rather than the awareness and description of feeling states.

May (1977) conducted a more specific analyses of the data generated by the two client-centered counselor client pairs. Although he found only partial support for six hypotheses related to client-centered theory, case grammar, and the concept of informative display derived from the model of psychological treatment presented above, he did observe, in each of the interactions, some patterns that are of interest. His most notable finding was that while both pairs demonstrated convergence of verb-type usage, the timing of that convergence differed. For example, the first counselor–client pair were semantically similar during the first third of each interview, but somewhat dissimilar in the final third. By contrast, the second counselor–client pair began each interview with a semantically divergent pattern, but decreased this divergence by the final third of the interview. In addition, the stylistic measures indicated idiosyncratic patterns for each counselor–client pair, yet each pattern led May to conclude that convergence was present. Thus, the first pair was similar across three measures of stylistic complexity, while the second pair demonstrated both convergence and divergence across three measures.

Two later studies (Meara, Shannon, & Pepinsky, 1979; Meara et al., 1981) using the CALAS were based on excerpts from the well known film series *Three Approaches to Psychotherapy* (Shostrom, 1966). In these films three famous therapists, Carl Rogers, Fretz Perls, and Albert Ellis, each conduct an interview with the same client, Gloria. The purpose of these interviews is to instruct the audience about the rationale and methods of therapy from the perspective of the three theoretical orientations espoused by these men. These orientations are: client-centered for Rogers, gestalt for Perls, and rational-emotive for Ellis. The Rogers interview is 35 minutes in length, that of Perls is 12 minutes, and the Ellis interview is 30 minutes. The middle three minutes and the final three minutes of each session were selected for analysis and comparison.

The first study using these data (Meara et al., 1979) compared the stylistic complexity of counselor–client language across all three interviews. There were four dependent measures of stylistic complexity: number of sentences, average sentence length, average block length, and average clause depth. These measures are discussed in detail elsewhere (Cook, 1979; Meara et al., 1979). The results indicated that the counselors were significantly different from each other across all four dependent measures, and these differences conformed fairly well to prior expectations. Ellis was by far the most complex on all four dependent measures; Perls was generally the least complex with brief frequent responses. Rogers's language was somewhat more complex than expected, but overall represented a relatively simple style.

The results for the client, Gloria, indicated statistically significant differences in her utterances across interviews on all four dependent measures. With some exceptions, her stylistic complexity varies in the direction of the particular counselor. In general, her speech is most simple with Perls and most complex with Ellis. Her interaction with Rogers is less complex with Ellis, but more complex than with Perls. Although cautious about generalizing from these data, Meara et al. speculate that these results (a) may be indicative of the social influence that counselors exert in counseling, and (b) suggest that modeling of linguistic style (i.e., linguistic concerted action via tracking and convergence) may represent an initial step in making possible substantive concerted actions in the form of commonly understood methods of speaking. Our psychological treatment model hypothesizes that such substantive concerted actions are necessary for effective psychological treatment.

The second study (Meara et al., 1981), using these same data from the film series, investigated semantic variables of counselor–client usage across all three interviews. The dependent measures were the frequencies of usage of the nine specific verb types derived from modifications of Cook's (1979) matrix model of case grammar. The results indicated that, for the most part, the counselors' speech, as measured by these semantic units, was similar to what one might expect, based on their theoretical preferences and stated intentions prior to the interview. Specifically, Ellis and Perls talk more about *action* than Rogers; Ellis used relatively more of the *action-basic* verbs (e.g., do), and Perls more of the *action-experiential* (e.g., say) verbs. Perls and Rogers use more *experiential* verbs (e.g., love) than Ellis, but Perls employs significantly more *action-experiential* verbs than the other two, and Rogers more verbs that are *state-experiential* (e.g., feel). Meara et al. (1981) suggested that these semantic units of informative display are reflective of counselors' policies about what ought to happen during treatment. In addition, we now suggest that semantic analysis may help us understand more explicitly the interactive policy-making process as it occurs in treatment.

In general, the client Gloria is remarkably consistent in her verb usage across all three interviews, suggesting the absence of social influence at the semantic or "deep structure" level of language. These results are consistent with those of Bieber et al. (1977), which demonstrated that clients are not influenced to change their semantic displays in an initial interview but may be influenced to do so in later interviews.

This preliminary work led us to expect that CALAS could provide a description of the discourse from which the ground rules of an interaction (i.e., policy) can be inferred. Other empirical and conceptual work in this area has been promising. For example, Pepinsky & DeStefano (1983) describe counseling, teaching, and the like as particular examples of interactive treatment. They interpret interactive talk during treatment as organizing behavior, and use as an example a case study in which DeStefano *et al.* (1982), analyzed the conversation rules in a desegregated first grade classroom of an inner city public school. The pattern of talk between teacher and students revealed the ground rules for their classroom conversations. These ground rules are conceptually defined as policy. For example, the analysis of the case study data revealed that the teacher not only determined who should talk to whom, but determined how they should talk to each other. The authors conclude that the treatment was "manifestly unilateral," since it was the teacher who exercised the greater amount of social influence. In analyzing the case study data, DeStefano *et al.* (1982) not only used the CALAS, but complemented their description of the interaction with other methods, most notably a method of cohesion analysis devised by Halliday and Hasen (1976).

Further descriptive work using elements of the model of psychological treatment has included a stochastic process analysis of the temporal relationships of interactive discourse (Friedlander & Phillips, 1984). This work was presented from a sociolinguistic perspective, using Discourse Activity Analysis System (Friedlander, 1984). It's purpose was to suggest how client and counselor establish a working relationship (Patton, 1984) in the early interviews by strategies of counselor talking which elicit ongoing client self-disclosure. The results of this sequential analysis were interpreted as "underscoring the reciprocal influence of client and counselor in establishing common understanding of the problem and defining their relationship" (p. 139). In Pepinsky and DeStefano's (1983) terms, these interactions were "bi-lateral."

The use of other category systems to code verbal responses (e.g., Classification System for Counseling Response [CSCR], Highlen, Lonberg, Hampl, & Lassiter, 1982, and the DAAS [Friedlander, 1984] in tandem with categories of linguistic structure) has been suggested by Highlen and Hill (1984) as a holding promise for future work. In addition to DeStefano *et al.* (1982) and Friedlander and Phillips (1984), whose work employed such category systems, Highlen, Hampl, Lonborg, Lassiter, and Williams (1982) have presented preliminary evidence suggesting an interface between stylistic complexity measures generated by CALAS and the CSCR. Friedlander's (1984) development of the DAAS from a social policy perspective might prove particularly useful in examining propositions related to our treatment model. In addition, if we are to conceptualize and execute empirical work related to our third level of meaning, such strategies that go beyond CALAS could be fruitful. This would be especially true if, through such methods, we could make more explicit what participants in interactive discourse take for granted.

RELATIONS BETWEEN LANGUAGE AND OTHER PHENOMENA OF PSYCHOLOGICAL TREATMENT

Although the foregoing descriptive work is essential and needs to be expanded, the potential pragmatic contribution of our work depends upon our ability to establish empirical links between our scheme of things and other "established" events of psychological treatment (Meara, 1983; Meara & Patton, 1984). Such links are suggested from the following illustrative hypothesis:

1. Different theoretically derived techniques of therapeutic intervention will exhibit different patterns of linguistic informative display.
2. Clients' linguistic patterns of informative display will change following the implementation of a specific therapeutic intervention.
3. Counselors whose linguistic patterns of informative display are different from each other will be perceived differently by observers.

Some initial work designed to empirically investigate and establish relations suggested by the first hypothesis has had mixed results. Wycoff, Davis, Hector, and Meara (1982) examined the use of empathy as a therapeutic intervention. They used as data 6 minutes of text selected from interviews conducted by six counselors with an angry client, who was a confederate. In three of the interviews, the counselors were judged to be high-empathic responders (HERS), and, in the other three, the counselors were judged to be low-empathic responders (LERS). The language of the two groups was compared with CALAS on selected stylistic and semantic measures. Some of the expectations were supported by the results; specifically, the LERS were more verbally productive, and used more *action* verb phrases, than the HERS. Significant differences were not found between the two groups on information block length (cf. ABL discussed above) or use of *state* verb phrases. In addition, low-empathic responders asked significantly more questions during the interview. After voicing appropriate cautions, the authors interpret these results as promising, in terms of linking language patterns to therapeutic interventions such as empathy. Thus, the authors suggest the use of systematic language training as part of teaching empathic responding to beginning students.

In another study related to the first hypothesis, Davis, Meara, and Moore (1984) analyzed statements made by a confederate trainee who was instructed to display resistance toward the supervisor, in an analogue of a single counseling supervision session. This session was videotaped and transcribed, and each trainee statement in the session was rated for verbal, nonverbal, and paraverbal forms of resistance by twenty experienced supervisors. The 10 statements for which the largest number of raters (16 or more) indicated the presence of verbal resistance were classified as high-resistance statements (HRS). The low-resistance statements (LRS) were identified as those 10 statements for which the fewest number of raters (five or less) indicated resistance. Selected stylistic and semantic attributes of the language contained in the HRS and the LRS were compared. The results indicated that the HRS were characterized by high verbal productivity and low self-disclosure about personal feelings. However, the unquestioned use of supervisors' ratings as a definition of resistance, and the analogue nature of the study, must be considered in interpreting these results.

An exploratory study related to hypothesis two was reported by Kidder (1984). Based on theoretical rationale derived from a client-centered approach to counseling, Kidder expected high rates of counselor-empathic responding to increase (a) client verbal productivity, (b) length of utterances, and (c) client expression of experiencing. These constructs were measured by selected stylistic and semantic output variables from the CALAS. He used as data four, 45-minute interviews conducted by two confederate counselors. After an initial 5-minute introductory period, the counselors alternated, in four 10-minute intervals, between (a) minimal reflection and (b) empathic responding. The results indicated that such alternating in therapeutic responding had no effect on any of the dependent variables. These results point out some of the limitations of CALAS that need to be addressed in CALAS-related studies. Since CALAS investigates the first and second levels of meaning in language use described above, one explanation is that these levels of analysis do not describe the influence that context has on their interaction. Second, other variables (e.g., probes, self-disclosures, nonverbals) known to relate to counselor empathic responding were systematically controlled in both conditions of responding. These variables probably contribute to the effectiveness of empathic responding, and thus, their control could have attenuated the effect of empathic responding.

Wyman, Hector, and Meara (1984) and Reed, Hector, and Meara (1984) attempted to look at related issues to illustrate hypothesis (3) above. The purpose of these studies was to investigate how the manipulation of selected stylistic and semantic attributes of a counselor's language affects perceptions of that counselor's perceived social influence, as measured by the counselor Rating Form (CRF) (Barak & LaCross, 1975) dimensions of *expertness, attractiveness,* and *trustworthiness.* The design of the two studies was similar, except for the population from which the subjects were selected and the procedures for random assignment. Wyman *et al.* (1984) used 88 females and 44 males who were selected from introductory classes in psychology. Reed *et al.* (1984) recruited subjects who were believed to be more knowledgeable about counseling. These subjects were 58 females and 14 male graduate and undergraduate students who had taken one or more courses in counseling.

Four audio tapes were developed from carefully prepared scripts, using an actor as counselor and an actress as client. Each tape purported to show excerpts from two interviews between counselor and client. The counselor's language was manipulated semantically and stylistically so that there were four experimental conditions: the use of language classified as (a) *state* simple, (b) *action* simple, (c) *state* complex, and (d) *action* complex. The client's language was identical across all four conditions. Results indicated no significant effect on the dependent measures, escept that the less knowledgeable subjects (i.e., those in the Wyman *et al.* study) perceived the counselor as more expert when he used complex language than when he used simple language. The results are similar to those found by Hurndon, Pepinsky, and Meara (1979), in which those who use complex language were judged to have a higher conceptual level than those using simple language. In some instances, it seems that stylistic complexity, a surface-structure variable, is related to how one is perceived by others. To this extent, language use acts as a social influence factor in person percpetion.

The last study we review is one by Warden and Wycoff (1984). These authors were interested in how experience level effected counselor language when counselors were encouraging their clients to explore feelings. This research approximates what might occur in a natural setting. Six counselors, two each from low-, medium-, and high-experience levels of similar theoretical orientation, met with two clients. Their task was to elicit client feelings that were stimulated by a guided fantasy conducted immediately prior to the interview. Entire transcripts of all twelve interviews served as the data set. Selected stylistic and semantic measures generated by CALAS were analyzed across experience levels.

Although there were differences of interest, they could not be attributed to experience level. It is noteworthy that in percentage of talk (i.e., amount of counselor talk versus amount of client talk) the two low-experience counselors were similar to each other and talked more than the medium-experience counselors. The medium-experience counselors resembled each other in their lower percentage of talk. The high-experience counselors were radically different from each other in percentage of counselor talk. One of these had the highest percentage of counselor talk of all six counselors, and the other had the lowest. The authors speculate that the high-experience counselors are confident enough to be idiosyncratic in their style and do not feel compelled to "go by the book." Warden and Wycoff (1984) call for a more contextual analysis to be completed, using this data set, the results to be reported in conjunction with the results obtained using CALAS. This suggestion is similar to the one by Highlen an Hill (1984) discussed above. Such analyses seem to be the next logical step in our empirical work, and are needed to test our newer conceptualizations (e.g., the third level of meaning).

CONCLUSION

The foregoing studies provide a description of some of the structural features of the language used by counselors and clients in counseling. We have inferred that the display of these semantic and stylistic features by each participant to the other is informative to them. It is informative, we further suggest, because it conveys meaning as a function of naming and relating. In turn, the operations of naming and relating reflect the use by each participant of grammatical schemes with which they may further understand (i.e., formulate) each other's talk.

These studies suggest some of the ways in which the elements of language serve as a "carrier" for the messages it transmits. Thus, as we construe it, the recognition that, in talking, another person is naming and relating names is minimally necessary for our further determination of what is being talked about in and through that naming and relating. Our next step is to try to make evident how counselors and clients formulate their developing discourse.

REFERENCES

Anderson, J. N. (1971). *The grammar of case: Towards a localistic theory.* Cambridge, England: Cambridge University Press.

Barak, A., & LaCrosse, M. (1975). Multitimensional perception of counselor behavior. *Journal of Counseling Psychology, 22,* 471–476.

Bieber, M. R. (1978). *A language analysis of three counseling series.* Unpublished doctoral dissertation, Department of Educational Psychology, University of Utah, Salt Lake City, Utah.

Bieber, M. R., Patton, M. J., & Fuhriman, A. J. (1977). A metalanguage analysis of counselor and client verb usage in counseling. *Journal of Counseling Psychology, 24,* (4), 264–271.

Brentano, F. (1955). *Psychologie von empirischen Standpunkt [Pyschology from an empirical standpoint].* Hamburg: Felix Meiner.

Chafe, W. S. (1970). *Meaning and structure of language.* Chicago: University of Chicago Press.

Cook, W. A. (1979). *Case grammar: Development of the matrix model (1970–1978).* Washington, D. C.: Georgetown University Press.

Davis, K. L., Meara, N. M., & Moore, K. B. (1984, April). A language analysis of resistance in psychological treatment. In M. J. Patton (Chair), *Research on language analysis in counseling.* Session conducted at the annual meeting of the American Educational Research Association, New Orleans.

DeStefano, J. S., Pepinsky, H. B., & Sanders, T. S. (1982). Discourse rules for literacy learning in a classroom. In L. C. Wilkenson (Ed.), *Communicating in the classroom* (pp. 101–129). New York: Academic Press.

Edwards, J. A. (1978). *Analysis of the relationship between grammatical structure and construct domains in counseling.* Unpublished master's thesis, University of Utah.

Filmore, C. J. (1968). The case for case. In E. Bach and R. T. Harms (Eds.), *Universals in linguistic theory* (pp. 1–88). New York: Holt, Rinehart & Winston.

Friedlander, M. L. (1984). Psychotherapy talk as social control. *Psychotherapy, 21,* 333–339.

Friedlander, M. L., & Phillips, S. D. (1984). A stochastic process analysis of interactive discourse in early counseling interviews. *Journal of Counseling Psychology, 31,* 139–148.

Garfinkel, H. (1967). *Studies in ethomethodology.* Englewood Cliffs, NJ: Prentice-Hall.

Garfinkel, H., & Sacks, H. (1971). *On formal structures of practical actions.* In J. C. McKinney and E. A. Tiryakian (Eds.), *Theoretical sociology: Perspective and developments* (pp. 337–366). New York: Appleton-Century-Crofts.

Garfinkel, H., Lynch, M., & Livingston, E. (1981). The work of a discovering science construed with materials from the optically discovered pulsar. *Philosophy of the Social Sciences, 11,* 131–158.

Goldstein, A. P. (1962). *Therapist-patient expectancies in psychotherapy.* New York, NY: MacMillan.

Goldstein, A. P. (1966). Psychotherapy research by extrapolation from social psychology. *Journal of Counseling Psychology, 13,* 38–45.

Halliday, M. A. K., & Hassan, R. (1976). *Cohesion in English.* London: Longman.

Highlen, P. S., & Hill, C. (1984). Factors affecting client change in individual counseling: Current status and theoretical speculations. In S. D. Brown & R. W. Lent (Eds.), *Handbook of counseling psychology.* (pp. 334–396). New York: John Wiley & Sons.

Highlen, P. S., Hampl, S. P., Lonborg, S. D., Lassiter, W. L., & Williams, D. A. (1982, August). *Convergence of content and structural approaches for analyzing the counseling process.* Symposium presented at the American Psychological Association Convention, Washington, DC.

Highlen, P. S., Lonborg, S. D., Hampl, S. P., & Lassiter, W. L. (1982). *Classification system for counseling responses (CSCR) manual.* Unpublished manuscript: The Ohio State University.

Hurndon, C. J., Pepinsky, H. B., & Meara, N. M. (1979). Conceptual level and structural complexity in language. *Journal of Counseling Psychology, 26,* 190–197.

Jaffe, J. (1964). Verbal behavior analysis in psychiatric interviews with the aid of digital computers. In D. M. K. Roch and E. A. Weinstein (Eds.), *Disorders of communication,* (Vol. 42). Baltimore, MD: Williams & Wilkins.

Kidder, D. W. (1984, April). Use of CALAS in a study of counselor empathy and client verbal behavior. In M. J. Patton (Chair), *Research on language analysis in counseling*. Session conducted at the annual meeting of the American Educational Research Association, New Orleans.

Kiesler, D. J. (1973). *The process of psychotherapy: Empirical foundations and systems of analysis*. Chicago: Aldine.

May, G. (1977). Psychotherapy and language: Linguistic convergence between therapist and client. Unpublished doctoral dissertation, Ohio State University.

Meara, N. M. (1976). A computer-assisted language analysis system for research on natural language. In H. B. Pepinsky (Chair), *Linguistic convergence of therapist and client*. Symposium presented at the Inter-American Congress of Psychology, Miami Beach.

Meara, N. M. (1983). CALAS: Conceptualizations and caveats in communicating and counseling. Paper presented at the American Psychological Association Annual Meeting, Anaheim, CA.

Meara, N. M., & Patton, M. J. (1984). Language analysis and policies of psychological treatment: An overview. In M. J. Patton (Chair), *Research on language analysis in counseling*. Session conducted at the annual meeting of the American Educational Research Association, New Orleans.

Meara, N. M., Shannon, J. W., & Pepinsky, H. B. (1979). Comparison of the stylistic complexity of the language of counselor and client across three theoretical orientations. *Journal of Counseling Psychology, 26*, 181–189.

Meara, N. M., Pepinsky, H. B., Shannon, J. W., & Murray, W. A. (1981). Semantic communication and expectations for counseling across three theoretical orientations. *Journal of Counseling Psychology, 28*, 110–118.

Oster, R. Q. (1979). *The identification of topical tracking in three counseling series*. Unpublished doctoral dissertation. Department of Educational Psychology, University of Utah, Salt Lake City, Utah.

Patton, M. J. (1969). Attraction discrepancy and responses to psychological treatment. *Journal of Counseling Psychology, 16*, 317–324.

Patton, M. J. (1984). Managing social interaction in counseling: A contribution from the philosophy of science. *Journal of Counseling Psychology, 31*, 443–457.

Patton, M. J., & Sullivan, J. J. (1980). Heinz Kohut and the classical psychoanalytic tradition: An analysis in terms of levels of explanation. *Psychoanalytic Review, 61*(3), 365–388.

Patton, M. J., Fuhriman, A. J., & Bieber, M. R. (1977). A model and a metalanguage for research on psychological counseling. *Journal of Counseling Psychology, 24*, 25–34.

Pepinsky, H. B. (1970). Psychological help-giving as an informed definition of the situation. In H. B. Pepinsky (Ed.), *People and information* (pp. 261–295). Elmsford, NY: Pergamon Press.

Pepinsky, H. B. (1974). A metalanguage for systematic research on human communication via natural language. *Journal of the American Security for Information Sciences, 25*, 59–69.

Pepinsky, H. B. (1985). A metalanguage of text. In V. M. Rentel, S. A. Carson, and B. R. Dunn (Eds.), *Psychophysiological aspects of reading* (pp. 263–325). New York: Gordon & Breach.

Pepinsky, H. B., & DeStefano, J. S. (1983). Interactive discourse in the classroom as organizational behavior. In B. A. Hutson (Ed.), *Advances in Reading/Language Research* (pp. 107–137). Greenwich: JAI Press.

Pepinsky, H. B., & Karst, T. O. (1964). Convergence: A phenomenon in counseling and psychotherapy. *American Psychologist, 19*, 333–338.

Pepinsky, H. B., & Patton, M. J. (Eds.). (1971). *The psychological experiment: A practical accomplishment*. Elmsford, NY: Pergamon Press.

Pepinsky, H. B., Weick, K., & Riner, J. (1965). *Primer for productivity*. Columbus: Ohio State University Research Foundation.
Pepinsky, H. B., Baker, W. M., Matalon, R., May, G. D., & Staubus, A. M. (1977). A users manual for the *Computer-Assisted Language Analysis System*. Columbus: Group for Research and Development in Language and Social Policy. Mershon Center, Ohio State University.
Percy, W. (1972). Toward a triadic theory of meaning. *Psychiatry, 11*(1), 29–64.
Reed, J. M. (1983). *Linguistic evaluation*. Unpublished paper. University of Tennessee, Knoxville.
Reed, J. M., Hector, M. A., & Meara, N. M. (1984, April). The effects of semantic and stylistic variations in language on perception of social influence characteristics in a counseling sophisticated population. In M. J. Patton (Chair), *Research on language analysis in counseling*. Session conducted at the annual meeting of the American Educational Research Association, New Orleans.
Rush, J. E., Pepinsky, H. B., Landry, B. C., Meara, N. M., Strong, S. M., Valley, J. A., & Young, C. E. (1974). *A computer-assisted language analysis system*. (Computer and Information Science Research Center, OSU-CISRC-TR-74-1.) Columbus: Ohio State University.
Schutz, A. (1967a). *Collected papers I: The problem of social reality*. The Hague: Martinus Nijhoff.
Schutz, A. (1967b). *The phenomenology of the social world*. Evanston: Northwestern University Press.
Shostrom, E. L. (Producer). (1966). *Three approaches to psychotherapy*. Santa Ana, CA: Psychological Films. (Film)
Strong, S. R. (1968). Counseling: An interpersonal influence process. *Journal of Counseling Psychology, 15*, 215–224.
Warden, K. W., & Wycoff, J. P. (1984, April). A linguistic analysis of counselor's affect-oriented responses across three levels of counseling experience. In M. J. Patton (Chair), *Research on language analysis* in counseling. Session conducted at the annual meeting of the American Educational Research Association, New Orleans.
Wycoff, J. P., Davis, K. L., Hector, M. A., & Meara, N. M. (1982). A language analysis of empathic responding. *Journal of Counseling Psychology, 29*, 462–467.
Wyman, E. A. (1983). *The effects of semantic and stylistic variations in language on perceptions of social influence characteristics*. Unpublished doctoral dissertation, University of Tennessee, Knoxville.
Wyman, E. A., Hector, M. A., & Meara, N. M. (1984, April). The effects of semantic and stylistic variations in language on perception of social influence characteristics. In M. J. Patton (Chair), *Research on language analysis in counseling*. Session conducted at the annual meeting of the American Educational Research Association, New Orleans.
Young, C. E. (1973). *Development of language analysis procedures with applications to automatic indexing*. Columbus: Computer and Information Science Research Center, OSU-CISRC-TR-3-2, Ohio State University.
Zimmerman, D. H., & Pollner, M. (1970). The everyday world as a phenomenon. In H. B. Pepinsky (Ed.), *People and information* (pp. 33–59). New York, NY: Pergamon Press.

8

Ethnography and the Vicissitudes of Talk in Psychotherapy

Roy D. Pea and Robert L. Russell

INTRODUCTION

Husband: I'm tired.
Wife: How are you tired? Physically, mentally, or just bored?
Husband: I don't know. I guess physically, mainly.
Wife: You mean that your muscles ache, or your bones?
Husband: I guess so. Don't be so technical.
            (after some delay)
Husband: All these old movies have the same kind of old iron bedstead in
            them.
Wife: What do you mean? Do you mean all old movies, or some of them, or
            just the ones you have seen?
Husband: What's the matter with you? You know what I mean.
Wife: I wish you would be more specific.
Husband: You know what I mean! Drop Dead![1] (Garfinkel, 1967, p. 7)

As observers of married life in American culture, we can specify what
the wife has done to exasperate the husband. We might satisfy ourselves

The order of authors has been arbitrarily determined because the chapter is an outcome of collaborative effort.
[1]This stretch of talk was a result in an experiment in which Garfinkel instructed his class to
ask for clarifications of the meaning of everyday statements, thus calling into question
common sense taken-for-granted structures shared by co-conversationalists. Had the
husband, and not the wife, been in the class, a similar breakdown in communication
could be expected.

ROY D. PEA • Educational Communication and Technology Program, 23 Press Building,
New York University, New York, NY 10003.   ROBERT L. RUSSELL • Department of
Psychology, New School for Social Research, 65 Fifth Avenue, New York, NY 10003.

with the "explanation" that for whatever characterization the husband produced in his speech, the wife, in a distinctly formal manner, proffers alternative characterizations, each of which is both more technical and precise than those whose place they are meant to usurp. The alternative characterizations do not appear to be fulfilling a clarifying, motive-neutral function (i.e., to circumscribe the referred-to state of affairs with less ambiguity); after all, the wife's procedures are occurring in a situation of the type which normally bars such specificity. But, what type of situation had been cognitively expected and had subsequently emerged for this couple? Presumably, the husband's background expectancies as to what should count as an adequate characterization in such a situation were erroneous. More importantly, since such expectancies were taken for granted to be shared with his wife, it appears that he could not legitimate her "attack" by connecting it, through a routine motive ascription, to his wife's biographical or current interactional relevancies. Thus, his telling exclamation: "Drop Dead," the meaning of which can at least be partially glossed as: "I cannot reconstruct, for ongoing practical purposes, the 'personage' of my wife, for I cannot, here, now, through my available set of motive ascriptions, render her behavioral displays as instances of bona fide social action." (Blum & McHugh, 1971; Mills, 1940.)

Besides considering characterizations, situationally constrained expectancies, biographies, and motives in our attempt to illuminate what transpired between wife and husband, sooner or later we would need to address the *processive* nature of their interaction—that, for example, only after repeated substitute characterizations did they become topics for the husband's critical comments. Our attempt to link the segments of the husband–wife interaction might well result in a construal of what had transpired in terms of rules, or situation-specific violations thereof. For instance, when addressed with a question, the husband initially acts "in accordance with"[2] the well-known discourse rule: "Unless such and so normative conditions are not met, a recipient of a question is obliged to formulate some response to it." Next, we might note that the relation of speaking turns to accomplished consequences (such as exasperating the husband) is not simply one to one: at the level of social action, one speaking turn can accomplish several acts at a time. Just as it seemed reasonable to suppose that speaking turns are explicable in terms of a set of sequencing rules, so too, the succession of accomplished social actions could be accounted for by reference to sets of action rules.

[2]The use of rules in understanding behavior has taken two radically different forms: (1) behavior can be said to result from its conformity to underlying rule structures, or (2) rules can be said to be actively indexed in participants' attempts to construct a sense of orderly conduct (see O'Keefe, 1979 for discussion).

Following all of the above lines of inquiry, in more or less detail (e.g., note the absence of any mention thus far of statuses, roles, power, solidarity, social structure, or even sex differences), would permit us to characterize what happened between this couple, and about why it happened as it did. Our characterizations would be, for the most part, easily comprehended. This ease in comprehensibility occurs just because the goings on between the husband and wife in this setting are already assimilable for us to a particular type of happening, formulable with a set of categories dependent upon, and growing out of, our everyday knowledge. Although the means introduced above to explicate the husband–wife interaction do not all address this fact (i.e., that our membership in American culture predisposes us *not* to question the facticity of an "interaction" occurring between a "wife" and a "husband"), an ethnography of this same event would have to specify what had taken place in terms of what had been created and understood by the participants, *and* to specify this in a manner which would make explicit the cultural context making the existence of this specific happening possible. That is, an ethnography of this event would seek to specify both the cultural conditions sustaining the possibility for, and the interactional procedures actually utilized in, the participants' work in creating this situation.

The readers familiar with developments in the ethnography of communication could discern several fields of inquiry ingredient in the above introduction. Work in such fields as linguistics, sociolinguistics, ethnomethodology, symbolic interactionism, speech-act theory, and cognitive anthopology are here interrelated to such an extent that there is reason to speak of a "new" ethnography of communication.[3] Even so, with many of the above fields developing only after the Second World War, the new ethnography has not congealed sufficiently to permit a programmatic presentation of its theoretical premises and empirically confirmed axioms. Thus, our presentation of an ethnographically inspired investigation of language use in psychotherapy is a research-inspired amalgamation. What follows, then, is not a consummate ethnography of talk in psychotherapy. Rather, through our brief (1) presentation of the various fields of inquiry figuring in the new ethnography, (2) overview of previous ethnographically inspired investigations of language use in psychotherapy, (3) summary of Labov and Fanshel's (1977) Comprehensive Discourse Analysis, and (4) suggestion of topics in need

---

[3] A "new ethnography" has been developed as ethnoscience (Sturtevant, 1974). Its emphasis on the "cognitive models with which a society operates" (p. 154) is meant to augment, not replace, the central tenets of ethnographic methodology. Our use of the epithet "a new ethnography" is similarly intended to underscore the influx of related methodologies into the arsenals of ethnography.

of further research, we will attempt to define some broad boundaries within which the theoretical work of creating an internally consistent ethnography can progress and be utilized in psychotherapy research.

Academic Fields and Styles of Analysis Contributing to the New Ethnography

At one extreme, the new ethnography of communication can be seen to incorporate so many ideas from so many distinct disciples that its likelihood of achieving an autonomous character would appear quite small. For our limited purposes, it will suffice to present two overarching approaches to the study of the social organization of communicative interaction [1] the normative approach, and [2] the interpretive approach),[4] along with the speech-act analysis developed by the ordinary-language philosophers J. L. Austin and John R. Searle. In considering the normative approach, special emphasis will be given to sociolinguistic research. In considering the interpretive approach, special emphasis will be given to ethnographic research carried out by researchers native to the cultural milieu that they are studying. This overview of the normative and interpretive approach, along with our treatment of speech-act analysis, is meant to provide a framework with which to approach the following presentation of an ethnographically inspired analysis of psychotherapeutic talk.

The Normative Approach and Sociolinguistics

Sociology and linguistics, as disciplines, did not form an alliance likely to span several generations of scholars until relatively recently. Several reasons for this state of affairs have been suggested. For example, with sociology seeking to discover a set of criteria capable of differentiating forms of social organization, language, possessed by all known societies, and thought to function similarly within them, seemed particularly unlikely as a robust criterion of sociological interest. Similarly, with the Saussurean distinction between language and speech, language became the ideal object of science independent of the social contexts in which everyday speech behavior occurred (Giglioli, 1972). Language was conceived as an abstract and ideal set of rules internalized by native speakers. What native speakers did when they conversed was not

---

[4]In using this dichotomy, we have drawn on the work of Wilson (1970) and Leiter (1980). Readers are referred to Leiter for an especially informative and readable introduction to the interpretive approach.

considered to consist of "instances" of language, and was relegated to a distinct sphere of scientific discourse concerned with speech.

As some sociologists explored such topics as social stratification, mobility, and the interaction between status-reciprocal and non-reciprocal members of society, the role of speech became of thematic interest. Conversely, to some linguists, the idea that a societal member who had a complete mastery of his/her native language could nevertheless be completely ignorant of the appropriate ways in which to deploy it in everyday situations appeared untenable. Consideration of this problem led to the development of the concept of communicative competence—what a speaker-hearer must know in order to deploy speech appropriately within the varying situations in his/her society (Hymes, 1968, 1972a,b, 1974). Thus, grounds for the convergence of work in sociology and linguistics were set.

The work in sociolinguistics is nevertheless tremendously varied. The overarching aim has been to describe systematic relationships between forms of language use and forms of societal structure. Typically, variations in forms of language use are conceived to be a function of variations in selected aspects of social structure. Such a conceptualization presupposes means to articulate varied forms of social structure and language use. Sociolinguistics has thus sought to identify relevant sets of sociological and linguistic variables and has exploited standard distinctions developed in sociology and linguistics proper. For example, such classic sociological variables as social class, status, role, power, solidarity, age, ethnic group, familial relations, sex, occupation, and formality have all been utilized. The main focus of investigation is, then, on the ways in which language behavior varies with respect to situations uniquely described by some small subset of the possible values of these variables. Such investigations have been considered the mainstay of descriptive sociolinguistics, and basic to the achievement of a more theoretically oriented science (Fishman, 1972).

A sociolinguistic variable is defined as "one which is correlated with some non-linguistic variable of the social context" (Labov, 1972, p. 283). An example of work in descriptive sociolinguistics is Labov's investigation of the sociolinguistic variable (th) (i.e., the phonetic form of the voiceless interdental fricative in *th*ought, *th*ink, etc.) as it varied with class and situational variables.[5] Review of the following figure will reveal that "(1) In every context members of the speech community are differentiated by their use of (th), [and] (2) . . . every group is behaving

---

[5]Labov's efforts have not been confined to this correlational approach, and he has been a leading figure in espousing the possibility of rule accounts of linguistic behavior (e.g., Labov, 1972, p. 71).

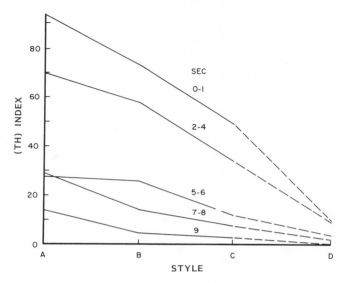

FIGURE 1. Stylistic and social stratification of (th) in *thing, three,* etc. in New York City. (Source: Labov, 1972, p. 284.)

in the same way, as indicated by the parallel slope of style shifting for (th)" (Labov, 1972, p. 285). On the basis of this study and others like it, sociolinguists have been able to describe the systematic effect variations in nonlinguistic situational factors have on speech productions.

Studies such as the above are distinguished, for example, by their choice of variables and their thoroughness, but not for their methodological innovation. Although sociolinguistic studies are routinely carried out using standard experimental methodologies, sociolinguistics as a whole certainly is not restricted to this method. Sociolinguistic methodology and forms of explanation also seek to explain language use in terms of invariant rules, rather than in terms of probabilistic laws. For example, in investigating the variations in the production of terms of address, Ervin-Tripp (1972, pp. 219–228; see also Grimshaw, 1980) has provided an analysis of the rules of address in America, nineteenth century Russia, and Yiddish. As one can see from the figure below, the rules are presented in the form of a flow chart:

Entering on the left, it is possible to pass from left to right, through a series of binary selectors, to a possible outcome in the form of one of the seven indicated forms of address. The determination of the form of address can be said to be a function of particular nonlinguistic aspects of the "situation" (e.g., whether the potential addressee is deemed to have the attribute "adult" or not). But, unlike the previous example, this

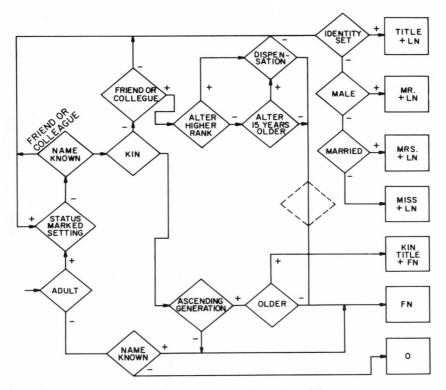

FIGURE 2. American address. (Source: Ervin-Tripp, 1972, p. 219.)

function cannot be described as a probabilistic one. The series of binary selectors in the flow chart express invariant constraints on the selection of an address term, given (1) an adult native speaker of English at the entry point, (2) the necessary applicability of one and only one selector at each choice point, and (3) a nonmetaphorical frame in which the address form outcomes might be appropriately situated (e.g., "look, _____, it's time to leave."). As a *logical* model of an American Address system, universal and necessary aspects are meant to be represented, not probabilistic outcomes based on empirical correlations. While the computer flow chart only implicitly embodies a series of formally stated rules, it should be clear that a shift in explicatory models has occurred in moving from Labov's study to Ervin-Tripp's rule-based grammar of American address terms.

Another shift is evident as well:

The diagram is not intended as a model of a process, of the actual decision sequence by which a speaker chooses a form of address or a listener interprets one. The two structures may or may not correspond. In any case, the task of determining the structure implicit in people's knowledge of what forms of address are possible and appropriate is clearly distinct from the task of studying how people, in real situations and in real time, make choices. The criteria and methods of the two kinds of study are quite different. (Ervin-Tripp, pp. 219–220.)

In Ervin-Tripp's analysis, unlike that of Labov's, explicit use is made of the competence–performance distinction (for discussion see Miller, 1975; Pylyshyn, 1973; Stone & Day, 1980), which allows for the disassociation of conditions of language use from the sets of constraints applicable in the construction of a logical model. If this distinction is expeditious in terms of facilitating the construction of abstract logical models of language, it at the same time reduces the power and scope of such models to explain or describe what humans do most characteristically: communicate through their speech. Thus, it has been thought possible to account for the selection of our address terms utilizing such variables as the role and affectional relationship between interlocutors and the setting (Grimshaw, 1980, p. 800). However, it is important to keep in mind that such variables, or values thereof, are at least as abstract, as competence-bound, as the model in which they are specified. At the extreme, the term "interlocutor" in such a model is related to a speaker of English with little more verisimilitude than a prime number. Such hypostatization effectively restricts the role of such concepts in the formulation of theory whose value rests in the degree to which it illuminates human processes (such as those involved in formulating an address to one another) presumably extant in time, if not in space.

However, rule accounts need not be concerned only with abstract structures, or competence. In fact, rule accounts of aspects of production and comprehension of discourse, constrained by processes unfolding in space and time, have been undertaken with some initial success.

Rule accounts of the processive nature of conversational phenomena are themselves "processive": rule applicability and the set of outcomes defined by successive rule orderings are limited by constraints formulated to capture the temporal course of conversations. For example, in accounting for the turn-taking organization of conversation, Sacks, Schegloff, and Jefferson (1974) develop a model composed of a set of rules, but which, unlike the model of the American address system, is processive in the above sense. Their model is composed of two components (a turn-constructional and a turn-allocational component) and a small set of rules. The turn-constructional component consists of the speaker's selection of a unit-type (e.g., a clause, a phrase, a sentence, etc.) with which to construct a turn. The first possible completion of the first unit type in the speaker's turn constitutes a point relevant for the selection of the next speaker. The turn-allocational component is composed of two groups of techniques: (a) those in which a next turn is allocated by the current speaker; and (b) those in which a next turn is taken by self-selection. The rules are as follows:

> For any turn:
> 1. At initial turn-constructional unit's initial transition-relevance place:
>   (a) If the turn-so-far is so constructed as to involve the use of a "current speaker selects next" technique, then the party so selected has rights, and is obliged, to take next turn to speak, and no others have such rights or obligations, transfer occurring at that place.
>   (b) If the turn-so-far is so constructed as not to involve the use of a "current speaker selects next" technique, self-selection for next speakership may, but need not, be instituted, with first starter acquiring rights to a turn, transfer occurring at that place.
>   (c) If the turn-so-far is so constructed as not to involve the use of a "current speaker selects next" technique, then current speaker may, but need not, continue, unless another self-selects.
> 2. If, at initial turn-constructional unit's initial transition-relevance place, neither 1(a) nor 1(b) has operated, and, following the provision of 1(c), current speaker has continued, then the Rule-set (a)–(c) reapplies at next transition-relevance place, and recursively at each next transition-relevance place, until transfer is effected. (Sacks, Schegloff & Jefferson, in Schenkein, 1978, p. 13)

At this point, there seems little that would distinguish this systematic rule-account of turn-taking organization from the account of the American address system: one could graphically represent the system of turn-taking rules in a form comparable to that of the computer flow chart. However:

> the ordering of the rules serves to constrain each of the options the rules provide. The fact that 1(a) is the first applying rule does not entail that its option is free of constraints imposed on it by the presence, in the set, of rules which would apply if 1(a) did not. Thus, for example, given the applicability of Rule 1(b)'s option if Rule 1(a)'s option has not been employed, for Rule 1(a)'s option to be methodically assured of use it needs to be employed before initial transition-relevance place. Thereby, the operation of Rule 1(a)'s option is constrained by Rule 1(b)'s presence in the set, independently of Rule 1(b)'s option actually being employed. Similarly, for Rule 1(b)'s option to be methodically assured of application given the presence in the set of Rule 1(c), it will need to be employed at initial unit's initial transition-relevance place, and before current speaker's option to continue—Rule 1(c)—is invoked. For if 1(c) is thus invoked, Rule 2 will apply, and the Rule-set (a)–(c) will reapply, and Rule 1(a)'s option will take priority over Rule 1(b)'s again. Thereby, Rule 1(b)'s operation is constrained by Rule 1(c)'s presence in the set, independently of Rule 1(c)'s actually being employed. Having noted that lower priority rules thus constrain the use of higher priority options, it should be recalled that the constraints imposed on lower priority rules by higher pri-

ority rules are incorporated in the rule-set itself. (Sacks, Schegloff, Jefferson,
in Schenkein, 1978, p. 13)

Thus, the reciprocally constraining functions of higher and lower
priority rules in effect incorporate the temporal dimension into the structure of the rule set, enabling it to "comprehend" the dynamic processive
nature of the phenomena of turn-taking organization. Admittedly, the
rule set is abstract, but it is meant to render the processive character of
turn-taking, and not the logical antecedents of hypostatized turn-taking
outcomes, comprehensible. Its aim is to provide a structural account of
actual constraints operative in everyday turn-taking behavior. In other
words, it is deeply concerned with "the task of studying how people, in
real situations and in real time, make choices" (Ervin-Tripp, 1972, p.
270). It is this latter task which Comprehensive Discourse Analysis un-
dertakes (Labov & Fanshel, 1977).

The Interpretive Approach

While ethnographers of communication seek to identify stable patterns in the social fabric of the community under study, and while their
conceptualizations have not been free from sociologistic formulations, a
discernable trend in the ethnographic approach has taken shape. The
most fundamental departure of the interpretive approach is its insistence that the "facts" of social life have situation-specific interactional
histories. In other words, the "facts," which we accept naively as facts,
ought to be seen as accomplishments achieved through the deployment
of "fact-production methods" by society's members, who are all con-
tinually engaged in the work of establishing and sustaining a sense of
social order for themselves and for others. The identification and description of such "fact-production methods" poses a problem for any
ethnographer, but especially for those who attempt ethnographic descriptions of the life of their own culture or speech community. This is so
precisely because of the culture's familiarity and the habit of cultural
members to suspend any doubt as to the factual character of its structure
and content. Nevertheless, the methodological prescription that under-
girds the interpretive approach recommends that the researcher attain a
position of neutrality with respect to whether or not everyday reasoning, and the facts which it engenders, are ontologically and epis-
temologically equivalent to the kind associated with "truly" scientific
knowledge. Of uppermost sociological import is the discovery of the
routine ways in which facts are co-constituted in everyday situations.
The aim, then, of this approach is to discover the sets of methods employed in producing the situation-specific shared recognition of, for ex-

ample, status differences and situational formality (for contrast, refer to Labov's study above). Rates and correlations, from this perspective, appear to simply pass over the category of phenomena most worthy of study. Variations in the form of speech productions do not result from the systematic interplay of abstract sociological rule sets, but rather are the achieved characteristics of situations that they have been instrumental in defining.

Thus, the interpretive approach does not establish the significance of language on an autonomous level independent of the contexts in which it is used. Rather than seek univocal structures and referential determinativeness as the conditions impelling consensus in language practices, the interpretive approach stresses the essential ambiguity of language and the essential interdependence of context and meaning. Thus, "definitions of situations and actions are not explicitly or implicitly assumed to be settled once and for all by literal application of a pre-existing culturally established system of symbols. Rather, meanings of situations and actions are interpretations formulated on particular occasions by the participants in the interaction and are subject to reformulation on subsequent occasions" (Wilson, 1970, p. 721). Language rules are not generating mechanisms of action; instead, societal members are seen to actively reference rules in the course of their attempts to construct a sense of orderly communication. Referencing rules is a method employed in constructing a sense of social order. Such indicating and referencing is as much an ongoing activity of the situation as any other aspect (O'Keefe, 1979).

Thus, the interpretive approach construes the actor and interaction so that emphasis is placed on the individual's capacity to act in a purposeful manner, one that takes into account the relevance of the individual's aims as well as his/her capacity to alter such aims after having considered the perspective of the other. The individual is considered to be sense-making, and to act on the basis of his/her understanding of the situation. Rather than be seen as an object of such social forces as status, power, and institutions, the actor is seen to actively confer motivational relevance on such forces. They (i.e., "status," "power," etc.) become speech categories referenced in an attempt to construct orderly situations. Interaction, then, is taken to be what transpires between individuals on the basis of their activities aimed at providing each other with a sense of social order. Thus, interaction and the social order it projects are not given "facts," but are *accomplishments* attained in the process of securing a shared belief in the objective character of individuals and society at large.

The above brief presentation of two approaches to the problem of language use and sociality is meant to serve as a roadmap for what follows. We hope that the reader is now in possession of enough of the landmarks to follow our presentation critically. Before presenting Labov and Fanshel's model, however, a brief sketch of Speech Act Theory will be attempted.

Speech Act Theory

The relation of *form* and *function* is a primary one in the analysis of discourse, in psychotherapy as elsewhere. A particular grammatical form may be used to express a variety of discourse functions, and as listeners we can recognize which function the speaker projects. How is this possible?

In one influential approach to the form/function relationship, the linguistic philosopher Austin (1962) presents an analysis of *How to Do Things with Words*. His account of speech acts introduced the concept of "performatives," sentences in which saying words count as the performance of an action of a particular type. For example, I may "promise," "warn," "estimate," "challenge," "argue," and so on by uttering certain words. To account for the ways in which "to say something may be to do something," he devised a tripartite distinction of the acts one simultaneously performs in producing an utterance:

> *Locutionary*—the act *of* saying something.
> > "He said to me 'shoot her' meaning by 'shoot' shoot and referring by "her" to her."
> *Illocutionary*—The act performed *in* saying something.
> > "He urged (or advised, ordered, etc.) me to shoot her."
> *Perlocutionary*—the act performed *by* or as a result of saying something.
> > "He persuaded me to shoot her." (Austin, 1962, pp. 101–102).

In the analysis of conversational interaction, something akin to these distinctions will be employed. Austin viewed the locutionary act as tied to *utterance meaning* and the illocutionary act as tied to *utterance force,* and each act as expressive of the speaker's intentions in producing the speech act. The perlocutionary act is, however, an *utterance consequence* and may totally surprise the speaker, being a function as it is of the history of the listener. "Your suit is appealing" may be intended with the illocutionary effect of a compliment, but have the perlocutionary consequence of making me sad, since that is exactly what my deceased friend used to tell me. Austin (1962), Searle (1965, 1969), McCawley (1977), and others (e.g., Cole & Morgan, 1975; Rogers, Wall, & Murphy, 1977) have devoted their analytic skills to specifying the conditions or rules which mark utterance tokens as successful performances of speech acts of a particular type.

As an example of analytic research in this tradition, Searle's (1969) formulation of the necessary and sufficient conditions for the successful execution of the act of promising are presented in abbreviated form below:

> Given that a speaker S utters a sentence T in the presence of a hearer H, then, in the literal utterance of T, S sincerely and non-defectively promises that p to H if and only if the following conditions 1–9 obtain:
> 1. Normal input and output conditions obtain. . . .
> 2. S expresses the proposition that p in the utterance of T. . . .
> 3. In expressing that p, S predicts a future act A of S. . . .
> 4. H would prefer S's doing A to his not doing A, and S believes H would prefer his doing A to his not doing A. . . .
> 5. It is not obvious to both S and H that S will do A in the normal course of events. . . .
> 6. S intends to do A. . . .
> 7. S intends that the utterance of T will place him under an obligation to do A. . . .
> 8. S intends (i-I) to produce in H the knowledge (K) that the utterance of T is to count as placing S under an obligation to do A. S intends to produce K by means of the recognition of i-I, and he intends i-I to be recognized in virtue of (by means of) H's knowledge of the meaning of T. . . .
> 9. The semantical rules of the dialect spoken by S and H are such that T is correctly and sincerely uttered if and only if conditions 1-8 obtain. . . .
> (Searle, 1969, pp. 57–61)

The surface forms of promises can differ and still fulfill the conditions of promising. With such formulations, it is clear that the lack of a one-to-one form–function relationship need not hamper the systematic study of speech acts.

Austin (1962) suggests that the number of illocutionary act-types is equal to the number of performative verbs (such as "state," "request," etc.) in the language, with his estimate between 1,000 and 10,000. If we include not only performative verbs listed in the contemporary lexicon, but the products of our creative propensities to make verbs from nouns (e.g., Clark & Clark, 1979), such as "He Reaganed her right to work" or "He was really Don Rickled after his performance," the list of performative verbs would be longer. Searle (1969) argues that some conditions are common to many performative verbs, so it is possible that there exist some basic illocutionary acts to which all or most others are reducible. This issue is a pivotal concern of many recent attempts at developing speech act taxonomies (e.g., Fraser, 1971, 1974; Hancher, 1979; Searle, 1976).

Austin's (1962) analysis of speech acts assumes that each speech act has a *unique* illocutionary force, but locutions can be multiply ambiguous. This problem of the polyillocutionary nature of speech acts is confronted in detail in Labov and Fanshel's (1977) Comprehensive Discourse Analysis. However, it is to earlier microanalytic studies of language in psychotherapy that we now turn.

Microanalytic Studies of Language in Psychotherapy

The importance of detailed studies of individual cases in elaborating psychological theories is well attested to (e.g., Davidson & Costello, 1969; Luria, 1968), and microanalytic studies of behavior have provided insights into *processes* of mental functioning not only in psychotherapeutic settings, but in studies of cognitive development (e.g., Langer, 1980). Linked to either frame-by-frame film analysis or video records, such microanalyses are a recent development that have yielded an understanding of the intricate structural and interactional complexities of conversational phenomena, whether in everyday settings such as classroom reading lessons (McDermott, Gospodinoff, & Aron, 1978; Mehan, 1979) or in psychotherapy.

The efforts of Pittenger, Hockett, and Danehey (1960) in their fine-grained behavioral analyses of 5 minutes of an audio-taped and filmed interview were revolutionary, both in the attention given to the context-determined meaningfulness of prosodic cues, voice quality and well-specified body motions, and in the nine general principles of interpersonal communication they derived from their study. They have provided a frame of reference for virtually all the subsequent studies in this tradition (e.g., McQuown, Bateson, Birdwhistell, Brosen, & Hockett, 1971; Labov & Fanshel, 1977). We present Labov and Fanshel's abbreviated version of the "Nine Principles of Conversational Analysis."

1. *Immanent Reference.* . . . No matter what else human beings may be communicating about, or may think they are communicating about, *they are always communicating about themselves, about one another, and about the immediate context of the communication.* (italics added)

2. *Determinism.* The only useful working assumption . . . is that any communicative act is, indeed, culturally determined: the indeterminate or "accidental" residue is nonexistent.

3. *Recurrence.* . . . Anyone will tell us, over and over again, in our dealings with him, what sort of person he is, and what his affiliations with cultural subgroups are, what his likes and dislikes are, and so on. . . . The diagnostically crucial patterns of communication will not be manifested just once.

4. *Contrast and the Working Principle of Reasonable Alternatives.* There is no way to understand a signal that does not involve recognizing what the signal is *not* as well as what it is.

5. *Relativity of Signal and Noise.* We communicate simultaneously in many channels, via many systems. Sometimes we may choose to focus attention on one channel, and as long as this focus is main-

tained, certain simultaneous events in other channels can validly be regarded *relatively* as noise.

6. *Reinforcement: Packaging.* Most of the signals that people transmit to other people are packaged: but in the normal course of events we are apt to respond only to some of the included ingredients, allowing others to pass unnoticed or to register on us only out of awareness. The phenomenon . . . is clearly related to what psychiatrists have traditionally called *over-determination.* . . . One observer may hear anger in a patient's delivery of a passage, while others detect remorse or depression or self-pity. They may all be right, in that the actual signals may reflect all these contributing factors in a particular varying balance. . . . The wise working assumption then is that always no matter how many possible contributing factors we have itemized, there may still be others that we have overlooked.

7. *Adjustment.* . . . Continuous recalibration of communicative conventions is always to be expected in transactions between human beings— . . . communicating and learning to communicate always go hand in hand.

8. *The Priority of Interaction.* A man knows what he is doing, what emotions he is feeling, what "choices" of response he is making, only by observing his own behavior via feedback. This input via feedback is subject to the same kinds of interpretation as is the input from the communicative behavior of other people.

9. *Forests and Trees: The Dangers of Microscopy.* There are important properties of things and events that are not invariant under change of scale. . . . Lengthy concentration of attention on the one event can easily blow up in significance far out of proportion to its original duration and its actual setting. One must not mistake the five-inch scale model for the fly itself. (Labov & Fanshel, 1977, pp. 21–22)

In this same tradition, McQuown *et al.* (1971), present an analyzed and interpreted corpus of linguistic, paralinguistic, and body-motion data from the microanalyses of a family psychiatric interview. Much of this effort was directed toward developing theoretical frames suitable for the interpretation of such rich interactional material. The general limitation the authors note was that the *generality* of use for the analytic and interpretational frames that they developed in the context of a single-family interview remained to be determined. Reservations cut across dialectical variations in English, the transcription and interpretation of paralanguage, and the transcription and interpretation of varieties of body-motion behavior, both across cultures and in other regional and social groups of the same culture. As Labov and Fanshel (1977) and others have noted, the sheer magnitude of McQuown *et al.*'s effort, and the lack of reduction of their procedures to a parsimonious presentation, barred other investigators from attempting the necessary replicatory work. While we cannot recount their findings here, they laid the foundation for current efforts by revealing that insights could be garnered concerning human interaction from microanalysis that would be glossed over by standard macroscopic, or content-analytic approaches. Labov and Fanshel's Comprehensive Discourse Analysis derives in part from these pioneering efforts.

COMPREHENSIVE DISCOURSE ANALYSIS

The problem addressed by Labov and Fanshel's (1977) procedure of speech act and conversational sequencing analysis concerns the relation between "what is said" and "what is done" in psychotherapy. Their Comprehensive Discourse Analysis is an integrative approach that both draws from and informs the work of psychiatrists, cognitive and social psychologists, philosophers of language, linguists, and sociologists. A central focus of the analysis is an account demonstrating the hierarchical nature of speech act sequencing in client–therapist speech:

> A conversation between therapist and patient or a reported conversation between a mother and daughter is an intricately woven fabric, and only part of it is visible at any one time. It cannot be treated like a string of beads, with linear connections that can be added and subtracted. (Labov & Fanshel, 1977, p. 272)

The sequence of steps in Comprehensive Discourse Analysis is presented in schematic form below.

Data Collection

Labov and Fanshel (1977) confined their analysis of language use in psychotherapy to an audio record. There are no inherent barriers to using video tape or film analyses with the methods of Comprehensive Discourse Analysis, but the observer effects of microanalysis may then be heightened (Labov & Fanshel, 1977), and choosing the units of behavioral analysis for nonspoken aspects of the interaction is complex. Studies by McQuown et al. (1971) and Scheflen (1973) of psychotherapy interviews have used film or videotape recordings, but to date studies utilizing only *audio* records have not been compared to studies using the same audio record supplemented by a visual record. It is not clear precisely what information is gained from the visual record, particularly with regard to the *interpretive* statements which answer "what happened"?. We would expect individual differences with respect to how much a visual record *changes* the analyst's account of "what happened." It is also not clear whether the *reliability* of the interpretative statements across discourse analysts would vary for audio and audiovisual records. These questions are all critical ones for those choosing a method of analysis, but it should be noted that kinesic and proxemic analysis, at the current time, are not readily assimilable to Comprehensive Discourse Analysis as practiced by Labov and Fanshel (see Birdwhistell, 1970 and Scheflen, 1973 for analyses of body motions).

Transcription

Few people who first attempt to accurately transcribe a conversation realize how much unconscious editing one carries out in writing down what is "heard" (Ochs, 1979). Words are interspersed with forms of hesitation, false starts, various pauses, and self-interruptions, all of which may bear significance. Getting the "right" text is an open-ended process. In the two-person psychotherapy conversation Labov and Fanshel (1977) analyze, "the text after four or five editings presents a reasonably objective input to the analysis" (p. 355). Tempo and pauses are captured in their transcriptions by the use of a set of well-defined transcription devices. For example, one dot is used for each ½ second of pause, and punctuation marks such as commas, dashes, hyphens, periods, question marks, and underscoring (contrastive stress) are all used, or specified utterance characteristics. Undecipherable words are represented by "xxx."

Defining the Situation

This step of Comprehensive Discourse Analysis makes clear the contribution of sociology to the understanding and production of talk. Labov and Fanshel's (1977) view that "conversation is not a chain of utterances, but rather a matrix of utterances and actions bound together by a web of understandings and reactions" (p. 30) was derived in part from a consideration of social and psychological propositions implicit in communications in the psychotherapeutic setting. In defining the situation, Labov and Fanshel employ some parameters of the roles of client and patient that "condition" interactions. As one example, the paradox of social stigma in psychotherapy is a consequence of the client *seeking out help* from the therapist, whereas the goal of the therapy is to foster *independence from help*. Labov and Fanshel (also see Turner, 1972) show how the client's early assertions of self-understanding through narrative anecdotes are reactions to this fundamental contradiction, and they document other forms of resistance (problem mitigation; total silence) which stem from the constraints imposed by roles in the psychotherapeutic situation. Labov and Fanshel do not claim the client knows that their speech actions are influenced by the roles defined in their situation, but they do find distinct *styles* of discourse during the client–

therapist interactions that are occasioned by the psychotherapeutic interview setting. Such styles are designated as "fields of discourse.".

Identifying Fields of Discourse

In the 15 minute conversation Labov and Fanshel (1977) analyze, they find four distinct fields of discourse. These fields are distinguished by stylistic features such as lexical choices and predominant paralinguistic cues. Fields of discourse are a critical component of Comprehensive Discourse Analysis, since Labov and Fanshel claim that they determine many of the linguistic forms that occur in them. Their main role is to act as *interpretive* devices that help *the analyst* focus on stretches of talk—the family style in this case—pervaded by paralinguistic cues that are of great emotional significance.

Other conversations in psychotherapeutic settings may draw on a different set of fields of discourse, possibly overlapping with these (Labov & Fanshel, 1977, p. 129). Dependent on the analyst's purposes, the fields might also be further refined, so that different family members might cue a different set of distinctive lexical items, emotions, and other discourse features. (Goffman [1974] has developed an account of frame

TABLE 1
Fields of Discourse

	Style	Abbreviation	Characteristics
1.	Everyday	EV	Continuous speech without pause, rapid level intonation. No emotionally colored or therapy-oriented language used. Few affective or evaluative expressions used.
2.	Narrative	N	Subvariety of EV. Account of events occurring in past. Typically begins without orientation to time, place, persons, and behavior characteristics of situation of narrative focus.
3.	Interview	IV	Many hesitations, long silences, false starts, creaky voice, falsetto, and volume. Vague pronominal references, and euphemisms regarding emotions. Topic of emotions/behavior as *objects* of talk.
4.	Family	F	Concentrated on bursts of expressing strong emotions. Special intonation contours carrying strong implication and affective meaning (some Yiddish in origin). Many idiomatic expressions of family use.

Compiled from: Labov & Fanshel, 1977, pp. 35–37, 128–130.

[field] shifts in conversation, and the notion of frames is discussed by Frake [1977]).

Identifying Episodes

In Comprehensive Discourse Analysis, an important structural unit of interactional analysis identified by Labov and Fanshel (1977, pp. 38–39, 328–331) is the *episode*. A general framework is provided for understanding "what goes on" within the session by the episode-parsing of the text. In Labov and Fanshel's work, the episode also provides a convenient unit for the structural analysis of interaction focused on a single topic.

For the reader, we present the authors' characterization of the five episodes comprising a single therapeutic session:

> Episode 1: Rhoda gives an account of how she "did the right thing" in calling up her mother and asking her to come home.
>
> Episode 2: In response to a question from the therapist about whether her Aunt Editha might help with the housework, Rhoda gives a narrative to show how her aunt would not help clean the house when she asked her and was altogether unreasonable.
>
> Episode 3: In response to a further question about whether Rhoda could arrive at a working relationship with her aunt, Rhoda gives another account of how her aunt would not prepare dinner even when she didn't work, and how Rhoda had to go out with her to eat.
>
> Episode 4: Rhoda returns to the problem of her mother's being away from home and gives an account as to how it came about.
>
> Episode 5: The therapist offers an interpretation to explain why Rhoda and her family are behaving in this way towards each other, drawing a parallel between Rhoda's mother staying away too long, and Rhoda's refusing to eat. (Labov & Fanshel, 1977, pp. 38–39)

The most compelling features distinguishing these episodes are the shift of topic for the conversation at the episode boundaries and the *therapist's initiatives* for conversation. Although shift of topic may be a general feature for demarcating episodes, Labov and Fanshel (1977, p. 331) indicate how the therapist's interventions are a consequence of the client's maintenance of the same topic *unless* interrupted, which may render this feature of episode boundaries of limited generality.

Transcription and Interpretation of Paralinguistic Cues

One of the most critical components of Comprehensive Discourse Analysis is assigning semantic value to paralinguistic cues. As any speaker knows, the prosody carried by a crisp "thank you" can override the complimentary meaning of the phrase to yield an insult. The deniability of these cues in conversational interaction is to the speaker's advantage, but the analyst's dismay. Nonetheless, the general *types* of cues which influence utterance meaning are not a focus of controversy; it is generalizable principles of interpretation that have eluded discourse analysts to date. The principal contributions of the method of Comprehensive Discourse Analysis in this domain are: (1) the insight that the co-occurence of shifts of cues in *patterns* may result in emergent semantic properties, and (2) the concurrent use of graphic displays with text for the reader's aid in interpreting subjective cues such as the *pitch* and *length* of specific utterances.

Types of Cues and Format of Transcription

The types of paralinguistic cues that play a role in Comprehensive Discourse Analysis are volume, pitch, length, breathing qualities, and voice qualifiers. It may surprise the nonlinguist that reliable methods of transcription for these cues—which are *perceptual constructs*—have not been developed. The physically measurable parameters of such gradient signals as amplitude, frequency, and duration do not directly map onto their subjective analogs—varying across different individuals—for volume, pitch, and length. Labov and Fanshel provide the heuristics of graphic displays of the acoustic signal of key utterances in order to represent hesitations and pauses, for the physical dimensions of *amplitude* and *duration* (shown in prints from a variable-persistence oscilloscope), and to represent pitch contours, for the physical dimension of *frequency* (shown in prints from a real-time spectrum analyzer). Voice qualifiers such as "breathiness," "glottalization" (creaky voice), and "whine" are also used by Labov and Fanshel as cues playing a supportive role in the interpretation of cue patterns. Laughter and suppressed laughter also seem to carry semantic value for this client–therapist pair.

Terms for the Meaning of Cues

Deriving meanings from configurations of paralinguistic cues is an art rather than a science even in Labov and Fanshel's approach. Their set of terms for the meanings of paralinguistic cues divide into five sets: (1) *Negative emotional states*—tension, tension releases, exasperation; (2) *Affective evaluations of speaker's interactional moves*—mitigation, aggravation; (3) *Affective evaluations of listener's interactional moves*—sympathy, derogation, neutrality; (4) *Style*—formal, informal; and (5) *Reinforcement*—nonspecific, noninterruptive listener contributions such as "mhm." But no unique set of cues yields any particular meaning in their system; instead, Labov and Fanshel's cue interpretations are based on recurrent *patterns of cues* that recur with certain textual themes. In the case of the patient whose talk they studied, the recurrent overlapping of hesitations, whines, and glottalizations with the theme of an inability to cope with the hurt from others' behaviors yields signals of *tension* indicating helpless anger (p. 191). Their research reveals the need for an account of the *general heuristics* for recognizing converging paralinguistic cues and textual themes for a given individual.

Expansion ("What Is Said")

This step of Comprehensive Discourse Analysis is intended to disambiguate "what is said" in the conversation by (1) a specification of unexplicit referring expressions; (2) the incorporation of *propositions* (or recurring themes) derived from the larger context of previous conversations and recounted events; and (3) the synthesis of text and a text-rendering of the meaning of paralinguistic cues. The goal of the expansion is to derive an ethnographically adequate understanding of utterances from the interactional context and history of the participants. Some parts of the expansion are at once difficult and controversial, particularly, as we shall see, the discovery of propositions. Expansion is also an open-ended process, without clearly defined limits, as Garfinkel (1967, p. 38ff), Clark (1977), and Labov and Fanshel (1977, p. 50ff) have observed.

The expansion of cues into text depends on the analyst's rendering of those paralinguistic cues that *alter* the meaning of the sentence into explicit text. Labov and Fanshel use, as we have noted, *patterns* of cues that converge on a semantic interpretation, and in the example below, cues said to register "tension" and "uncertainty" are supported by a theme of uncertainty in the text itself:

TEXT	CUES
1.1 R: I don't . . know, whether . . . I—*think* I did—the right thing, justa-little . . situation came up . . . an' I tried to uhm. . . . . . well, try to . . . . use what I—what I've learned here, see if it worked.	Tension: hesitation, self-interruption; uneven tempo: condensation and long silences, 3 and 4 sec.

EXPANSION

I am not sure I did the right thing, but I claim that I did what you say is right, or what may actually be right, when I asked my mother to help me by coming home after she had been away from home longer than she usually is, creating some small problems for me, and I tried to use the principle that I've learned

from you here that I should express my needs and emotions to relevant
others and see if this principle worked. (Labov & Fanshel, 1977, p. 119)

A major task in the expansion consists of making explicit the knowledge shared by conversational participants that is packed into vague
proforms and pronouns, such as "the right *thing*" in example 1.1 above.
In this case, the discourse analysts had to hear the patient's entire narrative to find out that "thing" referred to "asking my mother when she
planned to come home." Other anaphoric references are filled in by
similar means.

A central tenet of Comprehensive Discourse Analysis, derived from
the foundational work of Bateson and the Recurrence Principle of Pittenger *et al.* (1960; see above), is that speakers repeatedly allude to
general propositions which concern them, but which they rarely state
explicitly. Although it is possible that some propositions pervade virtually *all* conversational exchanges (e.g., X wants others' respect), Labov
and Fanshel find in their case study that the key propositions arise in the
patients' family interaction, (e.g., "[AD-X]" is the abbreviation for the
proposition that "X is an adult member of the household") and in the
therapeutic setting itself (e.g., [S]: One should express ones' needs and
emotions to relevant others). The importance of such propositions in
expansions of "what is said" cannot be underestimated, for many utterances only have *relevance* to the conversational context on the condition
that propositions are anchor points of talk.

Labov and Fanshel generally discover propositions in their corpus
of data by seeking out *explicit* formulations of the propositions at some
point in the conversational text, and by seeking out what issues underly
family disputes. In an important sense, it is the participants' *negations* of
propositions that make the conversational analysts aware of the propositions. There are, of course, many general propositions that are not a
focus of dispute and never arise in analyses but which, if they were to be
challenged, would emerge as themes of concern (see Footnote 1, p. 303).

The taxonomy of propositions Labov and Fanshel found necessary
for constructing coherent links between conversational transactions is
too complex for review here, but the procedures of discovery they out-
line (1977, p. 57ff., and numerous examples) make clear the need for an
approach based on the participants' points of view (also see McDermott
& Roth, 1978), which are fundamental to any ethnography of conversation. Such an ethnography will inevitably depend on future attempts at
working out the influence of *higher-order* propositions invoking such
social units as institutions, organizations, and government on conversational transactions (Cicourel, 1979, p. 170). In Labov and Fanshel's set of
propositions, such notions as "roles" and "obligations" are mentioned,

but the considerable philosophical (e.g., Rawls, 1972) and sociological (e.g., Gross, 1959; Turner, 1974) work on these concepts is not integrated with their approach.

Discourse Rules for Speech Acts, Interactional Analysis, and the Synthesis of the Sequence of Acts in the Flow of Conversation

"Doing things with words" is a fundamental concept of Comprehensive Discourse Analysis, derived from speech act theory (e.g., Austin, 1962; Searle, 1969, 1976). But the philosophical analysis of utterances as speech acts has, in its concentration on linguistic structure only, not yielded great insights into the sequential coherence of speech acts. Labov and Fanshel (1977, pp. 58–59) argue that this limitation is understandable because

> the crucial actions in establishing coherence of sequencing in conversation are not such speech acts as requests and assertions, but rather challenges, defenses, and retreats, which have to do with the status of the participants, their rights and obligations, and their changing relationships in terms of social organization.

As we noted, speech act analysis has been constrained in this respect because of its assumption that each utterance represents only *one* illocutionary act, whereas Labov and Fanshel show how the patterns of conversational interaction are only rendered as coherent sequences if one assumes that each utterance may simultaneously express a number of different actions at various levels of depth in a hierarchy of speech actions.

Four hierarchical levels of speech acts are proposed, and an utterance may simultaneously carry out actions on each of the levels. The speech acts that they found in this therapy session are presented below:

The first level of *meta-actions* has to do with the regulation of speech, with the turn-taking and alternations between speakers that characterize conversation (Sacks *et al.*, 1974). The second level of *representations* are acts that have often been thought by analytic philosophers (e.g., Russell, 1940) to be *the* function of utterances. They index information or emotions as states of affairs, either biographical (A-events) or disputable (D-events) in nature. The third level of *requests* are acts integrally tied to the speech situation and further acts of the two speakers, A and B. At the deepest level, acts are *challenges* that are "any reference (by direct assertion or more indirect reference) to a situation that, if true, would lower the status of the other person" (Labov & Fanshel, 1977, p. 64). At the same level, although not listed, would be *supports*, just the opposite of *challenges*. (It should be noted that the set of speech acts listed are only

SPEECH ACTIONS
(Verbal Interactions)

1. Metalinguistic

initiate interrupt redirect	continue respond repeat reinforce	end signal completion withdraw

2. Representations

A-events (in A's biography)

A	B	
give information express F demonstrate refer	reinforce acknowledge	

D-events (disputable)

A	B	A
assert give evaluation give interpretation give orientation	deny agree support give reinterpretation	contradict support

3. Requests

A	B	A
request X	give X [carry out] X put off	acknowledge reinstate redirect retreat mitigate
	refuse with account refuse without account	renew accept reject withdraw in a huff

4. Challenges

A	B	A
challenge question	defend admit huff	retreat mitigate

X = action
    information
    confirmation
    agreement
    evaluation
    interpretation
    sympathy
	F = belief
	    uncertainty
	    exasperation
	    deference

FIGURE 3. Speech actions referred to in the interactional statements. (Source: Labov & Fanshel, 1977, p. 61.)

those *happening to occur* in the therapy session Labov and Fanshel analyze, yet many other speech acts such as flattery, promises, threats, boasts, excuses, and so on are possible. The voluminous and growing literature on speech acts could provide the interested reader with analyses of other acts used in psychotherapy.)

So far, only individual utterances have been considered. Yet the construction of utterances that are *somehow* cohesive in sequence is a remarkable feat of which mature speakers are obviously capable. Discovering these connections is at the heart of Comprehensive Discourse Analysis. The connections linking speakers' speech actions into a coherent web are said to be mediated by *rules*, often quite abstract in nature.

Two planes of conversational behavior are distinguished in Labov and Fanshel's (1977) analysis. In one plane is "what is said" (the text as expanded by cues, referent specification, and implicit propositions); in the other is "what is done," a hierarchy of speech acts that comprise their interactional analysis. They represent their analysis by means of a three-dimensional rectangle. The two-way arrow on the bottom right side represents *rules of discourse* that connect the two planes of conversational behavior, and these rules are said to mediate the *interpretation* and *production* of speech actions that are ingredient to the conversational interaction. The coherency of the speech actions in the conversational interaction is explained via the workings of *sequencing rules,* relating the cross sections of a discourse to one another. Sequencing rules explain the horizontal, sequential coherency of the abstract actions performed via talk, while rules of interpretation and production explain the vertical relations between the surface words spoken and the underlying actions carried out for cross-sections of the stream of conversation.

Rules of Production and Interpretation

The rules of production and interpretation which Labov and Fanshel have developed are said to enable a speaker to create, and a listener

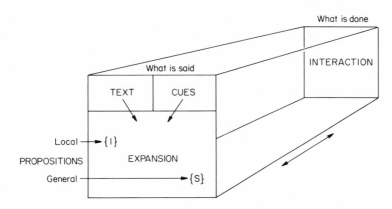

FIGURE 4. Discourse analysis: Cross section. (Source: Labov & Fanshel, 1977, p. 68.)

to understand, the actions that the surface linguistic forms convey—in other terms, the rules determine "what is heard," as well as "what is said." The discourse rules presented focus on *requestive, challenging,* and *narrative* conversational structures.

How do Labov and Fanshel "discover" such rules? As linguists, they could initially rely on their intuitions for constructing and evaluating conversations and attempt to formalize them as a rule, or like some ethnomethodologists (e.g., Schegloff, 1979) they could infer rules by relying on carefully transcribed texts of *naturally* occurring conversations. Labov and Fanshel utilize both tacts, also employing all the *contextual* information they have available. The rules formulated, they stipulate, must not be specific to the client-therapist under study but be as generally applicable as possible.

The Rule of Requests is one example that may briefly convey the format of a discourse rule. Taking the imperative grammatical form as the clearest formulation of the directive function of language, which requests also express, they formulate the Rule for Requests in this way:

> If A addresses to B an imperative specifying an action X at a time T_1, and B believes that A believes that
>
> 1a. X should be done (for a purpose Y) [*need for the action*]
>   b. B would not do X in the absence of the request [*need for the request*]
> 2.   B has the *ability* to do X (with an instrument Z)
> 3.   B has the *obligation to do* X or is willing to do it.
> 4. A has the *right* to tell B to do X,
>   then A is heard as making a valid request for action. (Labov & Fanshel, 1977, p. 78)

This rule screens out insults such as *up yours,* and other nonvalid requests, but as Labov and Fanshel note, many requests are made very indirectly, requiring other discourse rules. In particular, their Rule for Indirect Requests captures many requests made in the therapy sessions, and they generally work by altering the imperative form of a request through a mention of the preconditions of a valid request, cited in the Rule of Requests.

> If A makes to B a Request for Information or an assertion to B about
> a. The existential status of an action X to be performed by B
> b. The consequences of performing an action X
> c. The time T_1 that an action X might be performed by B
> d. Any of the preconditions for a valid request for X as given in the Rule of Requests
> and all other preconditions are in effect, then A is heard as making a valid request of B for the action X. (Labov & Fanshel, 1977, p. 82)

As examples of variants of the following indirect request actually made in the therapeutic session: "Wellyouknow, w'dy'mind takin' thedustrag

an' just dustaround?" Labov and Fanshel give the following alternatives:

a. Existential Status:	Have you dusted yet?
b. Consequences:	How would it look if you were to dust this room?
c. Time Referents:	When do you plan to dust?
d. Other Preconditions:	
Need for Action:	Don't you think the dust is pretty thick?
Need for the Request:	Are you planning to dust this room?
Ability:	Can you grab a dust rag and just dust around?
Willingness:	Would you mind picking up a dust rag?
Obligation:	Isn't it your turn to dust?
Rights:	Didn't you ask me to remind you to dust this place?

Labov and Fanshel formulate similar rules for putting off requests,
relayed requests, requests for information, embedded requests, delayed
requests, repeated requests, reinstating requests, and more interactively
critical speech actions, such as challenges. They find that many requests, such as those of the wife in our introduction, are used for ul-
terior purposes, very often confronting social and emotional relations of
the conversational parties (p. 93).

It is through the investigation of such rich discourse phenomena as
these conflict eliciting speech actions that the hierarchical nature of
speech actions becomes clear. As illustrative of the depth of the actions
executed by a single utterance, Labov and Fanshel cite the following
example. Here we first present the text, cues, and expansion, and finally
the interactional statement to convey the set of actions accomplished in a
single utterance:

TEXT	CUES
1.3 R.: $_N$An-nd so—when—I called her t'day, I said, $_F$"Well, when do plan t'come *home*? $_F$ $_N$	Exasperation: *plan to,* 'implication of deliberation'; contrastive stress on *home.*

EXPANSION

R.: $_N$When I called my mother today (Thursday), I actually said, $_F$"Well, in
regard to the subject which we both know is important and is worrying me,
when are you leaving my sister's house where (2): any obligations you have
already have been fulfilled and returning home where (3): your primary
obligations are being neglected as (4) you should do as (HEAD-Mo) head of
our household?
$>_F >_N$

INTERACTION

R.: R. continues the narrative, and gives information to support her assertion ⎯1⎯ that she carried out the suggestion [S]. R. requests information on

the time that her mother intends to come home and thereby requests indirectly __4__ that her mother come home, thereby carrying out the suggestion
[S], and thereby challenging her mother indirectly ⟨?HEAD-Mo⟩ for not
performing her role as head of the household properly, simultaneously admitting ⟨STRN her own limitations and simultaneously asserting
again __1__⟩ that she carried out the suggestion [S]. (Labov & Fanshel, 1977, p.
160)

Recall that the brackets and capital letter subscripts denote fields of
discourse. The bracketed numbers and abbreviations refer to local and
general "propositions," respectively:

LOCAL: [1] "I think I did the right thing"—Rhoda carried out the
            basic suggestion [S] correctly.
            [2] Mother has fulfilled her secondary obligations to
            Household 2.
            [3] Mother has neglected her primary obligations to
            Household 1.
            [4] Rhoda requests her mother to come home immediately.
General: [HEAD-X] X is a competent head of the household.
                    [In this case "X" is "Mo(ther)".]
[STRN] X's obligations are greater than his capacities.
[S]   One should express one's needs and emotions to
relevant others.

Finally, a "?" prior to a proposition, such as ?HEAD-Mo ,is a symbol
meaning that the proposition is being questioned and challenged in the
act. Similarly, propositions may be asserted, referred to, denied, or re-
fused $^{(\sim)}$. The directionalities of the arrows in the interactional
statement

> indicate the relations to the actions performed . . . to the sequencing rules
> that may be operating, connecting one cross section with another. Thus
> *reference* is characteristically a leftward- or backward-operating action, which
> does not contain in itself immediate consequences for the next action to be
> performed. Assertions . . . are forward-looking in just the opposite sense.
> Questions characteristically include both the act of reference to some pre-
> vious event or statement and a demand for a reply. Challenges are double-
> faced in the same way. (Labov & Fanshel, 1977, p. 127)

The arrows in their analysis very clearly indicate how the interdependence of different speech actions ensures that what had been called an
individual speech act in fact points forward or backward in time, and
constrains the set of appropriate or likely future speech actions. Labov
and Fanshel represent the hierarchical structure of speech actions carried out in R's utterance as represented in Figure 5.

   Thus far, we have presented only a *cross-section* of the therapeutic
interview. These cross-sections must be synthesized into a sequence.

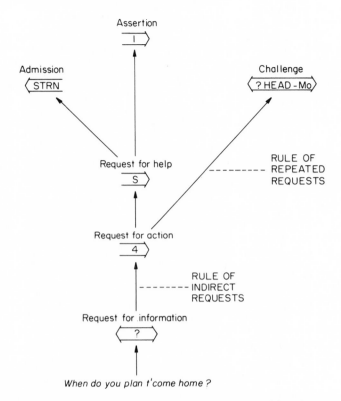

FIGURE 5. Interactional structure of 1.8. (Note: Propositions: {1} = R. carried out {S} correctly. {STRN} = R.'s obligations are greater than her capacity. {4} = R. requests her mother to come home. {?Head-Mo} = Mother is a competent head of the household [questioned]). (Source: Labov & Fanshel, 1977, p. 66.)

Labov and Fanshel refer to this analytic procedure as "assembly," and a look at how Rhoda's mother responded to 1.8 will serve as an example of such assembly. In essence, by "simply" saying "Oh, why"? in response, Rhoda's mother answers Rhoda's 1.8 at a number of different levels of abstractions. First, we present the text, cues, expansion, and interactional statement for the mother's response.

1.9

TEXT	CUES
R.: $<_N$So she said, $<_F$ "Oh, why?" $>_F >_N$	Surprise: *Oh*, 'contrary to expectation', Heavy implication: 2 1 2 information, There's more to this than meets the eye.

EXPANSION

R.: $<_N$So my mother said to me, $<_F$"Oh, I'm surprised; why are you asking me when I plan to come home, and do you have a right to ask that? There's more to this than meets the eye: Isn't it that [~AD-R] you can't take care of the household by yourself and I shouldn't have gone away in the first place, as I've told you before"? $>_F >_N$

INTERACTION

Mother asks R. for $\langle\underline{\ ?\ }$ further information which she already has, thereby putting off R.'s requests for action and for help $\langle\underline{~4, ~S}\ $ and asserts indirectly that she knows that the answer to her own question is that R. is asking for help because she cannot perform the obligations of household, thereby $\langle\underline{?AD\text{-}R}\rangle$ challenging R.'s status as an adult member of the household. (Labov & Fanshel, 1977, p. 166)

We have encountered the general proposition [AD-X] before; it represents the proposition that X, here Rhoda, is an adult member of the household. This proposition is at issue following Rhoda's complex speech actions of 1.8. Labov and Fanshel argue convincingly that "why"? as a response to "when do you plan to come home"? is not a coherent response at the surface syntactic level, because it doesn't follow from any regular ellipsis rule. By utilizing the unusual paralinguistic cues, their discourse rules of production and interpretation, and R's restating of this verbal encounter at a different point in the interview as "So she said, '*See* I *told* you *so*' " (i.e., that you couldn't hold status as an adult member of the household, and in fact need my help), Labov and Fanshel shows the coherency of the mother's response as one which hooks up to deeper levels of speech action that were expressed by Rhoda in 1.8, as depicted in Figure 6.

Rhoda's mother *puts off* Rhoda's request for action and request for help by a request for information herself. Rhoda's admission that $\langle\underline{STRN}\ $ —her obligations are greater than her capacities—and her challenge to her mothers competence$\langle?HEAD\text{-}Mo\rangle$are each answered by her mother's challenge in return, to Rhoda's status as an adult member of the household$\langle?AD\text{-}R.\rangle$The subsequent response by Rhoda, not discussed here, is to *apologize* to her mother, rather than taking, for example, the options of insisting that her mother respond to Rhoda's request for action, or of challenging her mother's challenge.

In summary, Comprehensive Discourse Analysis requires the use of two types of rules. *Rules of Production and Interpretation* are said to enable a speaker to create, and a listener to understand, the actions which the surface linguistic forms convey. These rules map surface forms onto actions of particular types, such as challenges, requests, refusals, and so on. *Sequencing rules*, on the other hand, generate all possible conversational sequences of speech act types (Labov & Fanshel, 1977, p. 110;

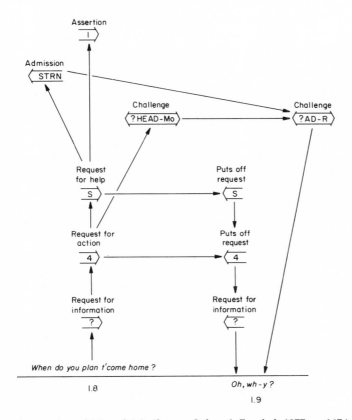

FIGURE 6. Sequencing of 1.8 and 1.9. (Source: Labov & Fanshel, 1977, p. 167.)

Sacks, Schegloff, & Jefferson, 1974; Sinclair, Forsyth, Coulthard, & Ashby, 1972), so that at any given point in a conversational interaction, one's choice of a speech-act type in production is constrained by sequencing rules setting out act types that are optional responses to the prior speech act type. Figure 3 provides an illustration of how the speech actions discussed by Labov & Fanshel are linked to one another. For example, a response to a *challenge* may be a *defense,* an *admitting* (Rhoda's choice in the previous example), or a *huff.* The rules of production and interpretation enable the analyst to derive "what is done" from the surface features of the utterances in conjunction with expansions, thereby yielding a cross-sectional analysis of the interaction that took place in the therapy session. These cross-sections are then assembled, by linking up the cross-sections into a sequence by means of sequencing rules.

POINTS FOR FUTURE DEVELOPMENT

Implicit throughout our discussion of the new ethnography of talk have been calls for a more systematic analysis of the *meaning* of paralinguistic cues, which, although making key contributions to the interpretation of both "what is said" and "what is done" in the talk of psychotherapy, are subjected to analyses much more intuitive than systematic in their approach. We must also critically note, as have others in their reviews of Labov and Fanshel (Cicourel, 1979, 1980; Grimshaw, 1979; Russell, 1979; Streeck, 1980) that the speech acts of "challenging," "defending," and "retreating," appeal to role obligations, rights, and status of the participants, but are not guided by a theory of status, roles, or obligations. Discourse analyses which require the invocation of such terms will ultimately need to make explicit the theories in which they are embedded. For example Labov and Fanshel (p. 59) want to characterize the tenor of interactional relations in terms of power and solidarity, but what these terms refer to in the maintenance of face-to-face encounters is not explicated sufficiently to be of much theoretical use.

In addition, we have seen that the overriding goal of Comprehensive Discourse Analysis is to "discover the connections between utterances" (p. 69), and that such discovery depends on adducing both general and specific "propositions" whose status is at issue in talk, and whose negotiation depends on high-level organizational phenomena such as status, rights and obligations. In what way is this "discovery" procedure related to the scientific understanding of conversation?

Labov and Fanshel talk very little about the place of their study in the context of the philosophy of science or of social science. They note their desire to "understand" conversation, argue that it is a "highly determined" phenomenon, and repeatedly imply that *parsimony* is required in their formulation of a theory which is accountable to all the data. This dictum—that parsimony and prediction are equally critical for a scientific explanation—is worth examining:

> It is not enough to understand the conversation; it must in some way be reduced to general principles that will make other conversations easier and quicker to analyze and report. (Labov & Fanshel, 1977, p. 27)

Two questions arise: (1) Is such a theory *predictive*, so that its explanation of the coherence of past conversational structures may be generalized in a specific manner to future ones? Or is this possible? (2) Can we have scientific understanding of conversation which is not *predictive* in this way?

With respect to the first question, Labov and Fanshel acknowledge that Comprehensive Discourse Analysis lacks *predictive* validity. For, although a given speech act constrains the set of permissible speech-act types that may follow it coherently, neither the precise act chosen by the conversationalist, nor the lexical items used, are dictated in their rules of sequencing. Instead, we note that the rules of discourse utilized in Comprehensive Discourse Analysis have the status of evolutionary laws in biology:

> The modern theory of evolution, like all historical theories, is explanatory rather than predictive. To miss this point is a mistake that theoreticians of history have often made. Prediction would require not only a knowledge of the main force—natural selection—but also a prescience of all future environmental conditions, as well as of future balances between the quasi-deterministic effects of the law of great numbers and the purely probabilistic role of genetic drift. (Luria, 1973, p. 23)

In this respect, Comprehensive Discourse Analysis falls short of predictive success, but fares relatively well on postdictive explanation, like the modern theory of evolution. Have they achieved parsimony in their postdictive account of discourse? Although an improvement over the mammoth text of McQuown et al. (1971), Labov and Fanshel still required several hundred pages to explain the connectedness of 15 minutes of talk. This is the cost of microanalyses today, and many social scientists argue that this inverse relation between explanation and parsimony is inherent to the study of human conduct in general (Campbell, 1972; Cronbach, 1975; Geertz, 1973; Jones & Konner, 1976; Kaplan, 1981), and by extension, to the study of discourse.

Obviously, much work is needed before Comprehensive Discourse Analyses such as Labov and Fanshel's contribute to an understanding of our therapeutic arsenal—comprised mostly of "mere" words. However, the employment of rule accounts and the explication of interaction from the point of view of commonly shared knowledge is bound to broaden researchers' perspectives on the complexity of language use in psychotherapy, especially its coherent sequential structure. It is hoped that this presentation of Comprehensive Discourse Analysis will spawn further interest in such microanalysis.

REFERENCES

Austin, J. L. (1962). *How to do things with words.* Oxford: Oxford University Press.

Birdwhistell, R. (1970). *Kinesics and context.* Philadelphia, PA: University of Pennsylvania Press.

Blum, A. F., & McHugh, P. (1971). The social ascription of motives. *American Sociological Review, 36,* 98–109.

Campbell, D. T. (1972). Herskovits, cultural relativism and metascience. In F. Herskovits (Ed.), *Cultural relativism.* New York: Random House.

Cicourel, A. V. (1979). Speech acts and conversations: Bringing language back into sociology. *Contemporary Sociology, 8,* 168–170.

Clark, E. V., & Clark, H. H. (1979). When nouns surface as verbs. *Language, 55,* 767–811.

Clark, H. H. (1977). Bridging. In P. N. Johnson-Laird, & P. C. Wason (Eds.), *Thinking: Essays in cognitive science* (pp. 411–420). Cambridge: Cambridge University Press.

Cole, P., & Morgan, J. (Eds.). (1975). *Syntax and semantics, vol. 3: Speech acts.* New York: Academic Press.

Cronbach, L. J. (1975). Beyond the two disciplines of scientific psychology. *American Psychologist, 30,* 116–127.

Davidson, P. O.,& Costello, C. G. (1969). *N = 1: Experimental studies of single cases.* New York: Van Nostrand Reinhold.

Ervin-Tripp, S. (1972). On sociolinguistic rules: Alternation and co- co-occurrence. In J. J. Gumperz, & D. Hymes (Eds.)., *The ethnography of communication* (pp. 213–250). New York: Holt, Winston.

Fishman, J. A. (1972). The sociology of language. In P. P. Giglioli (Ed.), *Language and social context* (pp. 45–58). England: Penguin Education.

Frake, C. (1977). Plying frames can be dangerous. *Institute for Comparative Human Development Newsletter, 1,* 1–5.

Fraser, B. (1971). An examination of the performative analysis. *Indiana University Linguistics Club.*

Garfinkel, H. (1967). *Studies in Ethnomethodology.* Englewood Cliffs, NJ: Prentice-Hall.

Geertz, C. (1973). *The interpretation of cultures,* New York: Baic Books. Giglioli, P. P. (Ed.). (1972). *Language and social context.* London: Penguin.

Goffman, E. (1974). *Frame analysis.* New York: Harper & Row.

Grimshaw, A. D. (1979). What's been done—When all's been said? *Contemporary Sociology, 8,* 170–176.

Grimshaw, A. D. (1980). Social interactional and sociolinguistic rules. *Social Forces, 58,* 789–810.

Gross, L. (1959). *Symposium on sociological theory.* Evanston, IL: Row, Peterson.

Hancher, M. (1979). The classification of cooperative illocutionary acts. *Language in Society, 8,* 1–14.

Hymes, D. (1968). The ethnography of speaking. In J. A. Fishman (Ed.), *Readings in the sociology of language* (pp. 99–138). The Hague: Mouton.

Hymes, D. (1972a). Toward ethnographies of communication: The analysis of communicative events. In P. P. Giglioli (Ed.), *Language and social context* (pp. 21–44). England: Penguin Education.

Hymes, D. (1972b). Models of the interaction of language and social life. In J. J. Gumperz, & D. Hymes (Eds.), *The ethnography of communication* (pp. 35–71). New York: Holt, Rinehard, & Winston.

Hymes, D. (1974). Ways of speaking. In R. Bauman, & J. Sherzer (Eds.), *Explorations in the ethnography of speaking* (pp. 431–451). London: Cambridge University Press.

Jones, N. B., & Konner, M. J. (1976). !Kung knowledge of animal behavior. In R. B. Lee & I. DeVore (Eds.), *Kalahari hunter gatherers* (pp. 325–348). Cambridge, MA: Harvard University Press.

Kaplan, B. (1981, June 1). *Genetic-dramatistic approach.* Paper presented at Developmental Psychology for the 1980's: Werner's Influences on Theory and Praxis, Heinz Werner Institute of Developmental Psychology, Clark University, Worcester, Massachusetts.

Labov, W. (1972). *Sociolinguistic Patterns.* Philadelphia, PA: University of Pennsylvania Press.

Labov, W., & Fanshel, D. (1977). *Therapeutic discourse.* New York: Academic Press.

Langer, J. (1980). *The origins of logic: 6 to 12 months.* New York: Academic Press.

Leiter, K. (1980). *A primer on ethnomethodology.* New York: Oxford University Press.

Luria, A. R. (1968). *The mind of a mneumonist.* New York: Basic Books.

McCawley, J. D. (1977). Remarks on the lexicography of performative verbs. In A. Rogers, B. Wall, & J. P. Murphy (Eds.), *Proceedings of the Texas Conference on performatives, presuppositions, and implicatures* (pp. 13–25). Arlington, VA: Center for Applied Linguistics.

McDermott, R. P., & Roth, D. R. (1978). The social organization of behavior: Interactional approaches. *Annual Review of Anthropology, 7,* 321–345.

McDermott, R. P., Gospodinoff, K., & Aron, J. (1978). Criteria for an ethnographically adequate description of concerted activities and their contexts. *Semiotica, 24,* 245–275.

McQuown, N. E., Bateson, G., Birdwhistell, R., Brosen, H., & Hockett, C. (1971). *The natural history of an interview.* Microfilm Collection of Manuscripts in Cultural Anthropology. Chicago: University of Chicago Library.

Mehan, H. (1979). *Learning Lessons.* Cambridge, MA: Harvard University Press.

Miller, G. A. (1975). Some comments on competence and performance. In D. Aaronson & R. W. Rieber (Eds.), *Developmental psycholinguistics and communication disorders.* New York; New York Academy of Sciences.

Mills, C. W. (1940). Situated action and vocabularies of motive. *American Sociological Review, 5,* 904–913.

Ochs, E. (1979). Transcription as theory. In E. Ochs & B. B. Schieffelin (Eds.), *Developmental pragmatics* (43–72). New York: Academic Press.

O'Keefe, D. J. (1979). Ethnomethodology. *Theory of Social Behavior, 9,* 118–219.

Pittenger, R. E., Hockett, C. F., & Danehey, J. J. (1960). *The first five minutes.* Ithaca, NY: Paul Martineau.

Pylyshyn, Z. W. (1973). The role of competence theories in cognitive psychology. *Journal of Psycholinguistic Research, 2,* 21–50.

Rawls, J. (1972). *A theory of justice.* Cambridge, MA: Harvard University Press.

Rogers, A., Wall, B., & Murphy, J. P. (Eds.). (1977). *Proceedings of the Texas Conference on performatives, presuppositions and implicatures.* Arlington, VA: Center for Applied Linguistics.

Russell, B. (1940). *An inquiry into meaning and truth.* London: George Allen & Unwin.

Russell, R. L. (1979). Speech acts, conversational sequencing, and rules. *Contemporary Sociology, 8,* 176–179.

Sacks, H., Schegloff, E. A., & Jefferson, G. (1974). A simplest systematics for the organization of turn-taking for conversation. *Language, 50,* 696–735. (Reprinted in Schenkein, J. [Ed.]. [1978]. *Studies in the organization of conversational interaction.* New York: Academic Press.)

Scheflen, A. E. (1973). *Communicational structure.* Bloomington, IN: Indiana University Press.

Shegloff, E. A. (1979). Identification and recognition in telephone conversation openings. In G. Psathas (Ed.), *Everyday language: Studies in ethnomethodology.* New York: Irvington.

Schenkein, J. (1978). *Studies in the organization of conversational interaction.* New York: Academic Press.

Searle, J. R. (1965). What is a speech act? In M. Black (Ed.), *Philosophy in America* (pp. 221–239). Ithaca: Cornell University Press.

Searle, J. R. (1969). *Speech acts.* Cambridge, MA: Cambridge University Press.

Searle, J. R. (1976). A classification of illocutionary acts. *Language in Society, 5,* 1–23.

Sinclair, J. McH., Forsyth, I. J., Coulthard, R. M., & Ashby, M. C. (1972). *The English used by teachers and pupils.* Final S.S.R.C. Report, Birmingham University.

Stone, C. A., & Day, M. C. (1980). Competence and performance models and the charac-
    terization of formal operational skills. *Human Development, 23,* 323–353.
Strawson, P. F. (1964). Intention and convention in speech acts. *Philosophical Review, 73,*
    439–460.
Streeck, J. (1980). Review of Labov and Fanshel, "Therapeutic discourse: Psychotherapy as
    conversation." *Language in Society, 9,* 117–126.
Sturtevant, W. C. (1974). Studies in ethnoscience. In B. G. Blount (Ed.), *Language, Culture,
    and Society* (pp. 153–176). Cambridge, MA: Winthrop Publishers.
Turner, J. H. (1974). *The structure of sociological theory.* Homewood, IL: The Dorsey Press.
Turner, R. (1972). Some formal properties of therapy talk. In D. N. Sudnow (Ed.), *Studies
    in social interaction.* New York: Free Press.
Wilson, T. P. (1970). Conceptions of interaction and forms of sociological explanation.
    American Sociological Review, 35, 697–710.

V
Conclusion

9

Psychotherapeutic Discourse
Future Directions and the Critical Pluralist Attitude

Robert L. Russell

As the contributions to this volume attest, important information about language use in psychotherapy can be discovered by distinguishing language-attribute dimensions or channels of communication and investigating each in isolation from the others. This is a time-honored strategy utilized in the natural and social sciences, and permits the reduction of what seems imponderably complex to more manageable levels. However, at some point, the dimensions that have been isolated through analysis must be resynthesized to gain an adequate comprehension of the process under investigation as a whole.

The use of language requires speakers and hearers to simultaneously coordinate scores of attributes into meaningful configurations that span variable durations of time. At some point, the dimensions or channels of communication that have been isolated from the totality of the communication process will need to be fit back together, so as to provide an account of language use in all of its obvious and not so obvious complexity. Thus, one recommended direction for future research is for the building-block categories presented herein (e.g., content categories, intersubjective categories, extralinguistic categories, case assignment categories, and so on) to be integrated into multidimensional coding systems. Such systems will enable researchers to ask and

ROBERT L. RUSSELL • Department of Psychology, New School for Social Research, 65 Fifth Avenue, New York, NY 10003.

provide answers to, more and more complex sets of empirical and theoretical questions.

The call for the construction of multidimensional systems for future research on client and therapist language use comports well with Kiesler's (1966) paradigm for psychotherapy process research. But in addition to this multidimensional emphasis, there are several other directions for future research that are likely to be worthwhile to pursue, even if they cannot be easily accommodated by Kiesler's paradigm. In fact, the inability to be accommodated by Kiesler's research paradigm may turn out to be an indication of the positive status of these new developments.

I present a brief sketch of some promising directions for the investigation of language use in psychotherapy. The directions that are outlined concern theoretical as well as empirical strategies that can or might have a direct influence on the conduct of research. Some of the directions have actually already been explored, and I summarize them in the belief that further exploration is likely to be rewarding. In concluding, I suggest that Kiesler's (1966) research paradigm cannot accommodate all of the new directions, and that, even at the level of description, a critical pluralist attitude may be better able to foster objectivity and scientific advance than the use of a single descriptive framework.

SEVEN FUTURE DIRECTIONS FOR RESEARCH ON LANGUAGE IN PSYCHOTHERAPY

Selection of Process End-Points Construed in Terms of Language Variables

Assessing the progress of patient and therapist language use in psychotherapy requires the selection of process endpoints or goals. If one is interested in the client's language use, or attributes associated therewith, as an index of adjustment or psychological well-being, then it is necessary to stipulate process endpoints or goals that are themselves construed in terms of clients' language use, or attributes associated therewith. This point has been advanced by Hertel (1972) with respect to psychotherapy process research in general, but it holds true for investigations of psychotherapeutic talk as well (Russell & Trull, 1986; see also Kaplan, 1966, 1967 for theoretical discussion). In the absence of a stipulation of some such endpoint or goal, it is difficult to see how changes in the patient's language or paralanguage could be assessed as therapeutic or regressive, adaptive or iatrogenic. Therapeutic changes in the client's language or language-related behavior are identifiable as those that result in bringing the client's communicative capacities into a closer approximation to the designated endpoint. Of course, other types of changes occur in psychotherapy, but unless they result in bringing the client's communicative capacities in closer approximation to the stipulated endpoint or goal, then they cannot be considered therapeutic.

Surprisingly, investigators of language use in psychotherapy have seldom explicitly stipulated process endpoints, which are construed in terms of client-communicative capacities. Adjustment, actualization, the expansion of ego control, and so forth, have all served as goals for psychotherapy, and their adequate operationalization has preoccupied scores of researchers. A corresponding investment of energy has not been spent in the construction of process goals in terms of language behavior. In fact, when stipulations of process endpoints, construed in terms of language or language-related variables, have been advanced, they appear rather simplistic. For example, from within the psychoanalytic framework, an increase in client-insight statements was taken as the endpoint toward which psychoanalytic therapy was to strive; from within the Rogerian framework, an increase in client disclosure or feeling-type statements was taken as the endpoint toward which Rogerian psychotherapy was to strive (e.g., Bergman, 1951; Dittman, 1952; Keet, 1948; Porter, 1942a,b; Snyder, 1945; Stiles, 1979). Although such increases may be associated with other factors indicative of therapeutic progress, the stipulation of the endpoint for client's communicative capacities in psychotherapy as simply an increase in insight or disclosure or feeling-type statements falls far short of dealing with the multivarious changes one could expect in clients' language usage, if significant development did in fact take place.

In attempting to formulate a more circumspect endpoint or goal for clients' talk in psychotherapy, it may be profitable to utilize a heuristic principle that has given direction to developmental investigations. The principle to which I refer is termed the orthogenetic principle and states: "Insofar as development occurs in a process under consideration, there is a progression from a state of relative undifferentiatedness to one of increasing differentiation and hierarchic integration" (Kaplan, 1966, p. 661). What this heuristic principle suggests is that the client's language or communicative capacities that approximate the designated endpoint will be characterized by a high degree of differentiation, and will be integrated with the successful pursuit of behavioral or interactional goals.

For example, suppose that it were possible to describe in detail the patterns of language use that constitute (or are associated with) the major interpersonal styles described by the different quadrants of the 1982 Interpersonal Circle (Kiesler, 1983). If it is true that clients seek therapy because of an extreme and/or rigid interpersonal style of communication, then progress in therapy would be marked by the client's adoption of differing communicative strategies and their integration into the client's verbal repertoire. The more differentiated and integrated the client's verbal repertoire became, the more the client's repertoire would approximate the stipulated endpoint for the development of communicative capacities (e.g., to have the capacity to appropriately deploy any interpersonal style of communication, so as to realize ethically justifiable personal or collective goals). In other words, the increase in the client's capacity to differentially respond in communication contexts having differing demand characteristics will be considered an index of therapeutic progress.

Naturally, to be of any real theoretical or empirical value, the stipulation of an endpoint or goal for the client's communicative capacities will need to be meticulously detailed and made relevant for all of the different communication channels. Such a project portends to be prohibitively time-consuming and difficult, entailing no less than the delineation of an exhaustive typology of communicative forms and functions, and a normative characterization of their relationship to types of communication situations. Progress in completing this task, however, will be likely to set the rate at which progress is made in assessing therapeutic changes in client verbal behavior.

Discriminative Sampling

Typically, studies of language use in psychotherapy have followed traditional methodological practices that have governed research on process as well as other clinical variables. This has meant that samples of the process of psychotherapy have been drawn on a random or structural basis (e.g., minutes 10–20 and 30–40 in a 50-minute hour), or complete sessions are used, when manpower and funding permit. That the significant processes of change are not evenly or randomly distributed throughout the therapeutic hour or over the course of therapy has had little impact on modifying sampling procedures. But, as Rice and Greenfield (1984) point out, "aggregating process as though all process during therapy is the same involves a uniformity myth from which psychotherapy has been suffering" (p. 10). By perpetuating this uniformity myth, true differences in the processes of psychotherapy can be easily overlooked, and the identification of curative factors can be unnecessarily encumbered.

An alternative discriminative sampling strategy has been gaining in popularity and may significantly hasten the discovery of the language processes responsible for, or at least associated with, therapeutic change. The strategy consists of three steps. The first step requires the process researcher to identify episodes in the hour that have had fairly obvious therapeutic value. The methods of identifying these episodes can vary—for instance, clinician ratings, client ratings, and/or expert observer ratings could be used. The idea is to accumulate a set of therapeutically significant episodes, preferably spanning across types of therapies, clients, and therapists. The second step involves submitting each of the significant episodes to a meticulous microanalytic study. The hoped-for result of this second step is the identification of process commonalities ingredient in each of the episodes. Presumably, this set of commonalities contains the processes responsible for the therapeutic progress evident in the episode. Once these commonalities have been identified and adequately operationalized ("manualized"), their role in achieving therapeutic change can be systematically investigated in controlled studies, the third step in the discriminative sampling procedure. This new approach, "which focuses on fine-grained process description of patterns in recurrent change episodes within specific contexts, can enable us to grasp the essential nature of the mechanisms leading to change, and thus to illuminate change across different therapeutic situations" (Rice & Greenberg, 1984, p. 14).

The emphasis in this newer approach on fine-grained description and analysis obviously comports well with the process-research tradition focusing on client and therapist communication processes, and can augment standard research practices, especially as a way to identify those language or language-related processes comprising the "curative" factors in change episodes. In this regard, the meticulous investigation of transitions between particular client states of mind (e.g., self-disgust, competitiveness, etc.), as expressed in and through language, promises to help illuminate both cognitive and emotional factors associated with change in the psychotherapeutic process (see e.g., Horowitz, 1979; Horowitz, Marmar, & Wilner, 1979; Marmar, Wilner, & Horowitz, 1984). In addition, this new approach dovetails with the recent renewed interest in single case studies of language use in psychotherapy, and sketches a reasonable strategy by which replication and validation can proceed.

Descriptive Statistics

The most frequently used descriptive statistic in investigations of client and therapist communication has been what can be termed the noncontingent frequency, that is, the frequency with which a specified verbal behavior occurs in the process sample, regardless of where in the sample the verbal behavior occurred. While this descriptive statistic can provide useful information about the rate of occurrence of specified verbal behaviors in psychotherapy, and can be used to compare types of therapies, therapists, and/or clients, its usefulness in providing information about therapeutic processes has been questioned (Gottman & Markman, 1978; Hertel, 1972; Russell & Trull, 1986). In particular, the near exclusive reliance on the noncontingent frequency as the basic descriptive statistic for studies of client and therapist communication stalls progress in discovering patterns or direction of influence in the therapeutic encounter. What has been recommended, in addition to the noncontingent frequency, are descriptive statistics which will enable researchers to better describe and assess the reciprocal influence patterns that transpire between client and therapist.

To launch a direct attack on the problem of influence patterns in psychotherapy, researchers have begun to use descriptive statistics which directly summarize the sequential relationships between language and language-related variables. These descriptive statistics have been elucidated under the rubric of *sequential analysis* (e.g., Gottman, 1979; Gottman & Markman, 1978; Russell & Trull, 1986) and are based on the contingencies, described in terms of conditional probabilities, between client and therapist talk. Combined with the growing number of statistical techniques to assess the significance of repetitive sequences of interaction (Allison & Liker, 1982), dominance in conversational exchange (Budescu, 1984), latent structures undergirding surface patterns of talk (Dillon, Madden, & Kumar, 1983), and cyclicity in conversations (Gottman, 1979), sequential analyses can provide a powerful strategy for deepening our understanding of client and therapist communication.

Unit Construction

Typically, the unit of communication (e.g., the clause, the sentence, the dysfluency, etc.) that has been coded to classification categories is defined in terms of a single speaker's output, and any other information that is used for coding purposes (e.g., the other speaker's responses) has been relegated to context. There is no necessity for the communication between client and therapist to be segmented in this fashion, and, in fact, reviewers of the field have often noted the absence of any theoretical justification for the selection of a segmentation or unit identification strategy (Marsden, 1965, 1971).

With the new trend in communication studies advocating a focus on reciprocal influence patterns, and on the interdependence between speakers' talk, there has come an innovation in the identification of the unit to be scored in language-classification systems. Basically, the newer strategy entails identifying the exchange between speakers as the unit to be classified. Thus, the conjunction of the two speakers' talk is identified and labeled as the principle scoring unit for study. In other words, it is the relationship between speakers' contiguous utterances that is being unitized and labeled, and which can be summarized over sessions using the sequential or noncontingent frequency strategies.

This focus on the exchange between speakers incorporates information about relationships at the classificatory level, and thus requires researchers to think in interactional terms. Currently, however, our research vocabulary is far richer when attempting to describe individual utterances than when attempting to describe different types of exchanges, interactions, or relationships. Kiesler's (1983) taxonomy of complementarity in human transactions is suggestive for descriptions of types of exchanges (e.g., complementary, anticomplementary, and/or acomplementary), and future "exchange" terminology will want to build on this promising start. This domain is relatively wide open, however, and one which will hopefully facilitate research progress on client and therapist talk.

Unit Size

The size of the language units that have been described and coded in studies of psychotherapeutic communication has varied considerably over the past forty years of research. If units of dysfluency are discounted, the smallest units have been phonemes and the largest units have been utterances (i.e., everything that one speaker says between the other speaker's consecutive turns at talk), or idea units or themes. Typically, the size of the unit has been a clause or a sentence, through which complete propositions can be communicated. As has already been indicated, the selection of the size of the units is not always or very often justified in terms of linguistic, communication, and/or psychotherapy theory. Focus has settled on the clause or sentence, probably because of pragmatic reasons (e.g., transcripts can be easily and reliably segmented into clauses or sentences), and because clauses and sentences are believed to be the carriers of propositions.

Interest in nonpropositional aspects of communication and cross-sentential relationships have spurred the exploration of other unit sizes. Larger units are becoming topics of theoretical and empirical focus. Of particular interest has been the exploration of the narrative or episodic description as a viable unit for process research (e.g., Russell, 1985; Schafer, 1980; Spence, 1982). The conjecture is that there are adaptive and nonadaptive styles of narration, just as there are adaptive and nonadaptive types of propositional usage (e.g., Beck, 1963, 1970), and the two different levels of organizing experience may provide independent or partially independent information. As the investigation of language use in psychotherapy proceeds, then, different and more varied unit sizes will need to be explored, and new strategies will need to be devised to objectively investigate the therapeutic relevance of such units as the episode description or narrative.

Sociological Specification of Context

Verbal behavior is learned and maintained in a social context. To deploy speech appropriately and effectively requires that speakers know what is expected and accepted in their society's various communication contexts. Typically, this knowledge concerns roles, statuses, traditions, and patterns of power and affiliation legitimized as constitutive of appropriate social behavior. While much of this knowledge remains tacit or implicit for the purposes of everyday communication, an account of the role of these sociological dimensions must be given in a circumspect explication of psychotherapeutic communication. In fact, talk has been described as taking place in accordance with *sociolinguistic* rules (e.g., Labov & Fanshel, 1977; Lakoff, 1982), rules the knowledge of which makes possible the appropriate deployment of speech, that is, speech which serves to constitute, and is constituted by, the evolving definition of specific social situations. This characterization of talk gives rise to three interrelated sets of questions: (1) What is the set of sociolinguistic rules which governs how speech is to be deployed to constitute and maintain the society's distinct types of social situations?; (2) Can maladjustment be adequately characterized as systematic violations of these sociolinguistic rules, and if so, what types of violation give rise to what types of psychopathology?; and (3) What distinct set of sociolinguistic rules—or violations thereof—characterize successful psychotherapeutic talk?

These questions are a long way from being answered. The concentration on intrapersonal constructs, in personality, psychopathology, and psychotherapy, has dominated psychology to such an extent that the systematic investigation of the correlativity of intra- and interpsychic processes has been relatively neglected. This has meant that the sociological dimensions that constitute the psychotherapeutic situation as a distinct type of social interchange have not been integrated into the analysis of the actions transpiring within psychotherapy, actions that include speech and speech-related phenomena. If the study of client and therapist communication can be successful only to the extent that it is investigated as a *social* situation, then the incorporation of sociological variables in future studies of process will be a requisite to continued progress.

Theory-Driven Research

Communication is a tremendously complex process, considered generally or in special contexts like psychotherapy. Even if it could be shown that science progresses from the bottom up, that is, from the working out of all possible empirical relations between phenomena and subsequently accounting for them by theoretical formulations, restriction on human and economic resources make it necessary to select only a limited set of phenomena for study, and this selection should be well-motivated by a defensible conjecture. But, as stressed earlier, theory is involved when making decisions about what units to use, how the units will be coded and classified, and how the relationships between the units will be formalized and reported. In fact, on one reading, the strategies of discovery presented in this volume can be seen as providing empirical methods whose theoretical worth will be evaluated in terms of their investigative payoffs, as hypotheses in need of confirmatory evidence. But further, it seems inevitable that, at some point, it will be necessary to reconstruct theories of psychotherapy in terms of communication processes, or conversely, to reconstruct available theories of communication and/or language behavior in terms applicable to the specific character of the psychotherapeutic situation. In either case, the reconstruction will need to be general enough to account for normal and abnormal development, so as to compete with theories which do not focus explicitly on language (e.g., classical psychoanalysis, behavior modification, etc.). In addition, of course, the theories will have to be able to account for change and development in just those substantive areas of continuing interest in clinical psychology—such as the relation of emotional and cognitive development to interpersonal adjustment. Following the articulation of such theories, hypotheses can then be derived and put to empirical test in the clinical situation. If science progresses by the empirical refutation of theoretical conjectures (Popper, 1959), then the development of theories of language use in psychotherapy should be a regular component of future process research.

Future Directions: The Critical Pluralist Attitude

In the introduction to this volume, Kiesler's (1966) skeleton of a communication research paradigm for psychotherapy process research was presented. Recall that Kiesler describes the psychotherapeutic process as a patient communication followed by a therapist communication, followed by a different patient communication or experience, and so on, with each communication being multidimensional and the patterning of this multidimensionability differing depending on the phase of treatment or patient population. Although the communication process can be seen and described as taking place in this fashion (i.e., a unit of speaker communication followed by a unit of listener communication, etc.), there is no necessity that it be seen and described in this manner. Segmenting the communication process in this way is, as we have seen, a result of a theoretical decision. Given the relevant theoretical training, the communication process could be seen and described differently. For example, the process of communication can be seen and described as taking place in and through exchanges, as that which transpires between, or as a result of, a therapist *and* a client utterance. Given training in this communication paradigm, a researcher would see and describe the same therapeutic encounter in very different terms than implied in Kiesler's model (see Hanson, 1958, for discussion).

I point out the theory-laden character of Kiesler's (1966) model not to disparage it, but to reiterate that even at the lowliest level of description, theoretical biases are at work, and favor certain types of perceptions, questions, and research methods. What is needed to ensure objectivity and scientific progress is the proliferation of, and clash between, such models. In other words, even at the lowliest level of description, pluralism is advisable, if pursued in a context of cross-model criticism. It is the development of this critical pluralist attitude which will ultimately ensure the progress of research on psychotherapeutic talk, and aid in the selection of promising strategies of discovery (Feyerabend, 1975).

REFERENCES

Allison, P. A., & Liker, J. K. (1982). Analyzing sequential categorical data on dyadic interaction: A comment on Gottman. *Psychological Bulletin, 91*, 393–403.
Beck, A. T. (1963). Thinking and depression. *Archives of General Psychiatry, 9*, 324–333.
Beck, A. T. (1970). The core problem in depression: The cognitive triad. In J. Masserman (Ed.), *Depression: Theories and therapies* (pp. 47–55). New York: Grune & Stratton.
Bergman, D. U. (1951). Counseling method and client responses. *Journal of Consulting Psychology, 15*, 216–224.
Budescu, D. V. (1984). Tests of lagged dominance in sequential dyadic interaction. *Psychological Bulletin, 96*, 402–414.
Dillon, W. R., Madden, T. J., & Kumer, A. (1983). Analyzing sequential data in dyadic interaction: A latent structure approach. *Psychological Bulletin, 92*, 564–583.
Dittmann, A. T. (1952). The interpersonal process in psychotherapy: Development of a research method. *Journal of Abnormal and Social Psychology, 47*, 236–244.
Feyerabend, P. (1975). *Against method.* London: Verso Editions.
Gottman, J. M. (1979). Detecting cyclicity in social interaction. *Psychological Bulletin, 86*, 338–348.
Gottman, J. M., & Markman, H. J. (1978). Experimental designs in psychotherapy re-

search. In S. L. Garfield & A. E. Bergin (Eds.), *Handbook of psychotherapy and behavior change: An empirical analysis* (Vol. 2, pp. 23–62). New York: Wiley.

Hanson, N. R. (1958). *Patterns of discovery.* Cambridge: Cambridge University Press.

Hertel, R. K. (1972). Application of stochastic process analysis to the study of psychotherapeutic processes. *Psychological Bulletin, 77,* 421–430.

Horowitz, M. J. (1979). *States of mind.* New York: Plenum Press.

Horowitz, M. J., Marmar, C., & Wilner, N. (1979). Analysis of patient states and state transitions. *Journal of Nervous and Mental Disease, 167,* 91–99.

Kaplan, B. (1966). The comparative developmental approach and its application to symbolization and language in psychotherapy. In S. Arieti (Ed.), *American handbook of psychiatry, Vol. III* (pp. 659–688). New York: Basic Books.

Kaplan, B. (1967). Meditations on genesis. *Human Development, 10,* 65–87.

Keet, C. D. (1948). Two verbal techniques in a miniature counseling situation. *Psychological Monographs, 62,* (7, Whole No. 294).

Kiesler, D. J. (1966). Some myths of psychotherapy research and the search for a paradigm. *Psychological Bulletin, 65,* 110–136.

Kiesler, D. J. (1983). The 1982 interpersonal circle: A taxonomy for complementarity in human transactions. *Psychological Review, 90,* 185–214.

Labov, W., & Fanshel, D. (1977). *Therapeutic discourse: Psychotherapy as conversation.* New York: Academic Press.

Lakoff, R. T. (1982). The rationale of psychotherapeutic discourse. In J. C. Anchin & D. J. Kiesler (Eds.), *Handbook of interpersonal psychotherapy* (pp. 132–146). New York: Pergamon Press.

Marmar, C. R., Wilner, N., & Horowitz, M. J. (1984). Recurrent client states in psychotherapy: Segmentation and quantification. In L. N. Rice & L. S. Greenberg (Eds.). *Patterns of change* (pp. 194–212). New York: Guilford Press.

Marsden, G. (1965). Content analysis studies of therapeutic interviews: 1954 to 1964. *Psychological Bulletin, 63,* 298–321.

Marsden, G. (1971). Content analysis of psychotherapy through 1968. In A. E. Bergin & S. L. Garfield (Eds.), *Handbook of psychotherapy and behavior change* (Vol. 1, pp. 345–407). New York: Wiley.

Popper, R. (1959). *The logic of scientific discovery.* New York: Basic Books.

Porter, E. H., Jr. (1942a). The development and evaluation of a measure of counseling interview procedures: 1. The development. *Educational and Psychological Measurement, 3,* 105–126.

Porter, E. H., Jr. (1942b). The development and evaluation of a measure of counseling interview procedures: II. The evaluation. *Educational and Psychological Measurement, 3,* 215–238.

Rice, L. N., & Greenberg, L. S. (1984). The new research paradigm. In L. N. Rice & L. S. Greenberg (Eds.) *Patterns of change* (pp. 7–25). New York: Guilford Press.

Russell, R. L. (1985). *Processive outcomes in psychotherapy: Toward a theory of narrative pluralism and change.* Paper presented at the Second European Conference on Psychotherapy Research, at the Catholic University of Louvain, Louvain-la-Neuve, Belgium.

Russell, R. L., & Trull, T. J. (1986). Sequential analyses of language variables in psychotherapy process research. *Journal of Consulting and Clinical Psychology.*

Schafer, R. (1980). Narration in the psychoanalytic dialogue. *Critical Inquiry, 7,* 29–53.

Snyder, W. U. (1945). An investigation of the nature of nondirective psychotherapy. *Journal of General Psychology, 33,* 193–223.

Spence, D. P. (1982). *Narrative truth and historical truth.* New York: W. W. Norton.

Stiles, W. B. (1979). Verbal response modes and psychotherapeutic technique. *Psychiatry, 42,* 49–62.

Index

Achievement Strivings scale, 55–56, 65
Acknowledgments (verbal response mode), 141
Advisements (verbal response mode), 139
Affect
    interviewer-interviewee interaction, 39–46
    language content measurement, 15–16
    plasma lipids and, 29–30
    rate of speech and, 16–17
    state versus trait measurement from speech, 58–60
Age level. *See* Children
Ambivalent Hostility scale, 46–47, 49, 65
Anxiety
    age and, 25–26
    classification of, 18–19
    hostility and, 27, 28
    intelligence and, 23–24
    interviewer-interviewee interaction, 39–46
    sex differences and, 24–25
    speech disturbances, 214, 215, 234–253
    subscale intercorrelations, 26, 28
Anxiety scale, 22–23
Anxiety scale examples
    emotion/plasma lipids, 29–30
    penile erection/REM sleep, 29
    plasma-free fatty acids, 30
    skin temperature changes, 29
Associationism, 277
Associative meaning, 74
Attentiveness (verbal response mode), 147
Automatic Vocal Transaction Analyser (AVTA), 207

Bound anxiety
    content-category analysis, 18
    See also Anxiety

Case grammar, 282–286
Castration anxiety. *See* Anxiety; Mutilation anxiety
Category
    commonality of meaning, 72–73
    speech disturbances, 216–219
    therapeutic interview (Snyder's classification), 109–113
    verbal response modes, 131
Children
    anxiety, 25–26
    concept analysis, 83–86
    normative scores, 60, 61–64
    speech disturbances, 248–251
Client-centered therapy
    natural language analysis, 290–295
    therapeutic interview, 116
    verbal response modes, 149–152
Client content categories, 110–111
Cognitive and Intellectual Impairment scale, 57–58, 64–65
Commonality (meaning), 72–75
Communication. *See* Ethnography
Comprehensive discourse analysis, 318–333
    cue meaning terms, 322–323
    cue types, 322
    data collection, 318–319
    defining of situation in, 319–320
    expansion, 323–325
    identifying episodes in, 321
    identifying fields of discourse in, 320–321